THE
HISTORY
OF
AMERICAN
NURSING

Edited by
Susan Reverby, Wellesley College

A GARLAND SERIES

NURSING
AND NURSING
EDUCATION
IN THE
UNITED STATES

The Committee for the
Study of Nursing Education

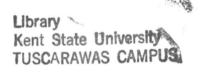
GARLAND PUBLISHING, INC.
NEW YORK • LONDON
1984

For a complete list of the titles in this series see the final pages of this volume.

This facsimile was made from a copy in the Yale University School of Nursing Library.

Library of Congress Cataloging in Publication Data

Committee for the Study of Nursing Education (U.S.)
  Nursing and nursing education in the United States.

  (The History of American nursing)
  Reprint. Originally published: New York : Macmillan, 1923.
  Includes bibliographical references.
  1. Nursing—United States.   2. Nursing—Study and
teaching—United States.   3. Nursing—Study and teaching
(Graduate)—United States.   I. Title.   II. Series.
[DNLM: 1. Nursing—United States.   2. Education,
Nursing—United States.   WY 18 N9742 1923a]
RT4.C56   1984   610.73′0973   83-49182
ISBN 0-8240-6506-9 (alk. paper)

The volumes in this series are printed on acid-free, 250-year-life paper.

Printed in the United States of America

NURSING AND NURSING EDUCATION IN THE UNITED STATES

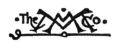

THE MACMILLAN COMPANY
NEW YORK · BOSTON · CHICAGO · DALLAS
ATLANTA · SAN FRANCISCO

MACMILLAN & CO., Limited
LONDON · BOMBAY · CALCUTTA
MELBOURNE

THE MACMILLAN CO. OF CANADA, Ltd.
TORONTO

NURSING AND NURSING EDUCATION IN THE UNITED STATES

REPORT OF THE

COMMITTEE FOR THE STUDY OF NURSING EDUCATION

C.-E. A. WINSLOW, DR.P.H., *Chairman*

MARY BEARD, R.N.
H. M. BIGGS, M.D.
S. LILLIAN CLAYTON, R.N.
LEWIS A. CONNER, M.D.
DAVID L. EDSALL, M.D.
LIVINGSTON FARRAND, M.D.
ANNIE W. GOODRICH, R.N.
L. EMMETT HOLT, M.D.
JULIA C. LATHROP

MRS. JOHN LOWMAN
M. ADELAIDE NUTTING, R.N.
C. G. PARNALL, M.D.
THOMAS W. SALMON, M.D.
WINFORD H. SMITH, M.D.
E. G. STILLMAN, M.D.
LILLIAN D. WALD, R.N.
W. H. WELCH, M.D.
HELEN WOOD, R.N.

JOSEPHINE GOLDMARK, *Secretary*

and

REPORT OF A SURVEY

by

JOSEPHINE GOLDMARK, *Secretary*

New York

THE MACMILLAN COMPANY

1923

All rights reserved

WYNKOOP HALLENBECK CRAWFORD CO.
Printing Headquarters
New York

MEMBERS OF THE COMMITTEE

C.-E. A. Winslow, Dr. P. H., *Chairman*
PROFESSOR OF PUBLIC HEALTH, YALE SCHOOL OF MEDICINE, NEW HAVEN, CONN.

Mary Beard, R.N.
DIRECTOR, INSTRUCTIVE DISTRICT NURSING ASSOCIATION, BOSTON, MASS.

Hermann M. Biggs, M.D.
COMMISSIONER OF HEALTH, NEW YORK STATE, ALBANY, N. Y.

Lillian S. Clayton, R.N.
DIRECTRESS OF NURSES, TRAINING SCHOOL FOR NURSES, PHILADELPHIA GENERAL HOSPITAL, PHILADELPHIA, PA.

Lewis A. Conner, M.D.
ATTENDING PHYSICIAN, NEW YORK HOSPITAL, NEW YORK CITY; PROFESSOR OF MEDICINE, CORNELL MEDICAL COLLEGE, ITHACA, N. Y.

David L. Edsall, M.D.
DEAN, HARVARD MEDICAL SCHOOL, BOSTON, MASS.

Livingston Farrand, M.D.
PRESIDENT, CORNELL UNIVERSITY; FORMER CHAIRMAN, CENTRAL COMMITTEE, AMERICAN RED CROSS

Annie W. Goodrich, R.N.
DIRECTOR OF NURSES, VISITING NURSE SERVICE, HENRY STREET SETTLEMENT, NEW YORK CITY

L. Emmett Holt, M.D.
PRESIDENT, CHILD HEALTH ORGANIZATION OF AMERICA; PHYSICIAN-IN-CHIEF, BABIES' HOSPITAL, NEW YORK CITY.

Julia C. Lathrop
FORMER CHIEF, CHILDREN'S BUREAU, WASHINGTON, D.C.

Isabel W. Lowman
MEMBER, CENTRAL COMMITTEE FOR PUBLIC HEALTH NURSING, CLEVELAND, OHIO

M. Adelaide Nutting, R.N.
PROFESSOR OF NURSING AND HEALTH, TEACHERS COLLEGE, COLUMBIA UNIVERSITY, NEW YORK CITY

Christopher G. Parnall, M.D.
DIRECTOR, UNIVERSITY HOSPITAL, UNIVERSITY OF MICHIGAN, ANN ARBOR, MICH.

Thomas W. Salmon, M.D.
FORMER MEDICAL DIRECTOR, NATIONAL COMMITTEE FOR MENTAL HYGIENE; PROFESSOR OF PSYCHIATRY, COLLEGE OF PHYSICIANS AND SURGEONS, COLUMBIA UNIVERSITY, NEW YORK CITY.

Winford H. Smith, M.D.
DIRECTOR, JOHNS HOPKINS HOSPITAL, BALTIMORE, MD.

E. G. Stillman, M.D.
PRESIDENT, HOSPITAL SOCIAL SERVICE ASSOCIATION OF NEW YORK CITY, NEW YORK CITY

Lillian D. Wald, R.N.
HEAD RESIDENT, HENRY STREET SETTLEMENT, NEW YORK CITY

William H. Welch, M.D.
DIRECTOR, SCHOOL OF HYGIENE AND PUBLIC HEALTH, JOHNS HOPKINS UNIVERSITY, BALTIMORE, MD.

Helen Wood, R.N.
DIRECTOR, TRAINING SCHOOL FOR NURSES, WASHINGTON UNIVERSITY, ST. LOUIS, MO.

CONTENTS

PAGE

INTRODUCTORY NOTE 1
REPORT OF THE COMMITTEE 7
REPORT OF THE SECRETARY 33

PART A. FUNCTIONS OF THE NURSE

I. PUBLIC HEALTH NURSING

1. *The New Trend in Public Health Work* 39
   Evolution of the Public Health Nurse 41

2. *Some Achievements in Public Health Nursing* 43
   School Nursing 43
   The Safeguarding of Motherhood and Infancy 46
   Prenatal Nursing 48
   Reduction of Maternal Mortality 49
   Reduction of Infant Mortality 50
   The Crux of Successful Public Health Nursing: Work in the
   Home 50
   Experience of the Metropolitan Life Insurance Company . . 52

3. *Scope and Method of the Inquiry: An Intensive Study* 53
   Some Determining Factors in Public Health Nursing 53
   Representative Nature of Organizations Studied 54
   Urban and Rural Agencies Included 54
   Geographical Distribution 55
   Public and Private Agencies Included 55
   Kinds of Nursing Service Included 55
   Focus of the Study: The Individual Nurse 56

4. *The Field of Public Health Nursing: Some Typical Days* . . . 57
   An Example of Rural Nursing 57
   Tuberculosis Nursing 57
   A Day's Visits 58
   Outside Activities: The County Fair 63
   The Establishment of Clinics 63
   The Expansion of a Nursing Specialty 64
   Nursing in a Small Town 65
   A Visiting Nurse in a Private Agency in a Large City . . . 66
   A Day's Visits 67
   Scope of the Day's Work 72
   Instruction in Bedside Care 72
   Calling in the Physician 72
   The Personality of the Nurse 73
   An Instructive Nurse under a City Department 73
   In the Welfare Station 74
   Home Visits 75

vii

PAGE

5. *Organization and Administration of Public Health Nursing Agencies* 76
   Types of Communities Served: City and Country 77
   Auspices of Agencies: Public and Private 78
      Advantages of Public Control 79
      Disadvantages of Public Control 79
      Some Safeguards of Public Control 80
      Advantages of Private Control 81
   Kinds of Service Rendered by 37 Agencies 82
      Number of Visits per Patient 89
      Number of Visits per Day 89
      Increase in the Number of Pay Patients 90
      Cost per Visit 91
   Differentiation between Public and Private Agencies: Preventive and Curative Work 92
   The Personnel of Public Health Nursing Agencies 93
      The Director 94
      Supervisors 94
      The Staff Nurses 95
      Students 96
      Persons Other than Nurses 96
        Clerical Workers 96
        Trained Attendants 97
   Size of Staff 98
   Requirements for Staff Candidates 99
      Hospital Training 99
      Special Training in Public Health Nursing 100
   Working Conditions in Public Health Nursing Agencies . . 101
      Salaries of Staff Nurses 101
      Salaries of Supervisors 102
      Vacations with Pay 103
      Working Hours 103
      Overtime 104
      Sunday Work 104
   Supervision of the Work 104
      Number of Nurses per Supervisor 105
      Accompanying Staff Nurses in Home Visiting 106
      Efficiency Records 106
      Written Instructions 107
      Reporting at Headquarters 107
      Meetings of the Staff 108
      Case Conferences 108

6. *Successes and Failures* 108
   A Rough Classification of 147 Nurses 109
      Varying Degrees of Success and Failure 109
      The Handicap of Poor Organization 110
   Teaching Ability: Examples of Failure 111
      A Parody of Public Health Nursing 111
      No Knowledge of Preventive Measures 114
      No Knowledge of Teaching Methods 115
      Ignorance of Emergency Measures 116
   Examples of Success 117
      Clear Cut Questions and Explanations 117
      Teaching in Communicable Diseases 120
   Relation to Relatives and Friends 121
      The Education of an Italian Husband 122

                                                                        PAGE
Other Examples of Assistance 123
Failure to Utilize the Assistance of Others 124
The Barriers of Language and Racial Customs 126
Relation to Physicians 127
Relation to Social Work and Social Agencies 130
  Examples of Failure 131
  Examples of Success 132
  Failure on the Part of Social Workers 133
The Relative Merits of Instructive Nursing and Bedside Nurs-
  ing Combined with Instruction 134
  Weaknesses in Generalized Nursing 135
  Weaknesses in Instructive Nursing Alone 136
Capital Importance of the Contact 136
The Vantage Ground of Generalized Nursing 137
The Handicaps of Poverty 138
Instructive and Generalized Work under Official Agencies . . 139
Some Contrasting Results of Generalized and Specialized
  Nursing 139
  Some Disadvantages of Specialization 141
  Demonstration of Special Needs by Specialist Organizations 143
  Tendency towards Greater Inclusiveness in Specialized
    Nursing 143
The Unit of Population Served 145
The Future Outlook 145
Educational Implications 146
  Need of Clinical Training 147
  Need of Special Public Health Training 148
  Length of Training 148

7. *Industrial Nursing* 149
Scope of a Brief Survey 149
Types of Work 150
First-Aid Work and Its Development 152
  Excessive Medication 153
Work with Employment Departments 153
Sanitation, Safety and Welfare Work 154
Lack of Records 155
Home Visiting 156
  Following Up Absentees 157
Education in Hygienic Habits 157
Training for Industrial Nursing 158
Use of Lay Workers 159

II. THE NURSE IN PRIVATE DUTY

Her Function 161
Differentiation of Care 162
Protection of the Public through Nurse Registration Laws . . . 163
The Need of a Subsidiary Group 164
Results of a Brief Survey 165
  Unnecessary Employment 166
  Kinds of Sickness Cared For 166
  Waste of Nurses in Various Types of Sickness 166
  Earnings of the Private Duty Nurse 168
  Seasonal Unemployment 168
  Living Expenses 169
Opinions of 52 Physicians in Private Practice 170

	PAGE
The Number of Trained and Untrained Nurses in the United States	171
The Standardization of a Subsidiary Group	172
Lessons in Home Nursing Care	173
Short Courses for Trained Attendance	173
Tendency to Disperse after Graduation	175
Primary Need of Licensing	177
The Place of Subsidiary Service in a Program of Nursing Education	178
Education of the Public	180
The Outlook for Persons of Moderate Means	181
Community Health Programs	182
Use of Hospitals for Acute Disease	183

III. THE NURSE IN INSTITUTIONS

1. *The Graduate Nursing Staff*	184
2. *Instructors and Administrators*	184

PART B. TRAINING OF THE NURSE

IV. THE HOSPITAL SCHOOL OF NURSING

1. *Present Status of the Training School*	187
Scope and Method of the Investigation	187
Basis of the Investigation: Hospital Training Schools Covered	189
Inclusion of the Best Schools in the Group Studied	190
Florence Nightingale and Nursing Education	192
The Dual Function of the Training School	194
The Conflict between Education and Care of the Sick: Records of Actual Experience	196
Causes of Irregular Assignments	201
The Dilemma of the Training School Superintendent	201
The Relation of Superintendent and Students	202
The Superintendent of the Training School and Hospital Organization	205
The Training School Committee	206
The Cost of the Training School	208
Financial Relation with the Hospital	208
The Balance between Cost and Services Rendered	210
The Objectives of Training	212
2. *Clinical Facilities in Hospitals of Different Type and Size*	213
Clinical Facilities Offered in 23 Hospitals Studied	214
Type and Size of Hospitals Studied	215
Municipal Hospitals	215
Private General Hospitals	215
Special Hospitals	217
University Hospitals	218
Conclusions	218
3. *Entrance Requirements*	219
Education	219
Age	221
Tuition Fees and Allowances	222
Previous Paid Occupations of Students	222
Number of Groups Entering Yearly	223
Credits for Advanced Standing	224

CONTENTS

PAGE

Credits for College Courses or College Degrees 225
Credits for Previous Experience 226

4. *The Period of Preliminary Instruction* 226
Disadvantages of the Apprenticeship System 226
The Preliminary Term 227
The Period of Probation 228
A Program for the Preliminary Term 228

5. *The Teaching of Nursing Procedures* 230
Their Central Importance 230
System of Teaching 231
Instructors 232
Assistance in the Use of Practice Material 233
Provision of a Demonstration Room 235
Equipment of the Demonstration Room 236
Adequacy of Supplies for Demonstration and Practice . . 237
Teaching Methods in the Classroom 238
Demonstration 239
Supervised Practice in the Classroom 240
Application of Classroom Instruction on the Wards . . . 242
Need of Prompt Application 242
Supervision 244
Examples of Successful Supervision 244
Examples of Inadequate Supervision 246
Lack of Co-operation 247
Inadequate Staffing 247
Other Methods for Securing Standard Technique 248
Use of Nursing Practice Card 248
Time Allowed to the Teaching of the Theory and Practice of
Nursing in 22 Schools 249

6. *The Case for the Basic Sciences* 249
General Benefits from Science Training 251
Need of Specific Sciences in Nursing Education 251
Why the Nurse Needs Anatomy and Physiology 252
Why the Nurse Needs Bacteriology 253
Why the Nurse Needs Chemistry 254
Why Scientific Teaching Should Precede Instruction in Disease 256

7. *Teaching of the Basic Sciences* 256
General Characteristics of the Science Courses 257
Lack of Well-Equipped Teachers 257
Lack of Laboratory Training 257
Inadequate Time 258
Anatomy and Physiology 258
Hours and Year When Given 258
Teaching Staff 259
Methods of Teaching 260
Use of Demonstration in Class 260
Obstacles to Good Teaching 260
Examples of Unsatisfactory Teaching 261
Examples of Resourceful Teaching 262
Lack of Demonstration 264
Equipment for Demonstration 264
The Essential Need of Laboratory Training and Equipment 265
Laboratory Facilities in the Schools Studied 266

PAGE

Use of Outside Facilities 268
Bacteriology 269
Hours and Year When Given 269
Instructors 270
Methods of Teaching 270
Facilities for Laboratory Work 271
Equipment 271
Examples of Good Laboratory Teaching 272
Demonstration by the Instructor Only 273
Chemistry 275
Hours and Year When Given 275
Instructors 275
Methods of Instruction 276
Cram Courses 278
Courses of Limited Scope 279
Chemistry as an Entrance Subject 280
Dietetics 281
Hours and Year When Given 283
Instructors 284
Methods of Instruction 285
The Need of Laboratory Training 285
Tendency to Over-Emphasize Cookery 286
Laboratory Equipment 287
Time Allowed to the Teaching of the Preliminary Sciences in
22 Schools 288
Laboratory Assistance in Science Teaching 289
Upkeep and Extension of Equipment 290
Science Requirements for Entrance and Credits for Science . . 291
Teaching of Preliminary Subjects outside the Training School 293
Use of the High School and the Vocational School 293
Use of the Junior College 294
Experiments in Central Teaching 295

8. *Practical Training* 297
Ward Training 297
The Gradation of Training 298
Examples of Graded Training 298
Use of Seniors as Head Nurses 301
Omissions in General Care 301
Examples of Ungraded Training 303
Staleness in the Third Year 304
Disadvantages of Specialization 305
The Combination of Graded and Ungraded Training . . . 306
Instruction and Supervision on the Wards 307
Examples of Success 307
Examples of Failure 310
Examples of Premature Responsibility 312
Lack of Good Management 314
Methods of Recording and Checking Ward Work 314
Use of Case Records 316
Private Service 317
Diet Kitchen 318
Diet in Disease 318
Training in Infant Feeding 319
Time Allotted to Diet Kitchen Service 319
Instruction and Supervision 320
Diet Kitchen Equipment 320

PAGE

Conditions of Valuable Training 320
Classroom Instruction in Diet in Disease 321
Need of Correlation with Classroom Instruction 322
Necessity for Practical Experience with Disease 322
Need of Correlation with Ward Cases 323
Some Instances of Effective Correlation with Ward Cases . 323
Examples of Valuable Training in the Diet Kitchen . . . 325
Provision of Kitchen Help 326
Instances of Conspicuous Failure 326
Compromises between Education and Service 328
Percentage of Students Admitted to Diet Kitchen Service . 328
Conclusions 329
Dispensary 330
Greater Number and Range of Cases 330
Preventing Sickness through the Dispensary 331
Social Problems in the Dispensary 331
Evolution of the Dispensary 332
Dispensaries Studied 333
Length of Assignments 333
Failure to Utilize the Dispensary as a Teaching Field . . 334
Correlation between Clinics and Ward Experience . . . 334
Correlation with Class Teaching 335
Absence of Planned Dispensary Instruction 336
Assignment to Clinics of No Educational Value . . . 338
Failure to Use Case Records 340
Time Wasted in Non-Educational Duties 342
Delegation of Non-Educational Work to Permanent Staff 344
Needed Changes in Dispensary Training 345
Length and Content of Student Assignments 345
Need of Dispensary Instructors 346
Conclusions 346
Time Wasted in Non-Nursing Duties 347
Non-Nursing Duties on General Wards 349
Duties on Special Services 350
Miscellaneous Duties 351
Duties of Daily Care 352
Waste Time in Individual Assignments 352
Examples from Another Hospital 355
Assignment of Seniors to Non-Nursing Duties 355
Head Nurseships 356
Total Time Wasted at a Representative Hospital 356
Total Time Wasted at Other Hospitals 359
The Solution: A Permanent Staff 359
Employment of Graduate Nurses 360
Employment of Other Paid Workers 360
Status of the Movement: Municipal Hospitals 361
Improper Use of Attendants 362
Private Hospitals 363
Efficiency and Economy Combined 364
Cost of a Permanent Staff 365
A Fixed Charge on the Training School 366

9. *Theoretical Instruction* 367
Different Forms of Disease and Their Treatment 367
The Physician-Instructor 367
Failure to Stress Prevention of Disease 369
Methods of Teaching 370

PAGE

Correlation with Ward Training 370
The Bedside Clinic 371
The Use of Quizzes 372
Failure to Correlate with Ward Training 375
Psychology 376
Time Allowed to the Teaching of Different Forms of Disease
  and Their Treatment in 22 Schools 378
Social Aspects of Disease and Its Prevention 378
Hours and Year When Given 379
Instructors 379
Training in Public Health Nursing in 22 Schools . . . 381
Disadvantages of Undergraduate Training 381
Lack of Teaching and Supervision 381
Inadequate Time 382
Training in Hospital Social Service in 22 Schools . . . 383
Some Examples of Present Training 385
Need of Special Postgraduate Training 387
Need of General Social Interpretation for All Students . . 388
Time Allowed to the Teaching of Social Aspects of Disease
  and Its Prevention in 22 Schools 389
Teaching of General Nursing Subjects 389
History of Nursing 390
Ethics 390
Time Allowed to the Teaching of General Nursing Subjects
  in 22 Schools 392

10. *Correlation of Class Teaching and Ward Work* 394
Correlation in the First Year 395
Correlation after the First Year 396
The Educational Loss 397
The Danger to Health 397

11. *Nursing in Three Special Branches* 399
Nursing in Tuberculosis 399
Nursing in Venereal Diseases 402
Nursing in Nervous and Mental Diseases 403

12. *Conditions of Work* 406
Day Duty 406
Excessive Length of Hours 407
The Necessity for 24-Hour Service 408
The Necessity for 7-Day Service 408
Irregularity of the Work 408
A Group above the Average 409
A Common Basis of Comparison 409
Standing of Hospitals Studied 410
Relation of Meals to the Daily Schedule 410
Relation of Class Work to the Daily Schedule 411
Time of Class Work 411
Tendency to Include Class Work in Hours of Duty . . . 412
Time Off Duty 413
Notification of Time Off Duty 414
Weekly Hours of Duty 415
Adherence to Schedules of Hours 416
Hours of Duty in Special Services 416
Ratio of Patients to Students 419
Annual Vacations 420

PAGE

Notice of Vacations 421
Relation of Hours to Health 421
Relation of Hours to Working Efficiency 422
Relation of Hours to Education 424
A Practicable Reduction 424
Eight Hours by Law 425
Night Duty 426
Comparative Educational Value of Services 428
Actual Assignments of Night Duty 428
Total Length of Night Duty Planned 431
Actual Duration 432
Length and Frequency of the Several Assignments . . . 434
Length of Intervals between Assignments 435
Hours of Night Duty 436
Provision of Sleeping Quarters 438
Provision for Class Hours 439
Ratio of Patients to Students 440
Length of Training before First Assignment 441
Supervision during the Night 441
Living Conditions 442
Living Quarters 444
Privacy: The Single Room 445
Toilet Facilities 446
Eating Arrangements 446
Home Life 447
Relaxation and Study 448
Social Life and Recreation 449
Social Relations with Medical Staff 450
Amusements and Exercise 450
Form of Government 451

13. *Conclusions and Recommendations* 452
Increased Cost of Training 453
The Need of a Permanent Paid Staff 454
A Proposed Curriculum 455
Differences between Schools 456
Affiliations for Small Schools 457
Entrance Requirements 457
Education 457
Age and Personal Qualifications 458
Hours of Duty 458
Reduction of the Present 3-Years' Course 459
Enrichment of the Present Course 460
Proposal for the Preliminary Term 461
Proposal for Practical Ward Training 463
Services Covered in the Proposed Program 464
Comparison with Actual Experience Records of Students . 466
Proposal for Theoretical Instruction during Ward Training . 469
Comparison of Proposed Course with Existing Curricula . . 470

V. TRAINING COURSES FOR THE SUBSIDIARY NURSING
GROUP

Capital Need of Regulation by a Licensing System 473
Places for Training 474

CONTENTS

| | PAGE |

Use of the Small Hospital 475
Limitations in the Use of Larger Hospitals Having Schools of Nursing 476
Length of the Course 478
Entrance Requirements 478
Practical Experience 479
Ward Training 479
Class Instruction 480

VI. THE UNIVERSITY SCHOOL OF NURSING

Evolution of the University School 485
Organization of the University Training Course 487
Standards 487
Field for Technical Training 487
Organization 489
Status in the University 489
  Financial Basis 491
  Financial Relations with Other Departments 491
  Financial Relations with the Hospital 492
The Curriculum 493
Hospital Training 495
Credit 497
Degrees 498

VII. POSTGRADUATE COURSES

1. *Public Health Nursing Courses* 499

  History and Development of the Courses 500
    Number of Existing Schools or Courses 500
    Courses Given prior to 1917 501
    Courses Organized since 1917 502
  Auspices and Financial Arrangements 504
    Tuition Fees 504
    Financing the Schools 505
  Administration 506
  Organization of the Course 506
    The Director 507
      General Education of Directors 508
      Professional Training 509
      General Standing 510
      Salaries of Directors 510
    Faculty 511
    Advisory Committees 511
  Entrance Requirements 512
    General Education 512
    Professional Education 513
    Previous Education of Students in 16 Schools 514
    Ages at Entrance 515
  Length and Number of Courses Offered 515

PAGE

Relation of Field Work and Class Work 516
Giving Field Work and Class Work Concurrently 516
Field Work Preceding Class Work 518
Class Work Preceding Field Work 518
An Introductory Period of Field Work 519
Apportionment of Work in Courses Studied 519
Relative Amount of Time Devoted to Class Work and Field
Work 520
Field Work 520
Technique of Bedside Care in the Home 520
The Family as Unit of Care 522
Relation with Other Social Agencies 523
Apportionment of Time and Services 523
Observation in the Field 525
Field Work in 16 Schools 526
Supervision 529
A Successful Teaching District 530
The Curriculum 532
Content of the Courses 535
Methods of Instruction 535
A Suggested Curriculum 537
Nursing Subjects 538
Social Subjects 538
Pedagogical Subjects 539
Scientific Subjects 539
2. Courses for Teachers and Administrators 540
The Teaching Staff 540
Ideal Requirements 540
Development in Recent Years 541
The Superintendent 542
Qualifications of the Superintendent 543
Academic Education 544
Assistant Principal and Superintendent 544
Instructors 545
Equipment and Training 545
Conditions of Work 547
Length of Yearly and Weekly Programs 548
Number of Subjects 548
Outside Duties 549
Salaries 550
Need of Standardization 550
3. Teachers College and Its Influence on Nursing Education . . 551
History of the Department 551
Facilities 553
Organization 553
Classification of Students 553
Curriculum 554
Required Courses 554
Electives 556
Future Possibilities 556
Inclusion of Public Health Nursing 557
Type of Students 558
The Larger Aim of Postgraduate Instruction 559
APPENDIX 561

NURSING AND NURSING EDUCATION
IN THE UNITED STATES

INTRODUCTORY NOTE

In December, 1918, at the invitation of the Rockefeller Foundation, a conference of persons interested in the development of public health nursing in the United States was called in New York. About 50 persons attended this conference,—physicians, representatives of public health agencies and public health nursing organizations, leaders in nursing education, hospital administrators, and other persons prominent in public health work. The primary object of the meeting was a discussion of the status of public health nursing in the United States and of the education desirable for training the needed personnel. On these two points all shades of opinion were expressed by those present; there was substantial agreement, however, that the usual three years' hospital training was not, in and by itself, satisfactory for preparing public health nurses.

Accordingly, by request of this initial conference and from nominations by ballot at the conference, a committee of seven was appointed by the president of the Rockefeller Foundation to study the questions raised and to prepare a definite proposal for a course of training for public health nurses, financial support for the investigation being provided by the Foundation.

The committee consisted of the following persons:

Miss Mary Beard, Boston
Dr. H. M. Biggs, New York
Miss Annie W. Goodrich, New York
Miss M. A. Nutting, New York
Miss Lillian D. Wald, New York
Dr. William H. Welch, Baltimore
Professor C.-E. A. Winslow, New Haven

In March, 1919, this committee, organized as the Committee for the Study of Public Health Nursing Education, elected as chairman Professor C.-E. A. Winslow, and added to its membership the following persons:

Dr. Livingston Farrand, Washington
Dr. L. Emmett Holt, New York
Miss Julia C. Lathrop, Washington
Mrs. John Lowman, Cleveland

1

Somewhat later, by the vote of the Committee as thus constituted, there were added to its membership:

Dr. David L. Edsall, Boston

Dr. E. G. Stillman, New York

The Committee was peculiarly fortunate in being able to place the actual conduct of its investigation in the hands of Miss Josephine Goldmark, whose eminent achievements in social research, as in the study which formed the basis of the decision of the United States Supreme Court in the Oregon case, and in more recent studies on industrial hygiene for the United States Public Health Service, peculiarly fitted her for such a task. Miss Goldmark was appointed secretary of the Committee in June, 1919, and in October began the actual organization of the investigations which form the basis of the following reports.

The Committee desires to make special record of its deep appreciation of the services rendered by Miss Goldmark in the conduct of her study of the difficult and complex series of problems with which she has had to deal. Such value as the report of the Committee may possess is primarily due to the tireless and skilful and constructive labor of its secretary; and the Committee believes that Miss Goldmark's detailed report, presented as a supplement to the brief report of the Committee itself, will prove of fundamental value in the development of nursing and of nursing education in the future.

It was originally decided to make a twofold inquiry; to study on the one hand typical examples of public health nursing and public health education carried on by persons other than nurses in various parts of the country, urban and rural; and on the other hand to study the education for such workers afforded by hospital training schools, graduate courses for public health nursing, and special schools of a non-nursing type.

In February, 1920, again at the invitation of the Rockefeller Foundation, a second conference on nursing education was called. At this second conference, discussion centered on the proper training of nurses engaged not in public health work, but within hospitals and on private duty. In effect, the entire trend of nursing education was considered. Following the conference, the Committee on the Study of Public Health Nursing Education was asked by the Rockefeller Foundation to widen its scope so as to include the entire subject of nursing education. In accordance with this request, and upon assurance of further financial support from the Foundation, the Committee agreed to widen its scope as requested and added to its membership six members including superintendents of hospitals and of nursing schools, a clinician and a representative of mental hygiene. The members added in June, 1920, were the following:

Miss S. Lillian Clayton, Philadelphia
Dr. Lewis A. Conner, New York
Dr. C. G. Parnall, Ann Arbor
Dr. Thomas W. Salmon, New York
Dr. Winford H. Smith, Baltimore
Miss Helen Wood, St. Louis

In the course of the investigation Miss Goldmark was assisted by the following staff:

During the first year of work, October, 1919, to October, 1920, Miss Anne H. Strong, R. N., director of the School of Public Health Nursing, conducted by Simmons College and the Instructive District Nursing Association, Boston, acted as assistant secretary of the Committee, and was in charge of the investigation of public health nursing and of the graduate training courses. She has continued her connection with the work as consultant.

During the second year of the work, the assistant secretary was Miss Carolyn E. Gray, R. N., formerly superintendent of nurses, City Hospital, New York, who has also continued in close touch with the work.

In order to secure disinterested and impartial opinions on controversial subjects, both nurse and lay investigators were employed in the field work.

The field work for the study of hospital training schools was carried on by Miss Elizabeth G. Burgess. R. N., inspector of training schools, of the New York State Department of Education; Mrs. J. B. Piggott, R. N., Maryland state inspector of training schools; Miss Carolyn E. Gray, head of the Department of Nursing Education, Western Reserve University; Miss A. H. Turner, professor of physiology, Mt. Holyoke College; Miss F. G. Gates, formerly dean of women, University of the State of Illinois. Miss Turner also made a study of postgraduate courses for teachers and administrators in schools of nursing.

In compiling data for the chapter on hospital training schools assistance was rendered by Miss Edith R. Hall, Mrs. M. P. Gaffney, and Miss P. K. Angell. Miss Hall also assisted in writing up various phases of the work. The statistical work was done by Mrs. S. Lowenthal. Various sections were written and much editorial revision done by Miss Mary D. Hopkins, who has had wide experience in teaching and research. Miss Hopkins is largely responsible also for the chapter on the university school of nursing.

For the study of public health agencies, the field work was carried on, for varying periods of time, by the following persons: Miss Grace R. Bolen, Miss Christina C. Miller, and Miss Elsa M. Butler, who were not nurses but were experienced in public health work, and Miss Helen Ross, experienced in industrial investigation; Mrs. B. A. Haasis, R. N., and Miss Janet R. Geister, R. N.., secretaries of the National Organization for Public Health Nursing, and Mrs. A. M. Staebler, R. N., secretary of the Massachusetts Committee on Health in Industry.

The statistical work for the chapters on public health nursing and on training courses for public health nursing was done by Miss Henriette R. Walter, who aided also in the preparation of these two chapters.

In the study of private duty nursing the field work was carried on by Mrs. J. David Thompson and Miss Adda Eldridge, R. N. Thanks are due to Miss Sara E. Parsons, R. N., for special assistance.

Owing to a special appropriation granted for publishing the Report of the Committee, the publishers are enabled to offer it at a substantially reduced price.

REPORT OF THE COMMITTEE
FOR THE STUDY OF
NURSING EDUCATION

REPORT OF THE COMMITTEE

Objects and Scope of the Investigation

The Committee which presents the following report was first appointed by the Rockefeller Foundation in January, 1919, to conduct a study of "the proper training of public health nurses."

It was, therefore, the pressing need for more and for better nurses in the field of public health that first suggested the desirability of such an investigation. It soon became clear, however, that the entire problem of nursing and of nursing education, relating to the care of the sick as well as to the prevention of disease, formed one essential whole and must be so considered if sound conclusions were to be attained. A year later, in February, 1920, the Foundation requested us to broaden the scope of our inquiry to include "a study of general nursing education, with a view to developing a program for further study and for recommendation of further procedure." We have attempted, therefore, to survey the entire field occupied by the nurse and other workers of related type; to form a conception of the tasks to be performed and the qualifications necessary for their execution; and on the basis of such a study of function to establish sound minimum educational standards for each type of nursing service for which there appears to be a vital social need.

The Rôle of the Nurse in Public Health

Since it was the obvious need for more adequate nursing service in the field of public health which brought to a head the demand for a comprehensive study of nursing education, long-felt and first voiced by the official organization of nurses, it seems natural to begin with a consideration of this phase of the broader problem.

It is obvious that the public health movement has passed far beyond its earlier objectives of community sanitation and the control of the contact-borne diseases by isolation and the use of sera and vaccines. Major health problems of the present day, such as the control of infant mortality and tuberculosis, can be solved only through personal hygiene—an alteration in the daily habits of the individual—and through the establishment of new contacts with the public, contacts which shall permit the application of the resources of medical science at a stage in disease when they can produce a maximum effect. Such changes in the daily habits of the people and in their relation to their medical advisers, can be accomplished by but one means—education. In its present phase of emphasis on personal hygiene, the public health movement has thus become during the past two decades pre-eminently a campaign of popular education.

The new educational objectives of the health administrator may be approached to a limited extent by mass methods. The printed page, the public lecture, the exhibit, the cinematograph, the radiogram, help to prepare the ground and to make success easier. The ultimate victory over ignorance is, however, rarely attained in such ways. Direct personal contact with the conditions of the individual life is essential to success in a matter so truly personal as hygiene. We have sought during the past twenty years for a missionary to carry the message of health into each individual home; and in America we have found this messenger of health in the public health nurse. In order to meet generally accepted standards we should have approximately 50,000 public health nurses to serve the population of the United States,—as against 11,000 now in the field. All public health authorities will probably agree that the need for nurses is the largest outstanding problem before the health administrator of the present day.

In view of this fact, public health authorities, both in this country and abroad, have naturally considered the possibility of finding a short way out of their difficulties by the employment of women trained in some less rigorous fashion than that involved in the education of the nurse. It was, therefore, to the question of the necessary and desirable equipment of the teacher of hygiene in the home that we first directed our attention. There are at present two distinct types of public health nursing practice in the United States—that in which the nurse confines herself to the teaching of hygiene, and that in which such instructive work is combined with the actual care of the sick. A third type of visiting nursing, in which bedside care is given with no educational service, may be observed in individual instances. It results, however, from temporary limitations rather than considered policy, since practically all visiting nurse associations, in theory at least, stress hygienic education in their official program.

The question whether the public health nurse should or should not also render bedside care has been hotly debated during the past few years. The arguments for purely instructive service rest mainly on two grounds, the administrative difficulties involved in the conduct of private sick nursing by official health agencies and the danger that the urgent demands of sick nursing may lead to the neglect of preventive educational measures which are of more basic and fundamental significance. Both of these objections are real and important ones. Yet the observations made in the course of our survey indicate that both may perhaps ultimately be overcome. Several municipal health departments have definitely undertaken to provide organized nursing service for bedside care combined with health teaching, while in other instances instructive nurses, under public auspices, combine a certain amount of emergency service with their fundamentally educational activities. So far as the neglect of instructive work is concerned it results from numerical inadequacy of personnel and can be avoided by a sufficiently large nursing staff.

On the other hand, the plan of instructive nursing divorced from bedside care suffers from defects which if less obvious than those mentioned above are in reality more serious because they are inherent in the very plan itself and therefore not subject to control. In the first place the introduction of the instructive but non-nursing field worker creates at once a duplication of effort, since there must be a nurse from some other agency employed in the same district to give bedside care. In the second place the field worker who attempts health education without giving nursing care is by that very fact cut off from the contact which gives the instructive bedside nurse her most important psychological asset. The nurse who approaches a family where sickness exists, and renders direct technical service in mitigating the burden of that sickness, has an overwhelming advantage, then and thereafter, in teaching the lessons of hygiene. With an adequate number of nurses per unit of population, we believe that the combined service of teaching and nursing will yield the largest results. Nurses employed by state health departments and others whose work is largely stimulative and supervisory in nature may not of course be in position to render direct bedside care.

There are other messengers who may be sent into the field to fulfil other functions. The task of the trained social worker, for example, is to diagnosticate and repair maladjustments in social relationships, a correlated but quite distinct vocational field. Even public health agencies may employ other field workers of an allied type, such as clinic messengers. It is obvious, however, that where health instruction is combined with bedside care the fully trained nurse is the only possible type of health educator; and such a combination represents the one type of service which it is feasible to supply in rural districts. Even purely instructive work, if conducted on the generalized district plan, calls for an ability to detect the early signs of contagious disease, to discern symptoms which suggest tuberculosis, to give counsel as to infant care or the feeding of older children, which can scarcely be attained without a wide training. The relative lack of nursing personnel in Europe has there led to the attempt to train health visitors of the purely instructive type for dealing with special individual problems, such as tuberculosis or child welfare, by training courses much shorter than those required for the preparation of the nurse. Opinion as to the result of such experiments in Europe varies widely; but for conditions as they exist in the United States we are convinced that the teacher of hygiene in the home should be equipped with no less rigorous training than that accorded to the bedside nurse, further supplemented by special studies along the lines of public health and social service.

Essential Qualifications of the Public Health Nurse

That an improvement in quality, as well as an increase in the number, of public health nurses is fundamental to the complete success of the public health movement, is a point on which we find all competent authorities to be substantially agreed. Miss Goldmark's report of an intensive study of the daily work of 164 public health nurses,[1] representing 49 different organizations, gives glimpses of women whose constructive service and compelling personal inspiration seems to touch the highest possibilities of social achievement. Such a nurse establishes herself in the confidence of her community, so that she becomes its trusted adviser and best friend, caring for the sick, securing medical aid, counselling as to hygiene, resolving difficulties of a hundred sorts with the touch of a practised hand.

[1] Exclusive of 24 industrial nurses omitted in this classification.

Nearly half of the nurses observed in our survey were classed as definitely successful in their work and less than one-fourth as definitely unsuccessful,—a showing perhaps better than would be made by a random sampling of most professions. Yet it remains true that either from a lack of knowledge of preventive measures or of teaching methods, from failure to effect contact with physicians or with social agencies, a substantial proportion of public health nurses do fail to realize the possibilities of their profession. Administrative policies, overloading and inadequate supervision, are sometimes at the root of the trouble; yet it is obvious that such a calling as public health nursing demands in the first place a high degree of natural capacity and in the second place a sound and a broad education.

We are convinced, therefore, that the teacher of hygiene in the home should possess in the first place the fundamental education of the nurse and that this should be supplemented by a graduate course in the special problems of public health. The latter point will be discussed in detail in a succeeding paragraph but we believe that the general considerations so far discussed warrant the following conclusion:

Conclusion 1. That, since constructive health work and health teaching in families is best done by persons:

(a) capable of giving general health instruction, as distinguished from instruction in any one specialty; and

(b) capable of rendering bedside care at need;

the agent responsible for such constructive health work and health teaching in families should have completed the nurses' training. There will, of course, be need for the employment, in addition to the public health nurse, of other types of experts such as nutrition workers, social workers, occupational therapists, and the like.

That as soon as may be practicable all agencies, public or private, employing public health nurses, should require as a prerequisite for employment the basic hospital training, followed by a postgraduate course, including both class work and field work, in public health nursing.

The Need for Nurses of High Grade in Hospital Supervision and Nursing Education

Before considering the basic demand for nurses to function in the routine care of the sick we must point out that it is by no means only in the field of public health nursing, that the need for women of high natural qualifications and fundamental training is now manifest. The modern hospital and the modern dispensary represent social forces of enormous and growing magnitude. The technical complexity of their operation increases with every passing year; and, aside from the problem of the staff nurses required for the ordinary routine of such institutions, which will be discussed in a succeeding paragraph, there is perhaps no more urgent problem for the hospital administrator than that of obtaining nursing superintendents and supervisors adequate for the performance of their difficult tasks. The development, both of public health nursing and of administrative hospital nursing, involves and demands a corresponding development in nursing education, which constitutes another inviting field for women.

The defective preparation and qualifications of many instructors in schools of nursing, in both theoretical and practical branches, is very marked. Yet in the training school the instructor is often called upon to teach six or eight different subjects, far more than would be demanded even of the teacher in a country high school. It should be noted, however, that the appointment of any full-time instructors is a very recent development, and has marked a signal educational advance.

With the development of nursing education which we visualize in the future, and particularly with the growth of university schools of nursing, to be discussed in a succeeding paragraph, the field for well-qualified teachers of nursing should prove an increasingly attractive one. We believe we may safely advance as

Conclusion 2. That the career open to young women of high capacity, in public health nursing or in hospital supervision and nursing education, is one of the most attractive fields now open, in its promise of professional success and of rewarding public service; and that every effort should be made to attract such women into this field.

The Problem of Nursing the Sick

We may pass next to the urgent and fundamental problem of providing nursing care for the sick of the community. Here we find far less unanimity of sentiment, in regard either to the quantitative or the qualitative adequacy of nursing service under existing conditions. An appalling shortage of nurses existed during the war; but conditions have materially changed during the past three years. The census reports show an increase in trained registered nurses, male and female, from 82,327 in 1910 to 149,128 in 1920, a truly phenomenal increase of 83 per cent. Some 11,000 of these are employed as public health nurses and approximately the same number in hospitals and other institutions, leaving over 120,000 for private duty service, of whom, however, many are not in the active practice of their profession. This 1920 figure gives us a ratio of one trained nurse to 700 persons for the country as a whole. The majority of trained nurses are concentrated in the larger cities so that the rural districts in many states are wholly lacking in service of this kind. The evidence is that at present in the cities the supply of trained nurses is adequate to existing demands in normal times. The reason why many persons who need nursing care in hospitals and in the homes of the poor fail to receive it is to be sought in economic factors, rather than in a shortage of nurses.

In regard to the quality of the nursing service available at the present day we find more radical differences of opinion. Private physicians frequently express the view that for ordinary nursing, even the graduate of the existing training school is "over trained," that the service which she renders is too costly, and that a woman with a very brief training in bedside routine would be as satisfactory, or perhaps more satisfactory, than the average registered nurse. As a result of this feeling there have been persistent and vigorous efforts in certain quarters to break down the standards of nursing education which have been laboriously built up during the past twenty years.

In so far as these efforts would remove the safeguards which guarantee to the patient suffering from acute disease, and to the physician caring for such a patient, the quality of service necessary for safety, we feel that they constitute a real danger to the cause of public health. Nurses, physicians, hospital authorities and legislators, in erecting these safeguards, have been inspired by a just sense of the vital dangers to life which may result from the unskilled nursing of a critical case and of the grave responsibility incurred by both the medical and the nursing professions when such malpractice occurs. We would therefore record our conviction in regard to this point as

Conclusion 3. That for the care of persons suffering from serious and acute disease the safety of the patient, and the re-

*sponsibility of the medical and nursing professions, demand the
maintenance of the standards of educational attainment now
generally accepted by the best sentiment of both professions and
embodied in the legislation of the more progressive states; and
that any attempt to lower these standards would be fraught with
real danger to the public.*

The Field for a Subsidiary Type of Nursing Service

When we find that certain private physicians, like the public
health administrators, demand nurses of a higher quality than
those now in the field, while others desire merely "hands for
the physician" with a minimum of education below the present
standard, it seems probable that there is reason on both sides
and that the apparent conflict is due to a difference in the objectives to be met. For the care of acute and serious illness
and for public health work it seems certain that we need high
natural qualifications and sound technical education; for the
care of mild and chronic illness and convalescence it may well
be that a different type of capacity and training may be
necessary.

It seems clear to the Committee, however, that, if two types
of nursing service are desirable, the distinction should be drawn,
not on economic grounds, but according to the type of illness
involved. We are even somewhat doubtful as to the possibility
of attaining very substantial economies by the introduction of
a subsidiary type of private duty nurse. Our survey of the situation does not indicate that the income of the private duty
nurse is at present generally an exorbitant one, when we take
into account the amount of unemployment,—amounting in a
typical group of 118 nurses to a week each month during the
busy winter season. If this factor be allowed for, the margin
between the average annual income of the private duty nurse
and that of the domestic servant is not so great as to permit
of the existence of an intermediate grade on a salary level very
much below that of the present registered nurse. The solution
of the economic problem which confronts the family of low
income must probably be sought along the lines of cost distribution through some form of community organization, or along
the lines of group insurance such as that being experimentally
tested in New York City.

In any event, a pneumonia case, a diphtheria case, a grave

cardiac case will require the highest grade of nursing obtainable, whether it occurs in a palace or a hovel. It is the mild and chronic and convalescent case which offers a field for the partially trained worker, and the exact extent of this field has never yet been fully surveyed. In our own study we have secured careful estimates from 118 graduate nurses which indicate that during a period of 3 months one quarter of their time was spent on cases which could have been cared for by an attendant of the partially trained type. A somewhat similar estimate was obtained from 48 practising physicians, 21 believing that trained nurses were unnecessarily employed for less than a quarter of their cases, 17 placing the figure between half and three-quarters, and 10 at over three-quarters.

In considering the problem of subsidiary nursing service it must be remembered that we are dealing with no new development. Of the 300,000 male and female nurses in the United States in 1920, slightly more than half were of grades below the standard of the graduate nurse. The "practical nurse," the "trained attendant," is an existing fact; and in the opinion of a large group of the medical profession who utilize her services she fills a real place in the complex problem of caring for the sick.

If we include with the trained and registered nurses (149,128) the student nurses in hospitals (54,953) and to these add the number of attendants and practical nurses (151,996), as constituting the entire body of persons occupied in caring for the sick, we have altogether one nurse, trained or untrained, to every 294 well persons. This would seem to give an adequate supply if numbers alone are considered, provided a proper distribution could be secured.

On the other hand the danger in the existence of a loosely defined and unregulated group of partially trained workers, in the same field as a more highly educated type, constitutes a real and a serious complication. The nursing profession has discharged a fundamental duty to the public in stimulating the development of registration laws which define and delimit the practice of that profession, and protect the community against fraud and exploitation by those who collect fees and assume responsibilities to which their qualifications do not entitle them. In addition to the registration of the trained nurse it is essential that the lower grade of nursing service should also be defined and registered; and the states of New York, Missouri, California, Michigan, and Maryland have taken definite steps in enacting legislation, toward this end. The name to be selected for the subsidiary group is a difficult problem. As is so often the case the root of disagreement lies largely in nomenclature. The title "attendant," embodied in three of the laws mentioned above, is distasteful to those who bear it and tends to discourage the enlistment of those who may desire to enter this field. On the other hand the term "practical nurse" assumes a most unfortunate antithesis between education and practice; and the splendid professional and public service rendered by "the nurse" in war and in peace, entitles her to the protection of her existing professional status. We are inclined to believe that the term "nursing aide" or "nursing attendant" best meets the need for clear differentiation, while providing the subsidiary worker with a suitable name.

With two distinct grades of service available, the individual physician would be responsible for the choice of a trained nurse or a nursing attendant or nursing aide in a given instance. The public can be safeguarded in these matters only by state legislation providing for licensing of nursing registries and requiring explicit statement as to the license qualifications of each nurse or nursing aide furnished. We believe that by this means the maximum increase of nursing service possible under existing economic conditions could be attained; and we would therefore recommend as

Conclusion 4. That steps should be taken through state legislation for the definition and licensure of a subsidiary grade of nursing service, the subsidiary type of worker to serve under practising physicians in the care of mild and chronic illness, and convalescence, and possibly to assist under the direction of the trained nurse in certain phases of hospital and visiting nursing.

The Hospital Training School

Our survey of the actual field of nursing service has thus led us to the conclusion that the good of the community demands: (a) the recruiting for public health nursing, hospital nursing, and the care of the acutely ill, of a larger number of young women of good natural capacity and the provision for such women of a sound and effective education; and (b) the development and standardization of a subsidiary nursing service of a different grade for the care of mild and chronic disease. We may next pass to the second part of our problem,—a consideration of existing educational facilities for the training of the two types of workers indicated as desirable.

So far as the trained nurse is concerned, whether she is to function in private duty, in public health or in institutional service, it is clear that her basic professional education must be acquired in the hospital training school. We have, therefore, devoted a major part of the present investigation to a somewhat detailed study of existing conditions and future possibilities in hospital training.

The development of the hospital training school for nurses constitutes a unique chapter in the history of education. In almost all fields of professional life education has begun on a basis of apprentice training. The first law schools and the first medical schools were the outgrowth of the lawyer's and the physician's office. In nearly all other fields than that of nursing, however, even in such relatively new professions as journalism and business advertising, education has outgrown the apprentice stage and leadership has passed into the hands of independent institutions, organized and endowed for a specifically educational purpose. The training of nurses, on the other hand, is still in the main, actually if not technically, directed by organizations created and maintained for the care of disease, rather than for professional education.

The progress which has been accomplished in nursing education, under such anomalous conditions, is such as to reflect high credit upon both hospital administrators and the leaders of the nursing profession. The hospitals have in many instances been inspired by a broad and constructive vision of training school possibilities; while the devotion with which nursing directors have labored for high standards, often against almost insuperable obstacles, calls for the warmest admiration. Yet the conflict of interests between a policy of hospital administration, which properly aims to care for the sick at a minimum cost, and a policy of nursing education which with equal propriety aims to concentrate a maximum of rewarding training into a minimum time, is a real and vital one.

The fact that a field so tempting as that of modern nursing, with its remarkable possibilities of service in public health, in institutional management, and in teaching, fails to attract students in the number, and of the quality, we should desire strongly suggests that there is some shortcoming in the established avenues of approach to the nursing profession. The hospitals themselves, depending as they do so largely upon student nurses for their routine operation, have in past years found themselves seriously handicapped by the small number of applicants, and many a superintendent will testify to the fact that the difficulty of securing a high quality of nursing is one of the gravest which he has to meet. The phenomenally rapid growth in the number of hospitals has created within a brief period a demand for a large number of students and the requirements for admission have therefore been kept at a very low level, thus resulting in a reduction in the proportion of well-educated applicants. For the good of the hospital, as well as for that of the nursing profession and of the public at large, a careful and dispassionate appraisal of the adequacy of the present day training school would seem to be urgently desirable.

Conditions Revealed by a Study of Typical Hospital Training Schools

An extensive survey of the vast field of hospital training schools (there are over 1,800 such schools in the United States) was obviously beyond the possible resources of our Committee. It was therefore decided to select a small group of schools, of reasonably typical character, for intensive study. Twenty-three such schools were finally chosen, representing large and small, public and private, general and special hospitals, in various sections of the United States. These schools were undoubtedly well above the median grade and their average may, we believe, be taken as fairly representative of the best current practice in nursing education. Each school was studied in detail by two types of investigators, one a practical expert in nursing education, and the other an experienced educator from outside the nursing field. By this means we aimed, on the one hand to secure competent criticism of nursing procedures, and on the other a broad view of general educational standards. The detailed results of this investigation as presented in Miss Goldmark's report, will, we believe, prove highly enlightening to the student of this problem.

The training of the nurse involves a certain basic knowledge of the fundamental chemical and biological sciences, theoretical instruction in the principles of nursing and, above all, supervised practical training in actual nursing procedures. In all three phases of this work Miss Goldmark's report reveals conspicuous successes and equally conspicuous failures; and the remarkable thing is that successes and failures so often appear side by side in the same institution.

Thus, we may find in a training school with a good ward service that the fundamental science courses fail because of wholly inadequate laboratory equipment. In another school, the theoretical instructor may show a hopeless lack of teaching ability (as in the case of class presentation which consisted in the dictation of questions and answers from a prehistoric notebook); or she may be so handicapped by other duties as to leave no time for the proper conduct of her classes. Lectures by physicians may be informative and inspiring in one department of a hospital; irregular in delivery, careless and dull in content, in another. Ward assignments are in many cases largely dictated by the need for hospital service rather than by the educational requirements of the students. This is clearly evidenced by the astonishing irregularity of the time spent on different services by individual students and by the marked deviation between all the time assignments actually performed and those scheduled in the official program of the course. Thus in one school where 7½ months were assigned to surgical service the members of a single class had actually worked on this service for from 7 to 13¾ months. Of the 23 schools surveyed by us one made no adequate provision for obstetrical service, while 5 gave no training in pediatrics, 7 no experience in communicable disease and 18 none in mental disease. In view of the difficulties in making affiliations in some of these subjects, notably in communicable and mental diseases, some of these omissions are scarcely to be wondered at.

The supervision of work on the wards was in certain instances notably inadequate. In only a few brilliantly exceptional cases was the ward work purposefully correlated with theoretical instruction. The lack of an intelligently planned progressive training was obvious in a large number of the hospitals studied, first year students often being found in positions of responsibility for which they were wholly unprepared, while seniors in another ward were repeating an educationally idle and profitless routine. Most striking of all, was the factor of time wasted in procedures, essential to the conduct of the hospital, but of no educational value to the student concerned. Hours and days spent in performing the work of a ward maid, in putting away linen, in sterilizing apparatus, in mending rubber gloves, in running errands, long after any important technique involved had become second nature, accounted in one typical hospital operating under the 8-hour system, where this problem was specially studied, for a clear wastage of between one-fourth and one-fifth of the student's working day.

The total amount of time assigned to ward service under the conditions which obtain in many hospitals is, in itself, a fairly complete obstacle to educational achievement. Our selected group of hospitals, surely in this respect far above the general average, shows a median day of between 8 and 8.5 hours on ward duty alone, exclusive of all classroom instruction. Irregular and excessive and unproductive night duty is the rule rather than the exception. Crowded and unattractive living conditions tend, in certain hospitals, to impair the morale of the student body; and an atmosphere of autocratic discipline frequently prevents the development of a psychological atmosphere favorable to effective co-operative effort.

The foregoing paragraphs present, we are aware, a somewhat gloomy picture. In presenting them, we would emphasize two points which are of major importance. In the first place, such shortcomings as have been pointed out are not fairly chargeable to deliberate neglect on the part of hospital authorities or nursing superintendents. In so far as they exist, they are due to the inherent difficulty of adjusting the conflicting claims of hospital management and nursing education, under a system in which nursing education is provided with no independent financial endowments for its specific ends. The difficulties involved in the task of resolving this conflict are perhaps illustrated by the fact that out of 144 registered training schools in New York State, 60 changed superintendents during a single recent year.

In the second place it is encouraging to note, by reference to Miss Goldmark's report, that every one of the shortcomings in hospital training discussed above has been corrected, with substantially complete success, in one or more of the training schools studied by our investigators. The difficulties are not insuperable. Each of them has been overcome in some schools and most of them in some of the best schools. Training schools exist today in which the student receives a sound and an inspiring education, with a minimum of sacrifice to the exigencies of hospital administration. Yet such schools are still the exception; and we are convinced that the progress we desire can come only through a frank facing of the truth. The following statement is, we believe, thoroughly justified by such facts as we have been able to obtain:

Conclusion 5. That, while training schools for nurses have made remarkable progress, and while the best schools of today in many respects reach a high level of educational attainment, the average hospital training school is not organized on such a basis as to conform to the standards accepted in other educational fields; that the instruction in such schools is frequently casual and uncorrelated; that the educational needs and the health and strength of students are frequently sacrificed to practical hospital exigencies; that such shortcomings are primarily due to the lack of independent endowments for nursing education; that existing educational facilities are on the whole, in the majority of schools, inadequate for the preparation of the high grade of nurses required for the care of serious illness, and for service in the fields of public health nursing and nursing education; and that one of the chief reasons for the lack of sufficient recruits, of a high type, to meet such needs lies precisely in the fact that the average hospital training school does not offer a sufficiently attractive avenue of entrance to this field.

Recommendations for the Improvement of the Hospital Training School

Miss Goldmark's study has not stopped short with a revelation of the defects which are commonly found in the conduct of nursing education. It makes clear that only the co-ordination and standardization of the best existing practice is necessary in order to place nursing education on the plane where it belongs.

In the first place we believe that a training school which aims to educate nurses capable of caring for acute disease or of going on into public health nursing or supervisory and teaching positions, must require for entrance the completion of a high school course or its equivalent. Nearly one-third of all the training schools in the United States now make this requirement; and with 150,000 girls graduating from high schools every year it should be possible for well-organized courses to attract an ample number of candidates.

The course should begin with a preliminary term of 4 months' training in the basic sciences and in elementary nursing procedures with appropriate ward practice but without regular ward service, as outlined in Miss Goldmark's report. The necessary teaching personnel and laboratory equipment for the former may in many instances be secured by the smaller hospitals through the establishment of a central training course or by co-operation with high schools, normal schools, or junior colleges.

There should then follow a period of 24 months (including 2 months for vacation) devoted to a carefully graded and progressive course in the theory and practice of nursing, with lectures and ward practice so correlated as to facilitate intelligent case study and with the elimination of routine duties of no educational value. Hospital and dispensary services in medicine, surgery, pediatrics, obstetrics, communicable diseases and mental diseases should be provided through appropriate affiliation. Teachers and equipment should be of such a grade as would be acceptable in a reputable college or normal school.

We regard it as fundamental that the working day for the student nurse, including ward work and classroom periods, should not exceed 8 hours. The working week should not exceed 48 hours and preferably 44 hours. Training school experience, as well as a comparison with that accumulated in other educational fields, makes it clear that a longer period of scheduled work for the student is incompatible, either with educational attainment or with the maintenance of health.

By such an organization of the course of study, and particularly by the elimination of unrewarding routine service, we are convinced that the period of training may be safely shortened from the present standard of 3 years to 28 months. Such a saving would mean an increase of over 20 per cent in the potential output of the training school through the saving of time alone. The shortening of the course would, in itself, prove an attraction to the prospective student; but the main consideration to be kept in view is that the shorter course projected would not imply a lowering but a raising of educational standards. Miss Goldmark's analysis of the situation makes it clear that the intensively-planned course of 28 months would involve no substantial sacrifice in a single service as compared with the actual median practice of the present day, and would supply other services now almost universally neglected. It is the experience in every other field of education that the way to attract students is to raise standards, not to lower them. In medicine, in law, in engineering, in teaching, the schools which raise requirements are the ones from which students must be turned away; and even in nursing the success of the better schools furnishes convincing testimony to the same basic principle. It is the higher standing of the course here outlined, quite as much as its lessened length, which we are confident would insure an increase in the number of students, as well as an improvement in their quality.

There are, we believe, two fundamental essentials to the success of a training school planned on the suggested lines. It must first of all be directed by a board or a committee, organized more or less independently for the primary purposes of education. The interests of hospital management and of educational policy must necessarily at times conflict, and unless the educational viewpoint is competently represented the training school will infallibly suffer in the end. In the second place it is fundamental to the success of nursing education that adequate funds should be available for the educational expenses of the school itself, and for the replacement of student nurses by graduate nurses and hospital help in the execution of routine duties of a non-educational character. A satisfactory relationship between school and hospital demands careful cost-accounting and a clear analysis of the money value of services rendered by the school to the pupil and the hospital, by the pupil to the hospital, and by the hospital to the pupil and the school. The cost of adequate education must in any case be a paramount consideration, to which we shall return in a succeeding paragraph. Assuming its essential importance, the following conclusion seems to us justified:

Conclusion 6. That, with the necessary financial support and under a separate board or training school committee, organized primarily for educational purposes, it is possible, with completion of a high school course or its equivalent as a prerequisite, to reduce the fundamental period of hospital training to 28 months, and at the same time, by eliminating unessential, non-educational routine, and adopting the principles laid down in Miss Goldmark's report, to organize the course along intensive and co-ordinated lines with such modifications as may be necessary for practical application; and that courses of this standard would be reasonably certain to attract students of high quality in increasing numbers.

Postgraduate Nursing Education

The course of 28 months discussed above would furnish the complete education for a student desiring to practise as a bedside nurse in private duty or in hospitals and other institutions; and its completion should entitle her to the diploma in nursing and to state registration. For the nurse who desires to specialize along either of the more advanced lines, of public health nursing, or hospital supervision and nursing education, a further period of postgraduate training is obviously desirable.

Teachers College in Columbia University has played the part of pioneer in preparing graduate nurses for hospital supervision and nursing education; and certain of the newer university schools of nursing are already offering attractive courses along the same line. The development of graduate courses in public health nursing has made even more notable progress. The first organized course of this type was offered in Boston in 1906, and by 1920 there were 20 such courses in operation, under the auspices of universities, public health nursing associations or schools of social work.

The activities of 16 of these schools of public health nursing have been studied in the course of our investigation, and the results achieved in this new field are in general deserving of high praise. The course is apparently in process of standardization at a length of about 8 months: 4 devoted to theoretical instruction in public health, public health nursing, educational psychology, and social problems; and 4 to supervised field work with a public health nursing organization. The courses at present offered are in many instances tentative and lacking in assured financial status. With the development of the university school of nursing (to be discussed in succeeding paragraphs), they may be expected to fall within its sphere of influence and to develop an increasing stability and usefulness.

Conclusion 7. Superintendents, supervisors, instructors, and public health nurses should in all cases receive special additional training beyond the basic nursing course.

The University School of Nursing

For advanced training the development of the University School of Nursing has been perhaps the most notable feature in the progress of nursing education during the past ten years. As long ago as 1899 Teachers College in Columbia University admitted properly qualified nurses to its junior class, thus giving 2 years of college credit for the 3 years of nursing training. Since 1916, no less than 13 different colleges and universities have provided combined courses, through which students may acquire both a nurse's training and a college degree.

The combined course in such a school, for example, involves 2 years of ordinary college work including, besides work of a liberal nature, certain of the fundamental sciences basic in nursing education. Then follow 2 years of intensive training in the hospital and, finally, a 5th year of postgraduate education in one of the higher specialties of nursing, public health, institutional supervision or nursing education. At the close of training the student receives a diploma in nursing and the bachelor's degree in nursing or in science.

This type of school of nursing should, in the judgment of the Committee, be a separate and independent department of the university, cognate in rank and organization with the school of medicine, or the school of law. It should have direct responsibility for all instruction given during the years of hospital training and the postgraduate nursing year.

A definite affiliation with one or more hospitals must in any case be established, along the line of the agreements now in force between medical schools and hospitals. The school supplies student nursing service and assumes a definite responsibility for a larger or smaller share of ward supervision and perhaps of graduate service. The hospital, on the other hand, provides maintenance for the nursing staff and conforms to the standards held by the university to be essential for the realization of its educational ideals. A university hospital will of course offer the most promising field for a university school of nursing; but in default of such an institution there seems no reason why a university school should not establish satisfactory working agreements with various adjacent hospitals, provided only that the maintenance of adequate standards in the practice field remains in its own hands.

If its present practical functions be clearly understood the university school of nursing possesses unique advantages in respect to both of the essentials for success in nursing education, to which reference has been made in a preceding paragraph. It possesses the power of independent educational leadership and is grounded on the solid foundations of educational ideals, to a degree which a training school committee, ultimately responsible to a board of hospital trustees, can seldom hope to realize; and it is likely to obtain financial resources to a more nearly adequate extent. Furthermore, through its university contacts the University School of Nursing has unique opportunities to attract students of the type so greatly needed for the fulfilment of the higher tasks in the nursing of the future.

It should be made quite clear that the Committee does not recommend that nursing schools in general should work toward the establishment of courses of a character that a university would accept for a degree. We realize that the numerical proportion of the nursing profession to be contributed by the university school will perhaps always be a relatively small one. Yet we believe that the importance of this portion of the educational structure would be difficult to overestimate. The value that we see at present in the university schools is that they will furnish a body of leaders who have the fundamental training essential in administrators, teachers, and the like. One of the greatest, if not the greatest, of the reasons for the imperfections in the present training of private duty nurses is that great numbers of schools have developed without any coincident development of adequate numbers of persons properly trained to guide the pupils during their course. Unless well taught they cannot be well trained. The university school of nursing should be the keystone of the entire arch. It will not only train leaders and develop and standardize procedures for all other schools. It will, by its permeating influence, give inspiration and balance to the movement as a whole and gradually but steadily improve the efficiency of every institution for the training of nurses of whatever type. We would therefore urge as

Conclusion 8. That the development and strengthening of University Schools of Nursing of a high grade for the training of leaders is of fundamental importance in the furtherance of nursing education.

Educational Provision for the Subsidiary Type of Nursing Service

We have pointed out in a preceding section of this report that there appears to be a real place for nursing service of a subsidiary type, to be used in the institution and in the home, for the routine care of patients suffering from disease of a mild or chronic type or in convalescence. We have also pointed out that this subsidiary service is an existing fact, whether we like it or no.

Existing facilities for the training of the subsidiary worker are today of the most limited type. It is obvious that courses in home nursing of a few weeks' duration, such as those conducted under the auspices of the American Red Cross, while most useful in disseminating the sort of knowledge which all girls and women should possess, in no way suffice as preparation for the practice of a profession. When they are advertised as adequate for this latter end, such courses may do far more harm than good,—as evidenced by the fact that "graduates" of such courses, after 48 hours of training, have practised as qualified nurses and received $5 a day for their services.

Courses for the training of nursing aides offered by the Household Nursing Association of Boston and by local Young Women's Christian Associations in various parts of the country and those stimulated by the Bureau for the Home Care of the Sick under the Thomas Thompson Trust are on a wholly different basis. The number of graduates from such courses is, however, small and their control after graduation, loose and unsatisfactory. Since the existence of the subsidiary nursing group is a concrete fact, and in view of the valuable results to be derived from the service of this group in a definitely restricted field, it seems obvious that specific provision should be made for the training of workers of this type.

The field for the training of nursing aides would seem to be an ample one. The special hospital not served by affiliation with a school of nursing, and the small general hospital whose facilities are inadequate for the maintenance of a nursing school of standard grade might be considered as training grounds. In the large general hospital whose opportunities are not fully utilized by student nurses there is no valid objection to the training of the subsidiary group, provided that it is conducted in separate and distinct wards so that the sacrifice of the interests of either of the two groups of pupils may be avoided. The requirement for entrance should be a grammar school course or its equivalent and the period of training approximately 8 or 9 months. Suggestions of great value in regard to the safeguarding of such a course for "trained attendants" will be found in a recent report issued by the Board of Regents of the University of the State of New York.

It is essential in providing for this new type of education that hospital patients should be protected from malpractice and students from exploitation by an adequate graduate nursing service for the care of acute illness and for supervision of the students. Again, therefore, we must assume a reasonable financial support before this, or any other, educational enterprise can be honestly undertaken. Furthermore, we believe that a useful development in the training of nursing aides can be expected only when the standards of the schools for such aides and their activities after graduation are controlled by a properly safeguarded system of state legislation, such as now exists in Missouri.[2] With these assumptions we would recommend as

Conclusion 9. That when the licensure of a subsidiary grade of nursing service is provided for, the establishment of training courses in preparation for such service is highly desirable; that such courses should be conducted in special hospitals, in small unaffiliated general hospitals, or in separate sections of hospitals where nurses are also trained; and that the course should be of 8 or 9 months' duration; provided the standards of such schools be approved by the same educational board which governs nursing training schools.

The Financial Problem

We believe that the educational plan which has been outlined above is, according to existing information, necessary and sufficient for the solution of the problems involved in securing an adequate nursing service of all essential types. The school for nursing aides would provide the subsidiary worker needed for the care of the mild and chronic and convalescent case. The hospital training school, with adequate funds and an independent educational organization, would attract more candidates and better candidates and would prepare them adequately for the nursing of acute disease. The university school of nursing would prepare the leaders in public health nursing, in hospital supervision, and nursing education and would inspire and standardize the entire movement. Progress must be made gradually, of course, building up for the future, step by step, upon the basis of existing facilities.

It is clear, however, that the attainment of these ends requires financial support, and requires it at all points along the line. The training of nursing aides will cost money; the training of

[2] The Missouri act is unusually effective in providing that "no person shall practise as a nurse for hire or engage in the care of the sick as an attendant for hire unless licensed by the Board as hereinafter provided."

nurses will cost more money; the university school will require endowment on a reasonably generous scale. The hospital, in its operation of the training school, has for generations been trying to make bricks without straw, in the upbuilding of an educational system on an apprentice basis and without independent educational resources. It has made every possible effort,—except the effort to secure educational endowment. It is time that the hospital should be relieved from the dilemma of exploiting student nurses on the one hand, or of diverting funds given for the care of the sick on the other, by the provision of endowment specifically devoted to the purposes of education.

We are well aware that many of those who have taken counsel with us in regard to this matter have cherished the hope that the Committee would find some magic pathway out of the maze of nursing education; but such hopes are vain. There is no short cut to the end which we all have in view. The establishment of a sound educational policy is the one essential to attracting students in quantity and of quality; and a sound educational policy requires specific financial support. If the community needs and desires the services of competent nurses for the care of the sick and the prosecution of the campaign of public health, it must pay for their education, as it pays for every other conceivable kind of education—either through taxes or through voluntary contributions or through the generosity of its great philanthropic foundations. No broadly conceived and systematic effort to obtain such financial support for nursing education has ever yet been made. When it is made we are convinced that it will not fail. In institutions where nursing education has been even partially endowed, as in the first school of nursing at St. Thomas' Hospital, London, and the Department of Nursing and Health at Teachers College, New York, substantial achievements in the better education of nurses have been rendered possible.

It is obvious that the plan recommended for improvement of the education of nurses cannot be adequately put into effect in any hospital training school without additional funds for this purpose. The strategic position which the university schools of nursing will occupy in regard to the whole movement indicates their development as of special importance. An adequate endowment for a group of such university schools would establish centers of influence which could safely be trusted to exert a profound influence upon nursing education. We, therefore, urge as the final conclusion from our study of this problem:

Conclusion 10. That the development of nursing service adequate for the care of the sick and for the conduct of the modern public health campaign demands as an absolute prerequisite the securing of funds for the endowment of nursing education of all types; and that it is of primary importance, in this connection, to provide reasonably generous endowment for university schools of nursing.

C.-E. A. WINSLOW, *Chairman*
MARY BEARD
HERMANN M. BIGGS
S. LILLIAN CLAYTON
LEWIS A. CONNER
DAVID L. EDSALL
LIVINGSTON FARRAND
ANNIE W. GOODRICH
L. EMMETT HOLT
JULIA C. LATHROP
ISABEL W. LOWMAN
M. ADELAIDE NUTTING
CHRISTOPHER G. PARNALL
THOMAS W. SALMON
WINFORD H. SMITH
E. G. STILLMAN
LILLIAN D. WALD
WILLIAM H. WELCH
HELEN WOOD

REPORT OF A SURVEY OF NURSING AND NURSING EDUCATION

BY

JOSEPHINE GOLDMARK, *Secretary*

REPORT OF A SURVEY

INTRODUCTION

The New Interest in Health and Nursing

The investigation on which this report is based was, in the first instance, prompted by the desire to obtain authentic, impartial information on public health nursing in the United States; to study its calibre and function in typical communities of our country, urban and rural; and to deduce, by scrutiny of workers in the field, the type of training needed for successful accomplishment.

The nurse as field agent of the great new movement for public health was thus the first object of inquiry. A study of her functions and her equipment led directly to the hospital training school, which has educated the nurse in public health work, as well as the older type of nurse who, after graduation, continues her activities within the hospital or in the ranks of private duty.

It soon became evident that a study of the training given for public health nursing necessarily involved scrutiny of that whole system of education for nurses which has, during the last half century, been slowly developing in wards and classrooms,—a teaching field of unrivalled potentialities in its congregation of clinical cases.

What, then, is the system of nurses' training evolved from such rich possibilities? What education, what preparation is being given today to the 50,000 young women in the hospital training schools of the United States? How are they being fitted for their ultimate destinations in one of the three branches of nursing, old and new: as public health nurses, as private duty nurses, or in institutions as teachers or administrators, or on the permanent nursing staff?

From being a special inquiry into public health nursing the scope of our study was thus vastly widened. Not only must we include all three branches of nurses, and seek to gauge their respective functions and needs, but we must go more deeply into the very heart of the problem, that is, the nature of the training school itself, its dual character as educational institution and provider of nursing service for the hospital. The relation, therefore, of the hospital and training school must be analysed and clearly set forth. It is only fair to say that such a fundamental study of nursing education has long been advocated and urged by the official organization of nurses.

This study of nurses and their training in the United States thus could not be a pure study in education or vocational training. For owing to the position of nursing in the world of education, as one of the few professions still actually in the stage of apprenticeship, the writer has of necessity been confronted at every turn by the genuine claims of service often in conflict with education. For a twofold reason the education of the nurse presents practical problems of the utmost delicacy and difficulty. It has shared, namely, with the continuous processes in industry, the problem of meeting a 24-hour service 7 days each week; while in rendering this service to the sick and helpless it has had responsibilities more solemn than any known to industry, shared only by the medical profession.

Whatever the future of the school of nursing,—and the history of vocational education gives promise of the final evolution of apprenticeship into an ordered educational system—the persistence of apprenticeship today must be reckoned with in any study of nursing as a highly influential if not still determining factor. Until the general public by taxation for public institutions, by endowments and gifts for those privately supported, makes the hospital independent of the school for its permanent nursing staff, the hospital must continue its paradoxical attempt to maintain a school without means; the school in its turn must remain in part at least crippled by work in excess of any possible educational program.

We have dwelt, in the following report, on the fatal error on the part of both hospitals and schools, of generally accepting as inherent and final the existing relationship between the two, and of having failed as yet even to give public expression to the inevitable consequences. To make clear this fundamental fallacy in the relationship of hospital and training school is in a sense the center and focus of our study.

For such a study the present moment is auspicious. At this time, and perhaps for the first time, various causes have contributed towards awakening a new live interest in health and in the work of nursing. It is not too much to say that health and, above all, public health has become a new reality in every-day life. Health terms and health activities almost unintelligible a decade ago are parts of our daily speech and acceptance. An epidemic of influenza or of infantile paralysis, the very threat of typhus, speaks louder than words the oneness of our common lot; and that democracy, which in politics and industry is still unrealized, in matters of health forces itself tangibly upon us.

This new concern, this preoccupation of large numbers of our people with the problems of health and disease is more than the reflection of a fear. It is more than the instinctive desire to protect one's own. It represents, whether consciously or not, a broader, more generous reaction from years of destruction and physical waste. Where war has left in political and industrial life chiefly stagnation or wreckage, and has closed the minds of men, in the field of health it seems to have released springs of interest and action. The horrors of war, the waste of young manhood, threw into relief as never before in peace the beauty and sacredness of normal physical health; never before was the preciousness of childhood so brought home to the hearts and minds of men. It has therefore been in accord with a genuine though dimly apprehended national interest that various large foundations have turned their huge resources to health programs; that community health work of all varieties has sprung up and made sensible progress during the last few years. Not the least index of this new interest is the increase in the number of public health nurses at work in the United States, which has more than doubled in the last six years, and for the study of whose work and equipment this inquiry was in the first instance undertaken.

From being a subject of special moment, therefore, only to the groups immediately concerned,—that is, the hospitals and the training schools, doctors and nurses,—the education of nurses and the problem of obtaining in sufficient numbers candidates of good calibre is now becoming a matter of concern even to the uninitiated. Almost suddenly, therefore, the apprenticeship system of training nurses, accepted as the only method of education, is on the defensive.

While this report deals necessarily with a great variety of more or less technical details—educational, medical, and administrative—it aims to be something more than a technical discussion for specialists. It aims to aid in the practical solution of the problem of supplying for the greatly widened sphere of the nurse in the modern world a personnel adequate in numbers, quality, and kind, and fitted for its proper work.

This practical problem needs, to do it justice, detailed discussion and analysis which is offered in the following report. Our final conclusions may, however, be very briefly summarized. From our field study of the nurse in public health nursing, in private duty, and as instructor and supervisor in hospitals, it is clear that there is need of a basic undergraduate training for all nurses alike, which should lead to a nursing diploma. Postgraduate training in any one of the three nursing specialties should be given after completion of the basic undergraduate course and should lead to a further diploma or degree. It is, moreover, clear that training is needed also for a subsidiary nursing group who shall be equipped to care for cases of nonacute illness and disability, for chronic and convalescent cases, in which the services of a graduate nurse are not necessary.

Safeguards for the training and employment of a subsidiary group are discussed in detail. The safety of the patient from incompetence must be the primary consideration; standards of nursing education already achieved must be in no way imperilled by the standardization of a secondary group. That both provisos can be met is the belief set forth in the following chapters. By the delegation to a subsidiary group of the appropriate cases, and by the improvements in nurses' training advocated in this report, the nursing profession will be the more surely enabled to play its part without which medical and hygienic science would be crippled in its beneficent purpose: the alleviation of mortal pain, the prevention and cure of disease, and the teaching of health.

PART A
FUNCTIONS OF THE NURSE

I. PUBLIC HEALTH NURSING

1. The New Trend in Public Health Work

The study which follows is essentially a study in personal relationships. The distinguishing mark of the new public health work is its emphasis on the individual—man, woman, and child; and their education in habits of hygienic living. So marked has been this new concentration on the individual, that, in the words of a leader in the field "what was 'the new public health' of fifteen years ago includes only the more conventional interests of the present day."[1] These more conventional interests center, broadly speaking, on factors of environment. Sanitation and the control of community infections, the achievements of the engineer, the bacteriologist, and the epidemiologist,—these have been and continue to be, fundamental to progress in public health.

Yet sole emphasis on factors of environment ignores the eternal interplay and interrelation of the twin forces which have moulded human destiny: the objective and subjective, external and internal. Without the intelligent co-operation of the individual, science fails to achieve its maximum benefits. Without the education of man, the conquest of environment is barren or of limited value. Hence a fundamental shift in the accent of modern public health work. The personal conduct of life! This is the new, yet age-old point of attack.

In the new programs of public health, for preventing disease, prolonging life, and promoting physical health and efficiency, education in personal hygiene thus emerges as a factor of supreme importance. In the campaign against infant mortality, for instance, it is not enough to provide pasteurization of milk, to eliminate flies, and to protect the baby from contact with infected persons.

[1] The Untilled Fields of Public Health. C.-E. A. Winslow, Professor of Public Health, Yale School of Medicine. Modern Medicine, March, 1920. Page 185.

"These are," says Winslow, "after all, incidents in a broad program which involves the education of the mother in the whole technic of infant care, feeding, clothing, airing and bathing. What we are really aiming at is a reform in personal hygiene."

Again, in tuberculosis, the main weapon is the weapon of personal hygiene; the aim, to find the early cases and teach each individual how to put into effect "a regimen of daily living that will make it possible for his own tissues to wage a winning fight against the invading micro-organisms."

It must be evident that, with this new accent in public health work, the organization of medical and nursing services for prompt diagnosis, preventive treatment, and education of the patient is one of the prime requisites.

During the past two decades a series of campaigns against preventable diseases have been organized by special national and local associations, and have achieved a varying degree of success. The campaign against tuberculosis was organized in 1902. About the same time the national movement on .behalf of the health of school children was initiated. There have followed movements to reduce infant mortality; to promote the health of children in the "pre-school" ages; against cancer and venereal disease; on behalf of dental hygiene and mental hygiene and health in industry.

For all these movements modern educational methods have been invoked in greater or less degree. Lectures, literature, graphic representations, travelling exhibits, moving pictures, advertising—the whole paraphernalia of publicity has been directed towards what is known in the jargon of the moment as "selling health to the people." But the critical question remains whether, in the first place, people wish to "buy," and, secondly, how far they put to use the new wares; how far, that is, they actually apply the excellent maxims, the precepts, the admonitions of the lecturer and the exhibitor. Invaluable as indubitably are these impersonal avenues of approach, something more is needed for that personal education which is effectually to impinge upon the consciousness of men and lead to action. A more intimate and tested relationship than that of the lecturer or the exhibitor to an audience is needed to help establish good habits of living, not only among wage-earning people, so often handicapped by the worst obstacle to hygiene, inadequate wages, but also among more prosperous people.

"The striking fact," writes M. M. Davis in his recent study of one important phase of public health, "apparent after a slight survey of these various movements, is their common dependence for practical success upon the field agent." [2]
Now the common field agent of these national health movements has been, for the most part, the visiting nurse.

EVOLUTION OF THE PUBLIC HEALTH NURSE

Visiting or district nursing, as understood today, dates from about the middle of the nineteenth century. In 1859, with Florence Nightingale's aid, William Rathbone of Liverpool founded the first district nursing association in that city, following earlier religious nursing associations. This kind of nursing, though newly organized, was of course no new thing, since tending the sick has been the age-long prerogative of women.

"Nursing as an art to be cultivated, as a profession to be followed, is modern," once wrote a great physician; "nursing as a practice originated in the dim past, when some mother among the cave-dwellers cooled the forehead of her sick child with water from the brook." [3]
Nursing has thus come down through the centuries, dating from far before the Christian era, becoming a tradition of many religious orders, to sink at last in the early part of the nineteenth century into degeneration, ignominy, and decay.

This is not the place to describe the new era initiated when Florence Nightingale, at the lowest ebb of a great tradition, first captured the imagination of the world on the Crimean battle fields, and then, while she reformed the whole administrative machinery of the British War Office and Poor Relief with relation to health matters, founded the modern secular profession of the hospital-trained nurse. Of this renascence of a great tradition in changed form, district nursing was a first fruit.

When, then, twenty-odd years ago, the first more popular public health campaigns were initiated in this country, visiting or district nursing—the care of the sick in their homes by trained nurses—was already established in the United States. Like the

[2] Immigrant Health and the Community. Michael M. Davis, Jr., Director, Boston Dispensary. Harper & Brothers, New York, 1921. Page 283.
[3] Aequinimitas and Other Addresses. Nurse and Patient. William Osler, M.D. Blakiston, Philadelphia, 1904. Page 163.

hospital training of nurses, the movement had come from England.

The first organized visiting nursing in this country was established in 1877 by the Women's Branch of the New York City Missions. But the scope of this work was limited to the congregations of the mission churches.[4] The first secular visiting nursing was initiated by the Ethical Society of New York City, which in 1879 placed in one of the city dispensaries a nurse who visited in the homes of the patients.

"For a number of years," says the historian of visiting nursing, "the extension of the movement was exceedingly slow. In 1890 there were but 21 associations in all of the United States, the greater number of these employing but one nurse."[5]

In 1893 a distinguished nurse, Miss Lillian D. Wald—since responsible for other great expansions in her profession, notably in school and industrial nursing—combined with district nursing the idea of the social settlement, thus adding a new emphasis on the improvement of standards of living, personal and civic, of first value in constructive health work. "Public health nursing" was the phase used to describe these extended activities.

By 1901 there were in the United States some hundred-odd nurses at work, maintained by 58 different organizations. Their growth in numbers since that date is shown by the following table:[6]

Year	Organizations	Nurses
1901	58	130
1905	200	400
1914	1,992	5,152
1919	3,094	8,770
1921	4,024	11,000

Here, then, there have been available a group of workers, insufficient indeed, but rapidly growing, who were already familiar visitors in the homes of the people, eagerly sought at need. These nurses the various movements for public health have in turn enlisted, to become bearers of the new gospel of prevention as well as cure, to become teachers of health.

The term "Public Health Nurse" thus does not necessarily apply only to nurses working under a public department of

[4] A Short History of Nursing. Lavinia L. Dock and Isabel M. Stewart. Putnams, New York, 1920. Page 195.
[5] Visiting Nursing in the United States. Yssabella Waters. Charities Publication Committee, New York, 1909. Page 13.
[6] Information furnished by National Association for Public Health Nursing.

health. Public health nurses are to be differentiated from institutional nurses, working in hospitals or other institutions, and private duty nurses who take care of private patients. The public health nurse is any graduate nurse who serves the health of the community, with an eye to the social as well as the medical aspects of her function, by giving bedside care, by teaching and demonstration, by guarding against the spread of infections, insanitary practices, etc. The object of our inquiry is precisely to determine how well she has carried out these functions, or what changes are needed in her equipment to enable her to do so more adequately in the future.

Before describing in detail the success or failure with which the visiting and district nurses have gradually taken over various educational public health functions, thus becoming generically known as public health nurses, we must first briefly indicate the field of their activities, and the need in behalf of which these activities are directed.

2. Some Achievements in Public Health Nursing

To most persons the extent and degree to which public health nursing has developed, will come as a surprise. It is in general vaguely conceived, if known at all, as an effort to nurse the poor in large cities. Of the part played by nurses in the larger movements for public health few persons have any knowledge; few know of the increase in the number of nurses in small towns and rural districts as well as in large centers of population. Experimental as is still this new profession, it has developed a technique and some definite standards of performance by which its work can be gauged. It has in a short space of time accomplished some specific results.

Of these results some of the most striking are the effect on the health of school children and the reduction of mortality, through skilled nursing care and instruction, in certain diseases and in the function of childbirth.

School Nursing

Thus, for instance, one of the earliest uses of the visiting nurse in distinctive public health instruction was in the public schools. The medical examination of school children was initiated in this country in Boston in 1894, to detect and exclude cases of communicable disease. But the exclusion from school of children suffering from many minor communicable diseases, such as skin affections and pediculosis, did not lead to their cure. Instead of securing treatment, the children were for the most part allowed to run about freely, infecting other children on the streets and being effectually given over to truancy.

Accordingly, it became apparent that some one must follow the child to its home, to secure the mother's co-operation and follow up the cure. The logical agent for this indispensable service was the visiting nurse. The experiment was successfully tried in London in 1901. In 1902 Miss Lillian Wald persuaded the Commissioner of Health of New York City to make a similar experiment, and lent a member of her staff to demonstrate the value of school nursing. So successful was the demonstration that within a month the first municipal school nurse had been appointed. Similar demonstrations were later made by visiting nurse associations in other cities until the municipal authorities themselves took over the school nursing. In Milwaukee, for instance, the visiting nurses assumed the work in 1908 and carried it until 1916 when the Board of Education accepted the responsibility.

Meanwhile the medical examination of children in the schools had proved that the number of acute infections were few compared with the preventable non-communicable physical defects which so seriously impair health and of the existence of which the draft figures have given sinister evidence; that is, defects of vision, of teeth, of hearing, enlarged tonsils and adenoids, weak foot arches or joint defects.

According to the best available estimates, it is believed that of the 22,000,000 school children of the United States:

> 5 per cent have defective hearing;
> 25 per cent have defective eyes;
> 10 to 20 per cent have weak arches or spines or other joint defects;
> 15 to 25 per cent have glandular defects;
> 50 to 75 per cent have defective teeth.[7]

All these defects, again, it is not enough for the school doctor or nurse to discover. Some one must see to it that they are

[7] U. S. Department of Labor, Children's Bureau. Publication No. 60, 1919. Standards of Child Welfare. Health Examinations and the School Child. Dr. Thomas D. Wood, Chairman, Committee on Health Problems in Education, National Council of Education. Pages 248, 250, 255.

corrected. This means explaining the child's condition to the mother or parents and persuading them to have the necessary remedial work done; that is, again, an appeal must be made to the home. The success of the school nurse is measured by the fact that without the nurse, corrections are made in from 15 to 25 per cent of the cases recommended. With the nurse, the percentage rises to from 75 to 90 per cent.

The practical effects of the school nurse's work is strikingly demonstrated by some statistics from Philadelphia given in Dr. Newmayer's standard book on medical inspection of schools.

"No amount of talk," he writes, "can give more convincing proof of the absolute need of school nurses than the following comparative study of the results obtained by medical inspection with and without nurses."

Without the nurse, to sum up these results, action was taken in only 21.1 per cent of the cases of defects found by a medical inspector; with the nurse, action was taken in 80 per cent of the cases.[8] In New York City, to quote a rise even more marked, the percentage of corrected defects rose with home visiting from 6 per cent to 83 per cent.[9]

But the care of the health of school children has developed beyond the salient points enumerated, that is, the cure of communicable diseases and of physical defects. We know also that of the 22,000,000 school children at least 20 per cent are suffering from malnutrition for which ignorance is probably as potent a cause as poverty. Five per cent have or have had tuberculosis; approximately one per cent, or 200,000, are handicapped by organic heart disease; another one per cent (250,000) are mentally defective.[10] To meet this huge problem of largely remediable ill-health or physical handicap it is now generally acknowledged that *no* conditions affecting health can be ignored; all must be envisaged, both in school and at home. To carry out so broad a program, to use the unequalled opportunities of the school for educating children in matters of health and en-

[8] Medical and Sanitary Inspection of Schools. S. W. Newmayer, M.D. Philadelphia Bureau of Health, Division of Child Hygiene. Lea & Febiger, Philadelphia and New York, 1919. Page 59.
[9] New York City Department of Health, Bureau of Child Hygiene. S. Josephine Baker, M.D., Director. Monograph Series No. 4, January, 1915. Page 99.
[10] U. S. Department of Labor, Children's Bureau. Publication No. 60, 1919. Standards of Child Welfare. Health Examinations and the School Child. Dr. Thomas D. Wood, Chairman, Committee on Health Problems in Education, National Council of Education. Page 250.

listing their spirit of competition, nation-wide publicity methods
have been successfully exploited.   In addition to doc⁺ ɔrs and
nurses, a host of workers are enrolled—teachers above all, nutrition workers, social workers of various kinds, etc.[11]

With this widened conception of health work among school
children, the school nurse's sphere of influence has also necessarily widened.   Persuasion of parents to have remedial work
done is no longer enough.   Home visits now must include consideration of all the factors that affect the child's life.

"Matters of home ventilation, cleanliness, conditions of
toilets, proper disposal of refuse, and all environmental
matters likely to affect the health of the child should receive
careful attention.   In addition, the home routine and hygiene
of the child should be outlined carefully so that the mother
may follow it out in detail."[12]

Thus the work of the school nurse, first enlisted to demonstrate one aspect of school nursing, has logically expanded into
a program in which the home shares equally with the school.

THE SAFEGUARDING OF MOTHERHOOD AND INFANCY

We have mentioned, among the concrete achievements of
public health nursing, the reduction of mortality by skilled
nursing care and instruction.   In no disease or physical disability has such a reduction of mortality been more notable,
indeed more impressive and moving, than in the decrease of
those premature deaths which make a unique appeal to every
normal human being,—the deaths of young mothers in childbirth.
How grave the danger of childbirth, how astounding the record
of our country in the protection of maternity, are facts which
are only beginning to force themselves upon the consciousness,
the surprised and reluctant consciousness, of the American
people.

That the United States has "a higher maternal death-rate
than any other of the principal countries," according to the latest
available statistics;[13] and that the nation lost in 1920 upwards
of 20,000 women in childbirth; that the rate has been 1 death in

[11] See publications of National Child Health Organization.
[12] Cleveland Hospital and Health Survey, Part III.   A Program for Child
Health.   S. Josephine Baker, M.D.   1920.   Page 306.
[13] U. S. Department of Labor, Children's Bureau.   Report of the Chief,
1920.   Page 9.

every 100 to 200 cases of pregnancy and childbirth;[14] that the death-hazard involved in childbearing is second only to that from pulmonary tuberculosis at these childbearing ages,[15] and is greater than that in mining coal or in railway service (two occupations which contribute the greatest number of industrial accidents),[16]—these facts, first given prominence in a remarkable series of reports beginning in 1917, by the federal Children's Bureau under Miss Julia C. Lathrop as chief, are as yet unknown to all but a small fraction of our people. The inertia of ages, almost a taboo, has lain upon the subject. Nothing has done more to inform the country than the agitation for the National Maternity Bill enacted into law by Congress in 1921.[17]

"Childbearing," writes a prominent obstetrician, "has long been regarded as merely the natural lot of women, and its hazards have been either neglected or accepted as inevitable. Can a function, however, that kills thousands of women annually, that cripples many thousands more, and that is responsible for a very large infant mortality, be called safe?" [18]

Moreover, there appears to be no reduction in maternal deaths. The census figures for the year 1916 indicated that "since 1900 no decrease in maternal deaths had yet taken place,"[19] and none has since been recorded for the general population. And the peculiar sting which lies in these figures of maternal mortality, representing perhaps the bitterest of human losses, and the disintegration and anguish of many thousand homes, year by year, is this: that they are in large part unnecessary; that they are not only preventable, but in certain favored communities, prevented.

[14] Mortality Statistics of Insured Wage-Earners and their Families. Louis I. Dublin, Ph.D. Metropolitan Life Insurance Company, New York, 1919. Page 213.
[15] U. S. Department of Labor, Children's Bureau. Publication No. 19, 1917. Maternal Mortality in the United States and Certain Other Countries. Grace L. Meigs, M.D. Page 16.
[16] Metropolitan Life Insurance Company Statistical Bulletin, April, 1920. Page 4.
[17] Under this law, during the next six years, annual appropriations are to be made by the Federal Government to the various states "for the purpose of co-operating with them in promoting the welfare and hygiene of maternity and infancy;" provided, that an equal sum has been appropriated for that year by the state.
[18] U. S. Department of Labor, Children's Bureau. Publication No. 60, 1919. Standards of Child Welfare. Maternity Centers in New York City. R. W. Lobenstine, M. D. Page 179.
[19] U. S. Department of Labor, Children's Bureau. Report of the Chief, 1918. Page 12.

We do not deal here with the whole medical organization of maternity services, and recent proposals for improved obstetrical facilities.[20] We deal here only with the results and records of what is known as prenatal nursing.

In prenatal nursing a visiting nurse is provided to teach and supervise the mother under direction of the physician, during pregnancy. Thus, nursing care and direction may be given in connection with one of the prenatal clinics or centers, which are being increasingly established in many cities under the department of health, or privately administered. Or prenatal nursing may be carried on in connection with private physicians, or in connection with midwives, if the patient wishes to have one and if she can be persuaded to co-operate with the nurse.

The main aims of prenatal nursing are to teach the pregnant mother the need of having medical examination and direction as early in pregnancy as possible; to help her arrange for care at the time of confinement if she has not done so; to teach her what to prepare for her baby; and to give her nursing care and instruction at regular intervals.

The best standards of prenatal nursing care, as formulated, for instance, by the Medical Board of the New York Maternity Center Association, require all patients to be seen by a nurse every two weeks up to the seventh month, and once a week or oftener thereafter. The nursing routine includes at each visit record of temperature, pulse, and respiration, urine analysis, blood-pressure, asking the patient about and looking for all the symptoms familiarly known as "the danger signals of pregnancy."

When prenatal nursing is carried on in connection with a clinic or center, the patients are usually asked to come there for as much of the medical and nursing supervision as possible. But they are not urged to come "if the visit would work a real hardship on the patient in the form of dragging with her several children under school age, or long-distance travel, or any real physical discomfort."[21] Visits of the mother to the center or

[20] A Suggestion for Improvement of Obstetrics. Stephen Rushmore, M.D. and Alonzo K. Paine, M.D. Boston Medical and Surgical Journal, November 30, 1919. Pages 615-618.
[21] American Child Hygiene Association, Transactions of the 10th Annual Meeting, 1919. The Work of the Maternity Center Association. Anne D. Stevens, R.N. Page 4.

clinic must in any case be supplemented by regular visits of the nurse to the home.

Reduction of Maternal Mortality

The results achieved by prenatal nursing have been so promising that during the past few years a considerable extension of this work has taken place.

Thus, for instance, in Boston the prenatal nursing of the Instructive Visiting Nurse Association reduced the maternal death rate for the year 1920 from 7 in every 1,000 births to 2 in every 1,000 births.[22]

In Cleveland a study of the records of 442 mothers receiving excellent prenatal care in a district of the city with highly unfavorable social and economic conditions showed a reduction in the maternal death-rate from 4 per 1,000 births for the city as a whole to 1.4 per 1,000 births.[23]

The Metropolitan Life Insurance Company, whose nursing services for its policy-holders are described in a later section (page 52), reports that during the period from 1911 to 1919, among women between the ages of 25 and 34, whom the nursing service especially served in maternity care, the mortality rate was reduced 20.5 per cent, while among women of these ages in the population as a whole, the reduction for the same period was 3.8 per cent.[24]

The remarkable growth of the prenatal work carried on by 12 privately supported visiting nurse associations with whom the Metropolitan Life Insurance Company has working agreements for nursing its policy-holders, is shown in a recent unpublished study by the Company.[25] Between 1916 and 1920 the percentage of cases given prenatal as well as postnatal care, of the total maternity cases visited by these 12 associations,

[22] Instructive District Nursing Association, A Review. Mary Beard. Boston, 1921. Page 14. 28,031 prenatal visits were paid during the year to 4,353 expectant mothers. 26 per cent of this work was carried on for patients of the Boston Lying-In Hospital in co-operation with the Harvard Medical School, 3 per cent for the Jewish Women's Maternity Service Association in co-operation with Tufts Medical School, and the remaining 71 per cent of the service for about 600 private physicians.
[23] Cleveland Hospital and Health Survey, Part III. A Program for Child Health. S. Josephine Baker, M.D. 1920. Page 274.
[24] A Decreasing Mortality Rate. Lee K. Frankel. The Public Health Nurse, February, 1921. Page 73.
[25] For access to this report acknowledgment is due to the Metropolitan Life Insurance Company.

50   NURSING AND NURSING EDUCATION

increased fivefold, from 8 per cent to 41 per cent. The duration
of such care increased more than two and one-half times, from
26.3 days in 1916 to 64.2 days in 1920.

Reduction of Infant Mortality

The result of prenatal care is as remarkably demonstrated in
the lessened death-rate of infants as of the mothers themselves.
In Boston the prenatal work of the Instructive District Nursing
Association in 1919, cut the death-rate of infants under 2 weeks
from 33.4 per 1,000 births, for Massachusetts as a whole, to 14.1;
and the still-births from 34.7 per 1,000 births to 22.7.[26] The
infant death-rate among cases which received postnatal care only,
was only slightly less than the city rate (32.0).

In the congested district of Cleveland mentioned above, the
mortality rate of babies under 1 month of age, was reduced to
24.8 per 1,000 births as compared with the city rate of 31.4.[27]
In New York City the Henry Street Settlement nursing service
reports a death-rate of 17.7 per 1,000 births under 1 month of age
as against 35 per 1,000 for the city as a whole.

According to a well-known public health physician:

"Reduction in the death rate of mothers and babies as
a result of prenatal care can be effected with mathematical
certainty. It is simply a question of providing the type of
care that has already been recognized and standardized." [28]

THE CRUX OF SUCCESSFUL PUBLIC HEALTH NURSING: WORK IN THE HOME

Now it is of first importance to note that in prenatal nursing,
as we have already seen in school nursing, and shall presently
see in practically every form of public health nursing, success
depends primarily on the nurse's work in the home, on her
ability to demonstrate and to have adopted the necessary preventive or curative measures.

"While medical advice can be given in an adequate manner
at the health centers, the value of the nurses' work is more

[26] Massachusetts House Document No. 1835. Report of the Special Com-
mission to Investigate Maternity Benefits. December, 1920. Appendix IV.
Page 85.
[27] Cleveland Hospital and Health Survey, op. cit. Page 273.
[28] Ibid. Page 274.

clearly shown in their home visits. Only in that way can they be sure that the proper routine is being carried out, that the directions of the doctor are being obeyed, and that the mother not only understands but actually puts into effect the essential methods of baby care."

So writes one public health physician; another puts the case even more tersely and strongly.

"Indeed, one may say paradoxically that the real work of the health center must be done by the nurses in the homes." [29]

This emphasis upon the home, on the rôle of the public health nurse as teacher and interpreter of hygienic rules and habits in the home, is of special significance in our present educational study. In order to determine what the training of the public health nurse should be, we have studied her work in the field and the results which she has thus far achieved. Our inquiry leads us to conclude that the distinguishing functions of the public health nurse which should determine her training are to teach habits of healthful living in the home, to see to it that the physician's instructions are intelligently carried out, to be on the alert for all that is suspicious or divergent from health. These functions differentiate the public health nurse from all the other workers—social workers and vocational workers, dietitians, clinic assistants, etc.—who also share in the manifold variations of public health work.

The nurse's success is not measured by figures of clinic attendance alone, invaluable though clinic attendance is for prenatal work, or for the tuberculous, or for well babies, etc. "Drumming up business for the clinics," and urging clinic attendance, which is sometimes held to be the nurse's chief objective,[30] is too narrow and inadequate a conception of public health nursing as it has developed and has achieved its best results in this country. For such work indeed any intelligent clinic messenger will suffice, but not for the wider demands and achievements of public health nursing as we have observed it at first hand in this investigation, and are to describe it in this report.

[29] U. S. Department of Labor, Children's Bureau. Publication No. 60, 1919. Standards of Child Welfare. Health Centers for Pre-School Children. Dr. Merrill E. Champion, Director, Division of Hygiene, Massachusetts State Department of Health. Page 198.
[30] Bulletin of the New York Charity Organization Society, 1920. Page 43.

It remains now, in this brief general survey of achievements, to give the main facts in what is the most extensive experiment in the field of public health nursing in this country, that is, the visiting nurse service established by the Metropolitan Life Insurance Company, already referred to.

EXPERIENCE OF THE METROPOLITAN LIFE INSURANCE COMPANY

Begun in 1909 in a single limited section of Manhattan through a working arrangement with the Henry Street Settlement nursing service on the initiative of Miss Wald, this work was started not only for a purely humanitarian object, but also for the legitimate business aim of saving money in death claims. From this experimental beginning, the Metropolitan nursing service has grown until, in the early part of 1921, it covered about 2,000 cities in nearly all the states of the Union, with a force of more than 500 individual and part-time nurses, besides having working agreements with 650 visiting nurse associations.

That the concrete results of this experiment have entirely satisfied the Company of its value is borne out by the fact that its scope has been steadily increased until it has reached these dimensions. In a word, it has paid. The expenditure by the Company during 1920 on visiting nursing and general welfare work for policy-holders was $1,412,596. During that year 23,910 fewer deaths occurred than if the 1911 death-rate had prevailed. This saving in lives is over and above that which was expected from the improvement in mortality in the general population of the registration area of the United States. The estimated saving in death-claims was $4,734,180. The saving in life has been greatest in those diseases on which the Company's nursing service has especially concentrated its efforts. Between 1911 and 1920, the death-rate for typhoid fever declined 71 per cent; for all diseases affecting children, 23 per cent; for tuberculosis (all forms), 39 per cent; in organic diseases of the heart, 18 per cent; for Bright's disease, 26 per cent. No decreases in any way comparable to these took place in the general population, as shown in the mortality figures for the registration area.

"After eleven years, it may be said," writes a prominent official of the Company, responsible for the experiment, "that the biggest public health nursing experiment in the world has been successful beyond all expectation. From the point of view either of economy or of humanity, it must continue." [31]

Such, then, are some of the palpable achievements of public health nursing and some of the outstanding needs. The accomplishments of the past few years are plainly merely indications, promises of what can be done in the future. With a larger and abler personnel, backed by a more cognizant and alert public opinion and with the coming expansions of public health work, the results obtained in a few favored communities and in limited fields may be many times multiplied.

3. Scope and Method of the Inquiry: An Intensive Study

We turn next to scrutinize the work of nurses in the field as observed and recorded by our investigators. For it is plainly only by intensive study of the individual nurse, by observing her daily contacts, her success or failure in concrete instances, that we can obtain light on the desirable equipment, personal and professional, of these field workers of health agencies, which is the special purpose of this study. Problems of organization and administration of health agencies were included only in so far as they necessarily affect the nurse's work.

Both lay and nurse investigators were employed for this part of our inquiry. The lay investigators were women of experience and proved competence in social work with sufficient knowledge of public health agencies to enable them intelligently to gauge the performance of the nurses visited. The nurse investigators supplemented our findings by more intensive professional criticism of methods and procedures encountered. In general it was apparent that the purposes of this inquiry were better served by an intensive study of a limited number of agencies than by cursory observation of a large number.

SOME DETERMINING FACTORS IN PUBLIC HEALTH NURSING

Three main factors determine the general character of a public health nursing agency and define its problems. These factors are the type of community which it serves, the auspices

[31] Sources for this section have been: A Decreasing Mortality Rate. Lee K. Frankel. The Public Health Nurse, February, 1921. Page 73; Lengthening Life Insurance Health Work. Haley Fisk. Metropolitan Life Insurance Company, New York, 1922; and an unpublished report of the Company.

under which it is conducted, and the kind of nursing services
which it renders. In other words, to judge a public health
nursing agency it is necessary to know whether its work is carried on in a large city or in a small town or in country districts;
whether supported privately or from public funds; and whether
it renders several kinds of nursing service or is restricted to
one field.

REPRESENTATIVE NATURE OF ORGANIZATIONS STUDIED

Effort was made to have the organizations studied, though
limited in number, representative of the main factors in public
health nursing stated above. Urban and rural, public and
private, agencies covering more than one field and agencies
restricted to one field only, were included. Forty-nine public
health nursing organizations employing field workers were
studied in 33 different communities.[32]

URBAN AND RURAL AGENCIES INCLUDED

Rural nursing is of very recent origin. It is natural that the
problems of health and disease in cities were first forced on man's
attention, and have long remained predominant. The cities
have absorbed a disproportionate attention because in the century and a half since the Republic was founded and on a wide-
spreading continent embracing almost half the globe, such has
been the movement towards urban life that half the population
lives in cities, half in the country. The greater acuteness and
conspicuousness of city problems, the greater incidence of communicable diseases and epidemics overshadowed the equally
important health problems of the country.

Only within recent years, and notably since the draft figures
revealed the physical defects of country boys, have the
always existing health needs of rural districts received more
effective notice.

Of the 49 agencies studied, 34 carried on their work in cities,
large and small, 15 in rural districts.

[32] Of these 49 organizations, 9 were separate bureaus in 4 departments
of health. Strictly speaking, these were not 9 separate agencies, but because
of their distinct organization, direction, and purpose, they amounted practically to separate organizations and have been counted as such. Should
each of these bureaus not have been counted as a distinct agency, the total
number of organizations included in the study would have been 44.

GEOGRAPHICAL DISTRIBUTION OF AGENCIES STUDIED

The public health nursing agencies included in this study were scattered in various parts of the United States; and one Canadian bureau was also covered. Ten agencies were located in New England, 14 in the Mid-Atlantic states, 20 in the Middle West, 3 on the Pacific coast, and 1 in a southern state.

In the urban group were cities as widely separated and varied in character as New York and Los Angeles; Boston and Portland, Oregon; New Haven and Chicago; Baltimore and Cleveland. In the rural group a conservative New England seafaring community stood out in contrast to a sparsely settled county on the northern part of the Pacific coast; a progressive little Ohio town in contrast to a small Rhode Island mill village. A Pennsylvania company mining town, a community centering around a naval training station, the wide expanse of one of our largest eastern industrial states, were some of the communities in which our field agents accompanied the public health nurse in her daily activities.

PUBLIC AND PRIVATE AGENCIES INCLUDED

Public health nursing agencies may be conducted under public control, federal, state, or municipal, or under private auspices. In a later section the respective advantages and disadvantages of these two types of control are discussed. Of the 49 agencies included in our study, 19 were under public control, and 30 were privately supported. Among the latter, 19 were city agencies and 11 carried on their work in small towns or rural districts. Among the organizations under public control, 15 were urban and 4 were rural agencies.

KINDS OF SERVICE INCLUDED

Another important distinction between public health nursing agencies is a distinction according to the different kinds of nursing service rendered. Some agencies give more than one type of service; others restrict themselves to a single field such as infant welfare, or tuberculosis work, or school nursing, etc. We defer to a later section discussion of these different types of organization. Of the 49 organizations included, 28 covered more than one field of service, 21 confined themselves to one field.

It is evident, therefore, that the agencies included in this study are representative of the various types of public health nursing activities and of the various parts of the country in which such activities have been developed.[33]

FOCUS OF THE STUDY: THE INDIVIDUAL NURSE

Our investigation centered on observation of the nurse's work in the field.   In each of the 49 agencies studied our agent accompanied the nurse in her daily activities in the schools, in clinics, in health centers, in industrial establishments, but chiefly in the homes to which her work took her.   Detailed information was obtained on the type of community visited, the scope of the nurse's work, etc.   The success or failure of the nurse in making personal contacts, in health teaching, or in co-operating with other social agencies were the main points observed.   An effort was made, also, to gauge the influence of the nurse's previous education or lack of education on the quality of her service.

In small agencies the work of only one nurse was observed; in larger organizations a larger number of nurses ranging from 2 up to 7 or 8 were accompanied in their activities.   The work of 164 nurses was studied in this way.   Twenty-four industrial nurses, employed in factories or stores, were also visited.

In addition, where opportunity offered, interviews were obtained with interested persons who could give a general and detached opinion of the local situation, and of the nurse's standing in the community.

To secure the necessary facts on the organization and administration of agencies as a background for the nurse's work, the heads of 38 organizations were interviewed.   In collaboration with these executives,[34] a schedule covering these facts was filled out during the interview.   In addition, information was secured from 377 directors, supervisors, and staff nurses, giving their schooling, their professional training and experience.[35]

Appreciation is also due the National Organization for Public

[33] For further confirmation of our findings, see Report of the Committee on Municipal Health Department Practice, the American Public Health Association.   The Public Health Nurse, October, 1922.   Page 514.
[34] See Appendix, Schedule II A and II B, Public Health Series.
[35] Responses to these questionnaires were secured in some instances during the visit of the investigator and in others by correspondence with agencies not covered in the field of study.

Health Nursing for making available certain confidential reports on public health nursing activities in several different communities.

4. The Field of Public Health Nursing:

Some Typical Days

To gauge the calibre and value of public health nursing we turn next to a description of the field. The accounts which follow have not been fitted together to make up a diversified pattern. They are the actual records of days spent with nurses by our field agents in various localities, and while they probably do not cover all the daily activities of the industrial nurses visited, they are nevertheless entirely typical of the work observed both in the country and in the city. They show the complex demands made on skill in nursing and teaching, on physical endurance, and human understanding.

An Example of Rural Nursing

Take first a rural tuberculosis nurse whose territory is a county, some 3,000 square miles in area, in a far western state with a scattered population of about 37,000. There are two small towns, one of them the county-seat, where, in the courthouse, the nurse has her office. The country is largely agricultural, but it has also lumber camps, mines, and canneries. One or two of the roads are excellent, but the majority are dirt, impassable with an automobile during much of the year owing to the heavy rainfall in this section, so that the nurse to reach a number of communities has often to walk or ride horseback. It is pioneer work, for not alone is she the only public health nurse in this county, but she is the first one ever employed and she has been at work only 18 months. Her work is supported by the county. Under the state law the expenditure of funds for public health nursing is restricted to tuberculosis nursing. She is therefore supposed to restrict herself to this specialty.

Tuberculosis Nursing

The function of the public health nurse in tuberculosis work has been well summarized by a public health authority in the following words:

"Next to the clinic and the sanatorium," writes C.-E. A. Winslow, "the public health nurse is the most vital factor in the anti-tuberculosis campaign. Her work is essential in the discovery of new cases and in bringing them in contact with the clinic and the sanatorium, in the active follow-up and bedside care of cases under the charge of the clinic, and in the after-care and continued instruction of discharged arrested cases." [36]

To gauge the performance of Miss C., the nurse in question, it will be most clarifying to analyse her work in detail, as observed and recorded by our investigator.

A DAY'S VISITS

The day started at 8:30 in the morning with a call at the office in the court-house to get mail, messages, bag, supplies, and the nurse's automobile. The story of the day's travels and encounters follows:

"Our first visit was to a woman with far-advanced tuberculosis, living on the edge of the county seat. The house was a comfortable bungalow, the housekeeper cleaning up after breakfast, children gone to school. The patient had been ill for two years, and had lately been sent home from a sanatorium to die. She was about 35, running high temperature, coughing and expectorating. As soon as she came home, Miss C., the nurse, started seeing her almost daily, giving her bedside care and helping her plan to get proper sleeping quarters. The bedroom, which had had but one window, had been transformed into a fine sleeping porch by putting in two more windows. Patient's mother now comes over almost daily from four miles away, and gives her a bath. Miss C. offered to give care, but patient stated that mother was coming. Patient using paper squares for expectoration and putting them in paper bag, as taught by Miss C. and sanatorium. Thermometer kept in carbolic solution in vaseline bottle, as directed by nurse. Nurse took away bag and fixed a new one in place. Took temperature and pulse, asked about husband and children, and complimented patient on her carefulness. The nurse was sympathetic, understanding and helpful, cheering patient.

[36] The Tuberculosis Problem in Rhode Island. C.-E. A. Winslow. Providence, 1920. Page 56.

"Our second visit was to a patient just aci oss the street, a young girl of 22 who has had tuberculosis for four years, spending one year in very good private sanatorium, and since then at home. Had open tuberculosis abscess in groin about six months ago, now healed up. The purpose of the call was first to show me the fine outdoor sleeping room occupied by patient and her sister, also to inquire about patient's last lung examination. Patient reported that doctor said she could work now several hours a day, and that she had secured employment in a doctor's office. Nurse stated that this girl had come home from sanatorium utterly afraid to make any effort; that the minute she had any temperature she would take to bed for a couple of weeks and let the family wait on her; and that she had had to put some backbone into her. This was one of the cases she visited mostly to give moral encouragement.

"Our third visit was to Mrs. H., 35 years old, bed case, moved to neighborhood of C. two months ago from Canada. Husband works farm and little boy goes to school. Miss C. had visited once before, soon after patient came, case having been reported by a previous patient. On that visit nurse said she got nowhere, patient would not let her do anything for her, refused to have a doctor, and seemed quite unapproachable. When clinic was held the week before, nurse had asked neighbor to see if she couldn't persuade Mrs. H. to come for examination and to bring little boy who had a cough. To her surprise, they came. Mrs. H. showed moderately advanced and little boy negative.

"When we called, we found Mrs. H. in bed in a little sleeping shack, but with stove going and curtains drawn so that little air got in. Patient seemed glad to see nurse, and when she offered care, said she would be glad to have her hair combed. This Miss C. did, and took her temperature. Told patient she was not satisfied with way she was keeping her thermometer, and explained again about keeping it in carbolic solution in a vaseline bottle. Promised to get her a vaseline bottle. After doing hair, we got patient up in a chair, Miss C. took all the bedding out to shake, turned the mattress, and made the bed, and we swept up the room. Nurse also changed paper bag and left fresh supply of paper napkins. Inquired about diet and gave good practical suggestions. Advised about little boy's diet, bedtime, etc. Nurse left patient and room tidy and clean; was friendly but firm in her instructions; washed her hands after finishing care; inquired about reading matter for patient and promised to bring her some magazines.

"Nurse told me after we left the house that she was delighted with the visit, as the last one had seemed so unpromising. In this, as in other cases where patient refuses to have doctor, Miss C. says, 'At least I can go on visiting, and advise about fresh air, hygiene, diet, etc., and in quite a number of cases I have had quite remarkable results.' She does her best, however, to get cases under doctor's care. In many instances this is required as prerequisite to any nursing care.

"Our next visit was to a two-room school house where the nurse had visited in the fall and introduced the Modern Health Crusade. One teacher was a young fellow of about 20, with a dirty shirt and collar but seeming rather a mild sort. The other teacher was a girl of about 18 or 19. The young man, with a perpetually hopeful smile, said he would be glad to have Miss C. speak to the children. Standing on one foot he bashfully asked her if she would also examine the children for physical defects."

Our field agent explains that the nurse had, however, found it a waste of time to examine school children for physical defects unless she was certain that the teachers would follow up her findings and get the children to the necessary doctors. Being a tuberculosis nurse, she gave that work her main attention. She always examined any special children whom the teachers reported to her, and advised what was to be done.

"The children of both rooms were brought together for the health talk, and it was quite evident from Miss C.'s handling of them, her handling of inattention, etc., that she was thoroughly at home in the schoolroom. She gave a talk, covering several points in the Health Crusade, and several others. She asked how many children were now bringing milk to school for lunch as she had suggested in a previous talk, and over a dozen held up their hands. She spoke of the necessity of keeping toilets clean; care of the teeth; ventilation; in fact she talked for 35 minutes to children varying in age from 6 to 16. On inquiry, several children reported that they had had eyes or teeth attended to, since her previous visit."

The fifth visit was to a lumber camp about two miles off the main road. The nurse had received a somewhat vague report from a doctor that a family with tuberculosis had recently moved there. After learning from the mill office where the family in question lived, a 15-minute visit convinced Miss C. that there was no history of tuberculosis in the family.

"We had lunch," continues our agent, "with a very nice farmer's family whose son-in-law Miss C. had cared for during his illness with tuberculosis several months before, and where she often takes a meal. They all seemed to think very highly of her, with respect as well as affection. Miss C. inquired for the widow, now moved away, and sent kindly messages to her. Mother of family was ill, and Miss C. went in to see her before we left. Found her flowing (46 years old) and depressed. Urged father to call a physician, and to have mother keep quiet in bed for a week."

On the way to the next house, Miss C. and our agent stopped in at a little one-room school. Miss C. had been there once before, had introduced the Health Crusade, and examined the children. She had just had a letter from one of the little girls reporting that she had had five teeth filled.

"As we went in, the children were at noon recess and the teacher told us that following Miss C.'s talk about bringing milk to school and making cocoa, they had for several weeks done this, making the cocoa over a bonfire in the yard. When the children saw us, they ran for the pump. One produced a piece of soap, and there was a general washing of faces and hands. Miss C. spoke briefly here, asking about the defects and finding that several had been corrected, one in the case of a girl who needed glasses, the rest in teeth cases; after which I gave a short talk on Crusaders. Miss C.'s attitude toward the children seemed excellent.

"About 20 miles from C. we stopped at a grocery store to inquire where several people lived, and how the roads were. Miss C. asked about one returned soldier, reported as arrested tuberculous, was told by the storekeeper that he was working on the farm, and that the road was not safe on account of mud. This case she postponed for another week. She also inquired about Indian Jake, reported to be tuberculous, and learned that he was well off, had a good farm three miles off the road, also impossible to visit until drier weather.

"An onlooker asked her who she was, and when she said
'County tuberculosis nurse,' he said, 'Well, you'd better come
over and see them Mays near us.' She asked what the
trouble was, and learned they were having flu, had a practical
nurse, and were in financial need. . . . Miss C. knew the
nurse on the case, knew that the nurse would call upon her
if even suspicious of tuberculosis and that she also knew
where to get relief if needed. Miss C. told me that she had
hard work not getting dragged into every home where there
was sickness or financial need, but that she felt that with
such a large territory, and such a definite purpose as her
work had, she simply had to refuse calls like this.

"We then drove about 10 miles through virgin forest, picking up a foot passenger and giving him a lift. The house we
reached was a comfortable one on a prosperous looking fruit
ranch about 30 miles from C. The patient was a returned
soldier, pronounced arrested tuberculous after several months
in the army sanatorium in Arizona. Miss C. had visited once
before, found patient sleeping alone in loft with windows
open, taking good care of himself, and very anxious for the
Federal Board for Vocational Education to get him to agricultural school. No cough or sputum. On this visit we found
that patient had gone to college but was finding climate of
eastern Oregon trying. Miss C. urged mother to advise him
to see doctor at once, take his temperature, etc.

"In the living room of this house," our investigator relates
further, "there was a baby asleep with his bottle. Inquiry
revealed that he was 18 months old but still could not drink
out of a cup. Miss C. talked to the mother about this bad
habit and advised her how to break it up with least difficulty.
She also inquired into the health of the rest of the family,
which seemed satisfactory.

"As it had rained all day and was getting pretty cold,
and the next case was a long distance on, we returned, reaching home about 4:45. In practically every house, in the
schools and in the store, Miss C. inquired whether they knew
of anybody in that vicinity who had tuberculosis, who had
a cough, or who was ill."

Analysis of the cases visited in the course of the day shows
in the first visit bedside nursing of an advanced case, and also
the results of excellent instruction, both in the outdoor sleeping
quarters provided for the patient and in the protective hygiene

which was being used to prevent infection of other members of the family. In the second case visited we see the general oversight of an arrested case, and, more important, the building up of moral stamina in the patient through the efforts of the nurse, without which little progress would be possible even in a hopeful case. All the other tuberculosis cases visited in the course of the day give evidence of the same effective teaching in the hygiene of the disease, and of efforts to prevent the spread of tuberculosis through the careful oversight of all contacts. We also see the nurse stopping in every village store, farmhouse, school, keen that in her efforts to cover the field no case of tuberculosis shall escape her.

OUTSIDE ACTIVITIES: THE COUNTY FAIR

Naturally, in pioneer work of this sort and in such a large territory, the nurse's hours of work are irregular and long. Often she cannot visit men patients who are still well enough to work until they come home after five o'clock. Often she takes occasion to speak on health matters in the evening at all sorts of meetings: school elections, school meetings, graduation exercises, picture shows, club or grange meetings, or at the county fair. All day Saturday she is on hand in her office in the court-house to see teachers, patients, and others who may wish to confer with her, and also to do her clerical work for the week. Her work at the fair showed so much ingenuity that it should be briefly described:

To stimulate interest in sleeping out-of-doors by both sick and well, she planned the erection of a model shack at the fair. Through her efforts, local mills donated the lumber and other materials, an architect drew up plans and the carpenters' union built the shack. Here she had posters and much special literature for distribution, and gave health talks during the entire fair week, thus enlisting active co-operation in her work among various groups in the county, and furthering health education in the entire southeastern part of the state whose inhabitants always come to the county fair.

THE ESTABLISHMENT OF CLINICS

Miss C. had come to this primitive western rural community from experience as staff nurse and supervisor in the efficient health department of a large eastern city. Her first months were full of difficult readjustment and discouragement, but she had persevered and had built up her work most successfully. The value of her experience in a well-organized agency was evident in the excellent method of record keeping and the state of the records, which were so well ordered, that were she to drop the work a new nurse would know just where to begin and what to do. Her knowledge of modern health and publicity methods was also a great asset. Finding none of the hospital or dispensary facilities to which city work had accustomed her, she arranged in co-operation with the state Anti-Tuberculosis Association for clinics to be held throughout the county for the examination of tuberculosis suspects. These clinics were held periodically by a specialist and a nurse in addition to the local nurse, whose chief function in this connection was to get people interested in coming to the clinics, either through their doctors or by direct invitation. In the week preceding our field agent's visit, clinics had been held in five places in the county, with an attendance of 42 people. Among these, 3 positive cases and 7 or 8 suspects had been found. Not alone are examinations made in these clinics, but lantern talks are given and public meetings held, and thus general interest in the possibilities of preventing tuberculosis is stimulated.

THE EXPANSION OF A NURSING SPECIALTY

The work of this nurse thus illustrates a combination of teaching and bedside nursing of a high order of excellence. But it illustrates more; that is, the necessary expansion of any good specialized work, such as tuberculosis nursing.

It has been well said by a specialist in tuberculosis that "the contributory factors of tuberculosis morbidity include anything and everything that adversely influence the health of man" [37] — a sufficiently inclusive range of possibilities! If this contention is true (and all recent research and experiment goes to substantiate it), how shall good tuberculosis work be confined to the narrow orbit of tuberculosis alone? For prevention as well as cure, it must inevitably take in other nursing specialties. Because of the enormous field she was covering, Miss C. was obviously unable to go into "anything and everything,"—witness

[37] The Larger Field of Tuberculosis. Allen K. Krause, M.D. Journal of the Outdoor Life, January, 1920. Page 6.

her refusal to make physical examinations in the school, or to visit the family of whose care under the practical nurse she was assured. But her work spread out almost automatically from the specialized field of tuberculosis into more general family health instruction.

While nominally restricted to anti-tuberculosis work by the terms of the state law under which she was engaged, her preventive work naturally started in the schools, teaching habits of health to the children, better nutrition by leading them to make cocoa in school, and the correction of defects so far as she was able. Thus, to be effective, the campaign against tuberculosis included school nursing. In the course of the day's home visits, the nurse's teaching as to diet and habits for the little boy with a cough (not tuberculous), for the year-old baby, and for the mother needing medical care, all developed naturally out of her family contacts. It is indeed a matter of course that the single nurse in the county must combine many functions which in larger communities devolve upon different individuals. Miss C. illustrates well how naturally the different phases of nursing care and health education interlock with one another and overlap,—a subject on which we shall have occasion to comment more fully in the course of this report.

Instances of such pioneering could be multiplied in the work of other rural nurses. This is the type of public health nursing which above all others calls for the utmost initiative, the utmost physical endurance, and the utmost devotion to the calling. Working alone, or practically alone in the field, the responsibility which devolves upon the rural nurse is far greater than that of her city colleague who needs but to go to the telephone to get almost immediate assistance in practically every emergency. The rural nurse shares in the romance of the pioneer.

Nursing in a Small Town

The nurse in the small town shares some of the difficulties of the rural nurse, and some of the advantages of the city nurse. Her patients live in greater proximity to each other than do those of the rural nurse; but, while she often has more adequate facilities in dispensaries and other health agencies, and rarely has to undertake all the public health nursing for the community single-handed, she cannot count on the wide range of medical and philanthropic agencies available for the nurse in the large city. The community spirit and fellowship so markedly characteristic of the small town in contrast to the large city, and in contrast often to the scattered rural community is, on the other hand, an asset to the nurse, both in establishing friendly relations with her patients and in finding new cases.

An excellent example of the constituency and influence which a nurse can win in this type of community during a period of years was found in a small middle western town adjacent to one of the largest cities. This town was populous and wealthy enough to have a hospital with an out-patient department, an infant welfare station, an associated charities, as well as the visiting nurse. The nurse herself had drifted into public health nursing quite by accident. One summer nearly 10 years before she had unwillingly undertaken the work of a summer substitute, and has continued ever since. While she has been very successful in her field, this has been due rather to gifts of personality and human understanding than to training or to background in the public health movement. Her work and her problems are not sufficiently different, however, from those of the rural and city nurses to warrant our analysing her work in detail. At this point we may merely indicate that between the two extremes of the rural nurse and the nurse in a great city, the nurse in the small town shares the advantages and the disadvantages of both of her colleagues.

A VISITING NURSE IN A PRIVATE AGENCY IN A LARGE CITY

At the opposite pole from the pioneer work of the far western county tuberculosis nurse, but characteristic of the wide ramifications of public health nursing and equally rich in human interest, are the daily activities of a staff nurse in a well-established general visiting nurse association in a large middle western city. This association has what is known as a "generalized" service; that is, each nurse serves a specified unit of population, giving whatever nursing care or instruction is needed in the families under her charge. The work of Miss L. is a good illustration of the growth of visiting nursing from the pure bedside care of its origin, to the broader family health work into which it is slowly developing, as nurses are becoming educated up to the newer inclusive view of public health nursing. In the city we have chosen for illustration, the population served by each nurse is within her capacity to cover, aggregating about 2,500 persons. The nurse is therefore not too hard pressed to give intelligent interest to the health problems of the families with which she is brought in contact.

Miss L.'s district lies in a crowded section, once the best residential district of the city. Its fine old houses have been transformed into tenements, and have acquired as neighbors cheap, poorly constructed three-, four-, and six-family houses. The section assigned to this nurse was so compact that she was able in the course of the day which our investigator spent with her to make 13 visits. An account of the most interesting calls of the day follows.

A DAY'S VISITS

"1. In two rooms lived parents and six young children. A third room is untenantable because of swaying floor, yet must be crossed in order to reach living room. The nurse will report this condition.

"This was the nurse's second visit to this family. Young infant, temperature 102° and very ill with broncho-pneumonia. Mother agreed with doctor and nurse in wishing to have baby sent to hospital, but father refused. Nurse took temperature; examined baby carefully; cautioned mother against sweeping with baby in the room; regulated windows; offered ice cap from loan closet; (this was called for at noon by neighbor's child). Without alarming mother unduly, she was urged to have doctor come soon. On mother's request nurse promised to 'phone for doctor at noon.

"Another child with hypertrophied tonsils, was examined. Father has refused operation but mother believes school nurse and nurse may perhaps persuade him to give his consent. A third child was restless and feverish and had a coated tongue. Nurse advised castor oil and gave directions as to mixing it with orange juice.

"(Later. Doctor and nurse conferred at noon. Doctor will call and again urge hospital care for baby. Next day nurse reported baby had died. Will start energetically now to help mother with other children and to improve home conditions.)

"2. Mrs. W., a chronic cardiac, had had recent acute attack, had almost died, now much improved, but still in bed. Pleasant home with conveniences to work with. Caretaker was doing both housework and nursing, during the day. At night husband and sons nursed patient. Nurse had called for seven or eight days. Twice a week gave complete bath; other days only partial care. Orders were left by private physician in attendance. . . .

"Patient, with appreciation, wished that every ill person in the world had such good nursing and 'such a friend, too.' Truly, no private duty relationship could have been gentler or nicer in every way.

"3. In basement of splendid old house lives the owner, a foreign Jew, with his family. Through rent of floor above and father's wages, family are trying to pay for this house. Through medical examination at health clinic, of mother and 3 younger children, all were found in need of tonsillectomy. By advice of the nurse, grandmother on top floor of this house will take baby, older girls will keep house for father under grandmother's supervision, while mother and three young children will all have operations performed at the same time, all being in Jewish Hospital for three days and paying a mere nominal sum for hospital care.

"Nurse also arranged with mother to have 5-year-old child taken to Children's Hospital dispensary for eye examination and to make possible arrangements for operation (strabismus).

"Father has consented to all this remedial work. Family are keen to attain good health, yet have no private physician; school nurse and visiting nurse have made all arrangements for them.

"4. At the next place visited, home conditions were good. Father earns comfortable living. Mother is intelligent and active in welfare of her neighborhood. Immediate reason of nurse's call: inquiry re husband's and younger daughter's health. Both had had flu recently. Nurse had called daily and instructed the mother to care for them. Father had badly diseased tonsils, presumably the cause of chronic rheumatism. Daughter had badly hypertrophied tonsils. Private physician in attendance recommended operation for both. Father demurred; 'was afraid.' Nurse reassured him and persuaded him; even offered to be with him during operation if necessary, because nose and throat work was her specialty. Father has great regard for nurse apparently. Mother promised nurse that he would 'phone her at the office to report final arrangements for operation for himself and daughter.

"Nurse also instructed mother in care of lodger, who is ill, probably with flu.

"A stop was made at this point for lunch. The entire staff have lunch at the headquarters of the Association where the meal is prepared for them. The lunch hour is a cozy, friendly time.

"5. Following luncheon," says our investigator, "the next call was to a woman whom the nurse had found very uncomfortable the day before, in bed in a dark stuffy room and in need of a bath. She had bathed her and suggested moving the bed into the light kitchen.

"On second visit, this had been done. Her two half-grown boys had moved her. One boy at work, other home from school caring for her. Nurse commended lad's ingenuity in shielding mother's eyes from light, and also his tenderness toward her.

"Call was brief, but friendly. Woman remarked, 'I've felt better ever since I found *somebody cared* yesterday,' and, 'You certainly are pleasant to have around a sick person.'

"Nurse took temperature. Because of slight fever woman was urged to stay in bed, . . . If fever continues, nurse will urge more strongly calling of a physician, although woman insisted that she never had a doctor. Always describes symptoms to the druggist, who prescribes without even seeing the patient.

"6. Another case where diagnosis of tuberculosis had been withheld by a doctor out of mistaken kindness. Man allowed to remain at home with family and to work up to a few weeks ago, although miserably ill. Nurse had been informed about case only after man was compelled to remain home from work. Then a few prompt calls were made, and partial support secured from the associated charities. In 10 or 12 days after first contact, the man was dead. Yet, in that brief time, entire family had been examined at health station. No active symptoms were found, but entire family showed predisposition to tuberculosis.

"Couple had been unusually devoted. Woman seemed crushed by suddenness of it all, and found it very difficult to decide as to future plans."

Our field agent then describes the nurse's treatment of a

difficult family situation. In order to have the children kept under medical supervision somewhat longer, the young widow was urged to remain in the city for a while instead of returning at once to her parents' home in the country, where medical resources were limited. The nurse also urged that the youngest child be promptly examined at the health station, on hearing from the mother of a recent convulsion. She examined him for possible paralysis, "asked definite, intelligent questions," and suggested a hot mustard bath as emergency treatment in case of another attack. Finally a dental appointment was made for the mother the next day at the health station. "The nurse," says our field agent, "was lovely in her understanding and handling of the entire situation." She explained that she had insisted upon the mother's exerting herself in these various directions, realizing from the woman's unwonted untidiness, soiled wrapper and uncombed hair that such habits must not be allowed to become fixed.

"7. The next visit was to a little 5-year-old girl with congenital dislocation of hips and shoulders, discovered by Miss L.'s predecessor during Children's Year house to house canvass.

"Family represented financially a group to whom the visiting nurse does not usually have access," says our field agent. "Family had accepted the dictum of their own private physician that child could never walk or use her arms, although he had not made correct diagnosis. Nurse finally prevailed upon family to consult orthopedic specialist, later to allow him to operate, which he did successfully. Later, for eight months nurse called daily to give massage.

"At present child can walk, although awkwardly and with difficulty. Shoulder condition can be little improved. Although she has a limited use of her hands, she will probably attend school next year. Because child seems slightly anæmic nurse advised re diet. She makes a monthly call. Family overwhelmingly appreciative of what she has done for them.

"8. Prenatal instruction had been given by nurse and followed by 17-year-old wife. Her grandmother, a practical nurse, was caring for her and the baby. Questions asked by nurse were cheerfully answered by the grandmother, who was naturally flattered by nurse's approval of patient's condition.

"This was a very brief call, since it temporarily interrupted a family party downstairs. Yet nurse spent a minute or two noticing each baby in the party and left behind her a veritable trail of good feeling.

"9. Here were two cases. Mother, an advanced case of laryngeal tuberculosis. All plans had been made through the tuberculosis society for her admission to sanatorium, when woman's private physician interfered, and she has remained at home, a menace to entire family. Nurse has been visiting for a year, with little result. Woman is ignorant, self-willed, and selfish. She makes and breaks numerous promises. Recently nurse succeeded in having 14-year-old daughter examined. Doctor asked for 4 p. m. temperature for a week. Today she showed slight fever which the nurse will report.

"Nurse noted several bad sanitary conditions, but spoke of only one or two. Although not very hopeful of medical results, nurse's effort was to make for more spontaneous and pleasant relationship between woman and herself, hoping to establish some slight influence over her for the little girl's sake."

After this full day's round of visits, which is entirely typical of other days, some time was spent in recording and in conference with the supervisor and other members of the staff. In addition, Miss L. has charge of a health clinic maintained by her organization two afternoons each week and two nights each month; she makes a weekly physical inspection of a private kindergarten in her district; she attends the children's clinic at the city hospital once a week; and occasionally she escorts her patients to the dispensaries or the hospital. Thus, though the responsibility and initiative of the nurse in a city visiting nurse association are perhaps not called upon to the same degree as are the rural nurse's, she has a great variety of duties and an infinite variety of problems in her daily work. Difficulties of transportation and exposure to weather are less; facilities for treatment are available; but because of the very advantages which she enjoys—the dispensaries, the hospitals, the social agencies, and various institutions to which her patients can be referred—her work is rendered more complex, and with the greater possibilities of adequate care, she must live up to more exacting standards than the rural nurse, who must often improvise facilities as best she may.

SCOPE OF THE DAY'S WORK

The day spent with Miss L. furnishes a good picture of the scope of generalized visiting nursing. In the course of one day she was called upon to give bedside care or make arrangements for several influenza patients, a pneumonia case, several tuberculosis patients and their contacts, to give infant welfare and prenatal care, to arrange for surgical cases such as the tonsillectomies and the strabismus operation, to supervise an orthopedic patient and a cardiac case. In one of the families visited during the day, she had first given maternity care at the birth of the last two children, she had placed a child predisposed to tuberculosis in a fresh air class, and she had later arranged dental care and tonsillectomies for other members of the family.

Instruction in Bedside Care

Not less important than the bedside care she herself gave was her education of other members of the family to give care between her visits, a test of effective public health nursing to which we shall recur in greater detail.

Calling in the Physician

Striking also is this nurse's initiative and success in getting her families under medical care. The woman who "always describes symptoms to the druggist who prescribes," the mother and children in one family, the father and daughter in another, needing tonsillectomies, the child taken for eye examination to the children's dispensary, the little girl with congenital hip disease brought under the care of a specialist, all, in the course of one day, testify to the reinforcement of the physician's scope and authority through the public health nurse. Far from interfering with the work of the physician or seeking to displace him, public health nursing is tested in one way precisely by the nurse's success in persuading her families to consent to the remedial and preventive work of the doctor. This means recourse to medical aid not only in acute illness when need arises, but recourse also before illness has become acute, for that prevention of illness which is the new development of medical science. To fit the nurse for this rôle, so that she may know the suspicious symptoms, suspect what is truly suspicious and dismiss what is trivial, her training must obviously be based on an adequate clinical training and the intelligent knowledge of disease. It is because of such future responsibilities in co-operation with the physician, in prevention as well as cure, that we have analysed in a later chapter the nurse's hospital training and shown its defects and strong points. Of the relation of the public health nurse with the medical profession we shall treat at greater length in a subsequent section and must not diverge here from the general description of the field which is the theme of this chapter.

THE PERSONALITY OF THE NURSE

Attention, however, should be called to the large part played in Miss. L.'s success by innate gifts of personality. When in the course of one day one patient says, "I've felt better ever since I found somebody cared yesterday," and another that she wished every sick person in the world could have "such a friend;" when a young widow is helped to re-establish not only health but courage and initiative, and men as well as women of the neighborhood have "great regard" for her, no further testimony is needed as to the qualities of the person in question.

But even the successful nurse has her failures and her difficult cases. The last case visited during the day showed not only failure to persuade a tuberculous mother to accept adequate treatment, but probable failure in protecting the other members of the family from the danger of tubercular infection. Ignorance and selfishness seemed impervious to persuasion. Yet the only hope of success in saving a 14-year-old daughter, already showing symptoms of infection, was to continue the effort of "hoping," as the nurse said, "to establish some influence over the mother for the little girl's sake."

An Instructive Nurse under a City Department

To illustrate another development of public health nursing of the first importance in the campaign against disease and for health, we will next pursue the work of a nurse attached to a municipal agency, the baby welfare station. Originally started merely for the distribution of pure milk, these stations, variously known in different cities as child welfare stations, infant hygiene centers, and the like, are now designed to furnish medical and nursing care and continued supervision of babies and young children.

In the case in question each nurse has her own district with a baby health station as a center for her activities, where a physician is in attendance several days per week. A lay assistant helps in the station work and the home visiting. Every morning from 9 to 1 the nurse holds consultations with parents and babies at the station. The babies are weighed and measured, and the parents confer with the nurse regarding feeding, teething, intestinal disturbances, and other matters of importance in baby welfare. The major part of the afternoon is spent visiting in the district, and the final hour of the day in writing up records. The work is largely with infants under 2; comparatively few children of pre-school age have so far come under the nurse's care.

The nurse, Miss O., has 408 cases registered. She tries to see every case once a month, and some of course more frequently. For this purpose she divides her cases into three groups: one, the malnutrition or bad feeding cases which she sees weekly either at the station or in the home; the second, the border line cases, seen every two weeks; and the third, the well babies seen once a month. Her district is a typical working-class neighborhood of a great city. The people, largely Irish, live in tenements, but there is less congestion and living conditions are somewhat better than in other parts of the city.

IN THE WELFARE STATION

Her morning consultations at the station average about 20 a day in the winter, but in the summer they run up to about 40. A description of this nurse's day in the clinic and in the homes of her district is given in the following extract from our field agent's report:

"All mothers came in to have their babies weighed. Those desiring to talk with nurse waited, but about half departed as soon as babies had been weighed. The conversations were very largely about feeding, teeth, intestinal disturbances, preparation of food. Nurse's instructions were good—they indicated a broad experience in feeding cases but not enough in hygiene.

"In our afternoon work we saw a number of children on the streets that had been 'brought up at the station' and their mothers attributed their splendid condition to Miss O. She and the station doctor have worked together a number of years and he permits her to prescribe feedings in his absence.

"All but one of the babies that came in to be weighed while I was there showed a gain and their records showed intelligent, intensive work on the part of the nurse.

"Some of the mothers made inquiries regarding their own health. The mother whose baby did not gain had been very much worried over illness in her family. The nurse's instructions to her were sensible and sympathetic, and bound to be of constructive value. The nurse related an instance of a mother who had casually made mention of her bad teeth. The conversation led to the discovery of a neglected breast abscess, which immediately received treatment.

"The nurse related other instances indicating that while the weighing of the baby had been the primary cause of the mother's attendance at the station, frequently the visit resulted in the discovery and correction of illness in other members of the family. One baby that up to 7 months had been progressing happily suddenly began 'falling off' unaccountably. The food seemed to agree with her and it seemed to be sufficient. The mother stated she (the mother) had heart trouble but an examination failed to reveal that this should affect the baby unfavorably. A call in the home, and coming in contact with the other children made the nurse suspicious of tuberculosis. The children did not seem to be thriving properly. 'Swellings' appeared on the baby. The nurse questioned the mother carefully regarding tuberculosis in the family but she was unable to find any trace of it anywhere in the history. After visits to several dispensaries the baby was diagnosed as tubercular and put on treatment that resulted in its ultimate recovery. As a result of the diagnosis other members of the family were examined and the father and two children were found to be well-advanced cases. The father died, but the two children are progressing favorably under open air treatment."

HOME VISITS

"Five calls were made in homes that afternoon. The nurse evidently has the friendship and affection of her people for she was warmly greeted wherever she went. Her instructions in the homes showed the same thorough-going knowledge of how to treat the sick or those below par, and the same half-knowledge of the principles of hygiene, that she showed in the station.

"1. Little girl, 5 or 6, chorea. Not at home. The nurse is carrying her because she appreciates the need of supervision of such a case. The family follow faithfully her instructions regarding diet, rest, play, and while the child does not get a great deal better she is certainly not growing any worse. The nurse did not know, however, modern treatment of chorea."

The next three visits were paid in homes where the babies had thriven, and showed unmistakable evidences of the nurse's constant instruction and watching. One mother said the nurse had been a "second mother" to her baby.

"5. Twins, 3 months old. Both artificially fed. Mother not strong—at 35 she had had 12 children. Nurse gave her excellent instructions, sensible and practical, regarding care of herself. The babies were making slow but steady progress on artificial food. They had just been given their bottles, which were filled and heated according to the nurse's instruction. Her teaching is evidently very thorough, for wherever we saw one of her cases on artificial feeding we found the milk carefully prepared."

5. Organization and Administration of Public Health Nursing Agencies

We have chosen, to illustrate some of the wide ramifications and established procedures of public health nursing, typical days encountered by our field agents in accompanying a successful county nurse in a primitive countryside, an able nurse giving generalized care under a private city visiting nurse association, and an efficient instructive nurse working under a municipal department. Naturally, among the 164 nurses visited, there were found also many mediocrities, many unsuccessful, and some glaring failures.

What, then, are the causes of success and of failure? Obviously, as in most human affairs, no one factor can alone be held accountable. Many factors are variously responsible, such as the nurse's personality and training, the conditions under which she works, the general support received in the community.

We have already indicated in the description of nurses accompanied by our investigators, the central importance of the nurse herself, her personality and training, in the success of her contacts. We shall subsequently analyse in greater detail the nurse's relations with the many different persons whom she must meet and work with in the community. But first we must make clear the main points in the organization and administration of the agencies under which she works, and their influence upon her performance. It is readily evident that whatever the native capacity or training of the nurse, her work is fundamentally affected by the way in which it is organized and directed.

Information as to the organization and administration of services was obtained for 37 of the 49 agencies whose work was observed in the field; that is, for something over four-fifths of the total number of organizations included. This is a sufficiently large proportion to afford data on the factors which lie for the most part beyond the nurse's control but which bear directly upon her work.

Accordingly, we consider next for the group of agencies studied the main factors bearing on organization of the work; namely, the type of community served, the auspices under which it is conducted, and the kind of nursing services rendered.

Types of Communities Served: City and Country

As we have already seen, the large city with its crowded tenements, its congested immigrant population, and on the other hand, its elaborate system of hospitals, dispensaries, social and other health agencies, brings an entirely different set of problems to the staff nurse of a large and prosperous visiting nurse association from those with which the nurse in a scattered rural community strives often single-handed to cope.

As we have also seen, in examining the work of Miss C. who was supposed to limit herself to the work of tuberculosis alone, it is inevitable that in country districts the nurse should be called upon for services of all kinds. It is obvious also, that with too large a district, she cannot do justice to such a rounded service. Various estimates have been made as to the size of the community which a public health nurse can successfully cover, ranging from 1,500 to 3,000 persons. These estimates are, however, rarely if ever met in rural nursing. They are more nearly approximated, as we shall see, in city organizations. With the recent introduction of public health nurses in country districts, the noteworthy fact is the extraordinarily rapid increase of their numbers during the past few years rather than the scarcity which as yet necessitates their covering territory far too large for adequate service.

Thus, for instance, the Red Cross Public Health Nursing Service, in promoting county nursing, reports that in the year between March 1, 1920, and March 1, 1921, the number of nurses employed almost doubled, rising from 701 nurses in 629 different places to 1,311 nurses in 1,200 different places.

"When one compares these figures," says the head of the Red Cross Public Health Nursing Bureau, "with those at the close of the war when there were only 97 nurses in this service, one is struck by its rapid growth." [38]

The great majority of these nurses are engaged in county-wide work, being employed by Red Cross Chapters whose jurisdiction covers the whole county. The rapid growth in rural nursing, through the new interest of the Red Cross and other local organizations, is reflected in reports from single states. Thus, for instance, a report from Texas says:

"Through our Chapters we are placing public health nurses in counties just as rapidly as we can secure the nurses. Last June we had one nurse doing rural public health nursing work in one county. Today we have 30 nurses in 28 counties, and 14 more that have been appointed and will be on duty by early summer. Many of our other counties are ready, have their money in the bank, and are waiting for their nurses to be assigned them." [39]

Of the 37 organizations dealt with in this section, 26 were located in cities large or small, and 11 were located in small towns, villages, or rural districts.

AUSPICES OF AGENCIES: PUBLIC AND PRIVATE

We have already seen in connection with school nursing how municipalities have taken over a nursing function whose value was first demonstrated by a private agency. Similar demonstrations in other fields have led to the assumption of other

[38] The Public Health Nurse, June, 1921. Page 321.
[39] Child Hygiene and Public Health Nursing. Ethel Parsons, Director, Bureau of Child Hygiene and Public Health Nursing, State Board of Health, Texas. The Public Health Nurse, June, 1921. Page 287.

nursing functions by public authorities, notably in tuberculosis and infant welfare work.

ADVANTAGES OF PUBLIC CONTROL

The advantages of state or municipal control of public health nursing are patent. No private organization has the continuous financial resources of a public agency. School nursing, for instance, could never have reached its present country-wide extent under private auspices. Infant welfare work, too, under municipal agencies is reaching numbers of babies and mothers hitherto necessarily untouched by private organizations.[40]

Besides the greater possibility of obtaining large funds, other advantages are inherent in state or municipal control of public health nursing. There is a definite gain, for instance, from having the bureau or division of public health nursing an organic part of the board of health, correlated with the other divisions having jurisdiction over sanitation, housing, the control of disease, etc. There is also gain in having the legal power to enforce certain hygienic regulations such as registering and supervising the tuberculous, quarantining persons suffering from communicable diseases, etc.

But more important than any of these advantages is the growing sense of community ownership evident in various localities where nursing services are under public control. In the country, for instance, particularly in the West, people feel a genuine satisfaction in having the public health nurse, like the school teacher, a part of the tax-paid town or county government, and rightfully available on equal terms for all. The future of public health nursing as an agency of preventive as well as curative science, may well be envisaged as developing on a par with public education.

DISADVANTAGES OF PUBLIC CONTROL

On the other hand, there are undoubted dangers in the present public control and administration of public health nursing. Chief among these is the danger of political interference. Where there are no civil service requirements, appointments are often made on purely political grounds and not on the basis of effi-

[40] Infant Mortality in New York City. Ernest C. Meyer, Ph.D., Director of Surveys and Exhibits, Rockefeller Foundation. International Health Board, New York City, 1921.

ciency, experience, and training. Often when the appointments are protected by the civil service, political influences still control the disposition of funds, of services to be developed, etc.

SOME SAFEGUARDS OF PUBLIC CONTROL

The best safeguard against such deterioration in publicly administered services, is some method of enlisting the continued co-operation of citizens and having them share in the direction of the work. Various methods have been employed in different cities to accomplish this result.

The experience of Cleveland may be quoted here in some detail owing to our special investigation of public health nursing in that city. In Cleveland there is a Central Committee composed of representatives of all the public health nursing agencies in the city, including those under both public and private control. It is not too much to say that the high rank of Cleveland in various branches of public health nursing is due in large part to the existence of this committee and the public interest which it reflects. The decisions of the committee are not mandatory but are presented in the form of recommendations to the organizations represented and have almost invariably been accepted and acted upon. Politics have been eliminated in the appointment of nurses, since all nurses are appointed by this Central Committee, those on the staffs of the municipal board of health and board of education, as well as those on the staffs of the visiting nurse associations and of other private organizations. The result of this method is shown in the unusually high calibre of the municipal nurses noted in the course of our investigation.

The assignment of applicants to the various staffs is determined by this committee on the basis of: first, expressed preference of applicant; second, urgency or emergency need; third, the date on which the request for additional nurses was filed by the superintendent. There has been no dissension among the superintendents over the assignments. Nurses are told of the work of all agencies and allowed to express preference, if they have any. They are assigned to the agency of their choice if there is a vacancy.

In other cities, notably in Los Angeles, Pittsburg, and Detroit, other co-operative arrangements have been put into effect whereby volunteer workers participate in the direction of public health nursing, both public and private. These experiments have now been in operation sufficiently long to prove that such joint control by representatives of the city government and representatives of the public is feasible, and tends to minimize, if it does not remove, political interference with the best ends of nursing.[41]

ADVANTAGES OF PRIVATE CONTROL

Yet it is undeniable that hitherto public health nursing under private control has, on the whole, and especially in cities, maintained higher standards of work than publicly administered agencies. The absence of political influence has, generally speaking, made for a better and more intelligent class of workers; there has been more freedom to improve the service by experimentation along various lines. The pride of ownership in nursing facilities, which may be a valuable asset of agencies under state or city auspices, has been fostered in privately supported visiting nurse associations by the appointment of local committees, responsible for local financing and details of management. This participation has resulted in a notable increase in interest and activity on the part of the community and thereby in an extension of the scope of the association's work.

Among the 37 agencies covered in this section of the study, 24 were private organizations and 13 were supported wholly by public funds. A few of the private agencies received partial support from public sources, but the control of the organization remained in each case in the hands of its private executive committee or board of managers.

Thus, for instance, in a small southern city the salary of the one nurse employed by the local visiting nurse association was $130 per month. Of this amount, $65 was paid by the association, $50 by the city, and $15 by the county. Again, in a village near a large eastern city, the $1,500 salary of the nurse of the local child welfare association was appropriated by the village board from local funds, while all other expenses of the work, such as maintenance of a baby welfare station, clinics, equipment, and overhead, were met by the privately supported association which had initiated the work and was still responsible for its continuance. Such instances of joint public and private support could be multiplied. It is illustrated on a nation-wide scale in the joint support by the American Red Cross, National

* Organization of Public Health Nursing. Annie E. Brainerd. Macmillan, New York, 1919. Pages 12, 13.

Tuberculosis Association, and various states, of state supervising nurses who give supervision and aid to local public health nursing in these states.

The public and private agencies were represented in practically the same proportion among rural and urban communities. Of the private associations, 17 were located in cities and 7 in country sections or villages; among the public bureaus 10 were urban and 4 rural.

KINDS OF NURSING SERVICE RENDERED BY 37 AGENCIES

Public health nursing agencies may be roughly divided into two categories: those which carry on several different kinds of nursing service and those which pursue only one specialty, referring all other calls to some other agency.

We have already seen how under the "generalized" system in a private society one nurse gives all kinds of nursing care and instruction in her own district (see page 66). We have also seen the remarkable increase in the scope of maternity services rendered by large visiting nurse associations (see page 49). In some societies offering various kinds of service (tuberculosis, child welfare, etc.), the different specialties are assigned to different members of the nursing staff thus forming a "specialized" staff. The arguments for a generalized or specialized staff will be later discussed. Here we are to consider the kind or kinds of nursing service rendered by the organizations as a whole.

It has already become evident that hard and fast lines cannot always be drawn and that, especially in the country, a single nurse or one organization may have to cover many different fields of service, since there are few or no other organizations to which to turn. Thus tuberculosis nursing perforce branches out into school nursing or infant welfare work. One tuberculosis committee visited was in process of developing mental hygiene clinics. In cities, too, similar expansions of work are found. Child welfare organizations find it necessary to provide prenatal instruction to mothers, etc.

In spite of these various kinds of procedure it is possible in a fairly accurate way to divide the 37 agencies here under consideration into these two groups. Of the entire number, 27 were by their own account covering several fields of service and 10 one special field. From our inspection it appeared later that of these 10 agencies only 3 were in actual practice restricting themselves to their one exclusive field.

As might be expected, the urban agencies show more specialization than the rural. Of the 26 urban agencies considered in this section, 8 confined themselves to one field of service, 18 or somewhat more than twice as many covered more than one field of service. Of the 11 rural agencies, 2 were restricted to one field of service; 9, or more than four times as many, covered more than one field. Table 1 shows the extent to which the various kinds of nursing services were covered by the 37 agencies in question.

TABLE 1

TYPES OF SERVICE INCLUDED IN THE WORK OF 37 PUBLIC HEALTH NURSING AGENCIES, BY TYPE OF AGENCY

Type of Service	Organizations				
	Private		Public		Total
	Urban	Rural	Urban	Rural	
General bedside nursing	13	6	3	..	22
Maternity nursing:					
Prenatal	16	4	4	1	25
Partum	9	4	1	1	15
Postpartum	11	4	3	1	19
Child welfare	15	6	6	4	31
School nursing:					
Public schools	4	6	5	4	19
Private and parochial					
schools	2	..	3	1	6
Tuberculosis	13	7	6	4	30
Venereal diseases	1	2	1	1	5
Control of other com-					
municable diseases	..	..	5	2	7
Mental hygiene	..	1	1	..	2
Industrial nursing	6	..	..	..	6
All other services	3	2	..	1	6
Total organizations re-					
porting	17	7	9	4	37

SERVICES INCLUDED IN TABLE 1

From this table it appears that tuberculosis and child welfare were the services occurring most frequently in the agencies covered in this study. Of the 37 organizations, 30 included tuberculosis and 31 child welfare. These two branches of public health nursing were most often covered because each represented a field commonly included in the work of the general agency as well as in that of a number of specialized agencies.

TUBERCULOSIS

Tuberculosis nursing usually included general supervision of all tuberculosis cases in the district covered by the agency, instruction in the hygiene of this disease, actual bedside nursing, suitable placement of patients in institutions or as the needs of the case might demand.[42]

CHILD WELFARE

The term "child welfare" connoted a wider variety of nursing activities. Among its many ramifications, the following were included:

Well baby clinics.
Clinics for sick babies.
Special nutritional clinics.
Milk stations.
Instruction to mothers regarding feedings.
General follow-up of all births.
Supervision of midwives.
Supervision of boarding homes.
Poliomyelitis after-care.
Special eye-work.
Physical examinations of the pre-school child.
Open air schools, etc.

PRENATAL CARE

Prenatal care was the service of next greatest numerical importance. In the majority of agencies in which prenatal care was given, postpartum nursing was also included; but the tendency was in some of these instances to leave actual obstetrical or partum care to a special agency. However, in the 15 agencies which had a confinement service both prenatal and postnatal care were given.

[42] Four of the agencies doing tuberculosis work did not include bedside nursing and one other did only "some," chiefly for demonstration purposes. Three agencies did not place their tuberculosis patients, and one state nursing bureau acted only as supervisor and advisor to local associations in their tuberculosis work.

GENERAL BEDSIDE NURSING

General bedside nursing was provided by all the privately supported agencies with the exception of 4 specialized city organizations and 1 rural tuberculosis committee. On the other hand, only 3 of the 13 public agencies maintained any bedside service, and these were all city organizations.

General bedside nursing does not always mean that all cases of sickness are accepted for bedside care. Most of these organizations refused one or more of the contagious diseases, such as scarlet fever, diphtheria, smallpox, and typhus. A few of the visiting nurse associations, however, accepted all cases referred to them, regardless of the degree of contagion involved.

COMMUNICABLE DISEASES

The control of communicable diseases in general was in the hands of municipal nursing bureaus whose nurses were responsible for establishing and terminating quarantine, placarding cases, taking cultures, and instructing in disinfection and other protective measures.

SCHOOL NURSING

We have already pointed out the extraordinarily wide possibilities of school nursing among the 22,000,000 school children of the nation. For the most part, school nursing as seen in the course of this study, when at all comprehensive in its scope, was carried on by publicly supported agencies. The public school work done by private city nursing agencies was, in one instance, only inspection for communicable diseases; in two others it was carried on in a few outlying districts of the county, while the work of the city proper was left to the municipal nursing bureau; and the fourth instance was found in a small southern city of 10,000 which had not yet developed enough civic spirit to support public health nursing as a governmental activity. In the rural agencies likewise, where there was no publicly supported agency to carry on the work, school nursing as well as all other branches devolved upon the privately supported rural nurse. In these instances school nursing frequently included only inspection of the pupils in the schools, owing to lack of time for follow-up of the school children in their homes. We have already pointed out the inadequacy of such classroom teaching alone.

Some agencies, both public and private, were carrying on a limited amount of school nursing in parochial or in private schools.

MENTAL NURSING

Only two organizations make special mention, among the fields of nursing, of mental hygiene. Yet it is evident that some knowledge of the principles of mental hygiene and of the resources that are available for dealing with mental illness and the mental factors in general illness must increasingly be a part of the public health nurse's equipment. With psychiatry definitely entering the field of prevention and attempting to make widely known the mental mechanisms that so largely control the emotional lives of human beings, it is apparent that the public health nurse, even to understand the drama of life enacted in the homes that she visits, must acquire some of the new knowledge of the deep springs of conduct. She can hardly be a witness to the disintegrating effects of psychopathic conditions in the family circle and remain content merely to observe the play of forces of which she is ignorant. She cannot be content to see a feeble-minded mother set the health standards of a home without wishing to possess knowledge of the avenues of instruction and encouragement that are open to the feebleminded.

The public health nurse is right in feeling that she must have the equipment, if it is obtainable, which will make some of the formidable mental problems encountered by her, challenges to helpful work rather than obstacles that justify surrender as soon as their nature is recognized. No one sees more clearly than she the social relationships of disease. She must not be forced, for lack of some additional training and a slightly different point of view, to be handicapped in this part of her work. She can not only render the most immediate and practical kind of aid if she has learned how to deal with "the facts of the mind as expressed in terms of behaviour" but, on account of her unique opportunities for observation, she can add to the stock of scientific knowledge concerning the social symptoms of mental diseases. "Hers," writes a wise psychiatric physician, "is the privilege of gathering the concrete facts from the stories of family and teachers, neighbors, physicians, employer, and priest." [48]

[48] Is Psychiatric Training Essential to the Equipment of a Graduate Nurse? Esther L. Richards, M.D., Associate in Psychiatry, Johns Hopkins University. American Journal of Nursing. May, 1922. Page 632.

Upon information gathered in this way will be decided many times issues of admission to or discharge from mental hospitals, accurate diagnosis in doubtful conditions, and determination of real causes when false ones seem more probable, that will mean success in treatment or rehabilitation and the future happiness of whole families as well as of individuals.

Let no one think that such situations will be rare in the daily experience of the public health nurse. Frank mental disease—dealt with by commitment to a public institution—is so prevalent that for instance (according to the estimate of Dr. Thomas W. Salmon) one adult out of every 10 in New York State enters a state hospital before he dies. This shows the extent of "insanity"—a term that is properly used only in conditions in which some legal step must be taken for treatment or other purpose. No one can correctly estimate the amount of mental disease not so designated that exists in the community. Feeblemindedness—to an extent that interferes with ability to acquire a common school education or to earn a living—exists in about 2 per cent of the population. The functional nervous diseases ("nervousness," "nervous breakdown," neurasthenia, or hysteria) are still more prevalent than the more serious conditions that have been mentioned and they are to be found at all ages and in every social environment. As complicating factors in other illnesses, they are responsible for an enormous amount of needless disability and needless prolongation of organic diseases. It goes without saying that to be successful, the public health nurse must not only be aware of these facts and vigilant to detect them, but she should be trained also to know whatever practical resources exist for dealing with them.

INDUSTRIAL NURSING

Owing to its importance as a new branch of public health nursing, a special study of industrial nursing was made in the course of this investigation, as described in a later section. We include industrial nursing in Table 1 so far as it was reported as part of the activities of general nursing associations.

A few of the urban visiting nurse societies did home visiting of employees for certain industrial firms on a contract basis. Some of these firms employed first-aid nurses whose entire time was devoted to work in the plant itself. Other firms had no nurse regularly in their employ and relied entirely on the visiting nurse association for whatever care they afforded their sick employees. An interesting new departure in industrial nursing here included is being made by a well-known public health nursing agency in one of our largest cities. One of the district offices of this association is established in a textile plant; the district nurse spends two hours each day in the first-aid room, attending to the needs of the workers in the plant; the rest of her time is spent in the usual neighborhood work. As most of the employees of this plant are drawn from the immediate neighborhood, the nurse naturally visits them and their families in the course of her home visiting. In this way these industrial workers are receiving nursing care and instruction without feeling under obligation to their employer for the service, since the firm provides only the office rent free, all other expense being borne by the visiting nurse association.

AREAS COVERED

In general the various services indicated in Table 1 were rendered by the organizations for the entire district within their jurisdiction. In certain cases, however, only a few selected districts were covered for certain special or new and experimental services. For example, an infant welfare society, newly undertaking prenatal work, was giving this care in only one of its many districts, until the best methods of conducting the service should have been evolved, with the ultimate purpose of having prenatal nursing carried together with infant welfare work in all districts. In another instance lack of funds made it necessary for a child welfare organization to limit work in 14 of its stations to children of 2 years or less, while in 6 of its districts it had been able to expand its work so as to cover all children of pre-school ages. These two causes, then, tend to restrict the development of new services to limited areas; namely, the necessity for pioneering and experimenting on a small scale to work out new methods and technique; and the limitation of financial resources.

TOTAL NUMBER OF SERVICES RENDERED

The number of different services rendered by one agency varied considerably. No one organization had established all 12 of the branches of work listed in Table 1. Nine was the largest number of services rendered by a single agency, and so large a number was found in only one large urban visiting nurse association. Seven agencies covered 8 different services, and an equal number included 7 fields of activity. The other 22 agencies included from 1 to 6 branches of nursing within their scope. Comparing the different types of organization, we find that the privately supported rural agencies average the greatest number of different services, the privately supported urban coming next, the public rural next, and the public urban agencies last.

NUMBER OF VISITS PER PATIENT

In the analysis of statistics from 12 leading city visiting nurse associations already quoted from the experience of the Metropolitan Life Insurance Company (see page 49), the average number of visits made per patient was found to be 7.2. This, then, may serve as a general standard of performance which is fairly approximated by the statistics of 17 agencies included in our study, for which figures showing number of visits per patient were available.[44] The average for rural communities was 6.1 visits per patient, for urban communities 7.6 visits per patient.

The number of visits per patient will, however, naturally vary in accordance with the kind of nursing service rendered. We have already seen the large increase in the number of visits per patient in maternity services, especially in prenatal work, owing to the need of keeping the patient longer under observation and care.

Within the general averages for the group of organizations studied, a surprising amount of variation was found. The visits per patient varied from 3.6 in a visiting nurse association in a far western city to 12.0 in an eastern child welfare society. The highest average for rural communities was 8.6 and the lowest 3.8. On the whole, fewer visits were made per case in rural than in urban communities. The higher average of visits per patient reported by two infant welfare societies follows naturally from the duration of time during which the babies were kept under observation.

NUMBER OF VISITS PER DAY

Figures were secured from 16 private agencies showing the average number of visits paid each day by each nurse on the

---

[44] Figures computed from statistics of total annual number of visits and total annual number of cases.

staff. Here obviously the difference between rural and urban agencies is marked. In her scattered territory and often without adequate means of transportation the rural nurse cannot be expected to visit as many persons as the nurse in a city organization who has a more or less compact district, and who has also the advantage of city transportation facilities. Of the 4 rural agencies for which figures were obtained, 3 had an average of 5 visits per day per nurse, and one an average of 6 visits. Among the 12 city agencies, on the other hand, the lowest average was 7 visits per day, and the highest 16. This high average was maintained in an agency operating in a selected district highly organized for community health and other social experimentation. Because of its compactness and the unique organization of its staff, a greater bulk of work was evidently possible for each nurse; although according to the best standards, this is too large a number of visits per day for the best work. One middle western visiting nurse association reported a daily average of 15 visits per nurse, and a large and efficient New England district nursing society came next with an average of 13. Only 2 out of the 12 city organizations had a record of less than 8 visits daily per nurse.

That the number of visits which a nurse can make in a day is dependent on the exact nature of her work is self-evident. The organizations which submitted these averages were almost entirely general visiting nurse associations and the differences in the character of their work were not marked enough to explain the considerable variation found in the daily average of visits per nurse. The differences are to be accounted for rather by differences in organization of staff or district, or by variations in the intensiveness of the work. One example may be quoted to show how the type of work affects the number of visits. An organization maintaining a maternity service will find that its nurses average about half an hour for prenatal cases after the first visit, about an hour for daily postpartum care, and about 3 or 4 hours in confinement cases.

INCREASE IN THE NUMBER OF PAY PATIENTS

One of the most significant developments of privately supported nursing associations has been the increase in the number of pay patients. The original purpose of most of these societies was to provide skilled care for the very poor, hence no charges were made. Gradually the scope of the work has widened; nursing care and instruction is beginning to be brought within the reach of persons of small means, at very moderate rates.

This development is of special importance in view of the reproach often levelled at the nursing profession, that nursing care is provided only for the very rich who can afford to pay the charges of the private nurse, or the very poor who have free services. The extent to which pay patients are beginning to avail themselves of the services of nursing associations is of more than passing interest in demonstrating the possibilities, with a larger personnel, of the community organization of nursing.

TABLE 2

PROPORTION OF PATIENTS PAYING IN FULL, IN PART, OR NOT AT ALL FOR VISITS FROM 13 PRIVATELY SUPPORTED VISITING NURSE ASSOCIATIONS DURING THE YEAR PRECEDING THIS STUDY *

Number and Type of Organization	Per Cent of Patients Visited Free	Per Cent of Patients Paying for Visits		
		Total	Paying in Full	Paying in Part
Urban:				
1	100.0	..	..	..
2	100.0	..	..	..
3	100.0	..	..	..
4	100.0	..	..	..
5	42.6	57.4	36.3	21.1
6	39.5	60.5	45.2	15.3
7	37.6	62.4	57.3	5.1
8	31.0	69.0	46.9	22.1
9	27.2	72.8	43.9	28.9
10	25.0	75.0	10.0	65.0
Rural:				
11	2.0	98.0	94.4	3.6
12	35.6	64.4	†	†
13	99.4	0.6	0.6	..

* These figures are based on reports submitted by these organizations. Visits made for the Metropolitan Life Insurance Company were counted as full pay visits. These were included in four urban societies' reports.
† Distinction between those paying in full and in part was not made in report given us by this organization.

COST PER VISIT

The cost of a nursing visit has been satisfactorily worked out in only a few nursing organizations. This cost must necessarily fluctuate with fluctuations in the cost of living, etc. In the year 1919-1920 when information was obtained on this point for 14

privately supported organizations, the cost per visit ranged from
42 cents per visit in a middle western city which had reduced
overhead expenses by consolidation with other public health
nursing agencies, to $1.00 per visit in another larger middle west-
ern city. The median cost was 60 cents per visit. Differences
in the method of computing overhead charges, etc., to some extent
invalidate these figures. A special national committee has recently (1922) been appointed to make an intensive study of
visiting nursing, including the "per visit cost." [45]

DIFFERENTIATION BETWEEN PUBLIC AND PRIVATE AGENCIES

Certain tendencies in regard to the fields of service covered
by publicly and privately supported public health agencies are
noticeable. Among the 24 private agencies, 4 specialized infant
welfare societies restricted their activities to work with well
babies, instructing mothers how to feed, bathe, and keep them
well, etc. The remaining 20 private agencies were giving bedside
care in every instance, usually in combination with hygienic instruction.

The public agencies, on the other hand, did not for the most
part include care but devoted themselves to instructive work
such as school nursing, following up all births, teaching mothers,
educative tuberculosis nursing, quarantine, communicable disease
work, etc.

This distinction has grown naturally out of the special nature
of each type of agency. The visiting nurse associations are, as
we have seen, privately supported agencies originally organized
to bring skilled nursing care within the reach of the poor and
those of moderate means. They have naturally retained their
original function together with the various nursing specialties
developed in the successive public health campaigns which we
have already described, tuberculosis, child welfare, etc. The
public agencies, having successfully taken over educational activities, the value of which was first, for the most part, demonstrated by privately administered organizations, have naturally
centered on these special educational activities.

Yet it is important to note that of the 13 publicly administered
agencies included in our study, 6,—that is, 3 urban and 3 rural
agencies,—gave some bedside care in addition to instruction.

---

[45] The Committee to Study Visiting Nursing, Dr. William F. Snow, Chairman; Miss Almena Dawley, Secretary.

This number included 3 large and efficient municipal nursing bureaus, recently reorganized.

Indeed the relative merits of curative and preventive work are hotly contested issues in public health nursing. In a later chapter the arguments on both sides of the controversy are assembled and an effort is made to present the conclusions to which this study has led.

THE PERSONNEL OF PUBLIC HEALTH NURSING AGENCIES

In accordance with the educational purpose of our study, organization of the staff is considered only so far as needed for an intelligent understanding of the work and in so far as it affected the work of the nurses observed.

It is clear that the character of the personnel of a public health nursing agency must vary in accordance with the size and type of the organization itself. A rural agency, for instance, is more likely than a city agency to have one general nurse who is superintendent, supervisor, and staff nurse all in one. The city agency on the other hand is more likely to have a large staff of nurses, each assigned to a small district for general service or to a larger district for a special service, and questions of organization and supervision play a large part. A state nursing bureau operating in rural districts may be giving bedside nursing, in which case it would employ general staff nurses; or it may be giving supervision and setting standards for locally supported nurses throughout the state, in which case it would doubtless employ nurses with executive experience who are specialists in particular lines.

Whatever the variations, there are, nevertheless, certain fundamental similarities in the personnel of different kinds of agencies—whether they be general visiting nurse associations, infant welfare societies, tuberculosis committees, or state or municipal nursing bureaus. Certain functions of direction, supervision, and home visiting must be assigned to different members of the staff.

The usual public health nursing agency has a paid professional staff composed of a director or superintendent of nurses, a certain number of supervisors,—the number depending on the size of the staff and the scope of the work,—and a group of staff nurses, who do the bulk of the home visiting. In many instances students, graduate or undergraduate nurses, form part of the staff.

THE DIRECTOR

The director is the responsible executive, who works out the policies of the organization and directs their application. In private societies the director acts in conjunction with the board of managers or the nursing or other committees; in publicly administered agencies, under the direction of the head of the department or of some designated bureau. The director frequently has authority over appointments and dismissals of staff nurses and sometimes of supervisors as well. In the agencies covered in this study she is known by the various titles of superintendent, director, executive, chief, and chief nurse. The two former are more common in private agencies, the two latter in public ones.

These positions as directors of nursing organizations offer, it should be pointed out, opportunities for women of executive ability of quite exceptional scope and authority. Comparatively few positions are open to women even in the business world involving the annual expenditure of a budget of upwards of $100,000, the direction of important policies and of a large staff of workers.

SUPERVISORS

Next in authority after the director are the supervisors. In small agencies there is often only one supervisor, in reality an assistant superintendent, who shares the direct supervision of the nurses in the field. On the other hand, in very large organizations there is sometimes, in addition to a staff of supervisors, an associate or assistant superintendent to assist the director in purely executive duties. The duties of the supervisor are to exercise direct oversight over the work of the staff nurses, to advise them on difficult cases, and to be generally responsible for the quality of the work done within her jurisdiction. In some agencies each supervisor is assigned to a certain district of the city, to oversee all work done in that particular section; in others she is assigned to the supervision of all work done in a certain field of nursing, such as tuberculosis, prenatal work, infant welfare, and the like; in still other agencies a combination of the two plans is used. Under the last plan, in addition to a supervisor for each district, a group of specialist supervisors is available for consultation and oversight of their particular specialties in all the districts. The district supervisor is the actual director of the nurses' work and the specialist supervisor is the consultant.

THE STAFF NURSES

The rank and file of the personnel is made up of staff nurses. They may be assigned to welfare stations or clinics or take part in various other special or experimental features of the agency's work. Their main duties, however, are to give nursing care and instruction in the homes of the community.

We have already referred to the organization of the staff under the "generalized" plan in which each nurse renders all types of nursing care and instruction in her district, and under the "specialized" plan, in which each nurse gives intensive care and instruction in one specialty. In a later chapter we will discuss the relative merits and defects of these two types of organization. Here it suffices to give the facts for the group of agencies studied. Both types of staff organization were exemplified. Several agencies were in process of transition from specialized to generalized staff, so that at the time of our visit, the staff was partly generalized and partly specialized. Such transitions were as a rule being gradually effected, one district at a time until the entire personnel should be placed on the new basis.

In still other agencies the major part of the staff was generalized but a limited number of special nurses were permanently retained. For example, one of the largest visiting nurse associations had a staff of 119 nurses, 114 of whom were assigned to general service, the other 5 being appointed to special experimental services that were in process of development. One of the 5 was assigned to a cardiac clinic and its follow-up work, 1 to a special intensive block experiment, 1 to social service and first aid in a health center, 1 to work with an industrial plant, and 1 to special work with contagious diseases. In another instance, an agency with a staff of 58 nurses, assigned 52 to generalized work, but reserved 6 for its maternity service, with its necessarily irregular hours.

Of the agencies which rendered general nursing service, by far the greater number had their staff also generalized or chiefly generalized. This was true of both private and public agencies. The specialized agencies, such as school nursing committees among the public organizations or infant hygiene societies among the private, naturally had an entirely specialized staff in keeping with their special purpose. The leaning toward generalization among the agencies studied, however, was sufficiently marked to justify its being considered a definite tendency in this direction.

A number of organizations also take student nurses for limited periods, to give them practice work in connection with public health courses conducted by some co-operating university or association. These student nurses are sometimes undergraduates in the senior year of their hospital training courses and sometimes graduate nurses who are taking a postgraduate course in public health nursing. Six of the private city agencies did not use any student nurses. Of the 11 remaining associations of this group, all had undergraduate nurses on their staffs at the time of investigation, and 7 had both graduates and undergraduates. In some organizations the students form a substantial proportion of the staff.

In the organization using the largest number of students, for instance, they formed almost 30 per cent of the nursing staff. Of these students, a little more than half were undergraduate nurses; the other half taking postgraduate courses. We defer until a later chapter discussion of the value and supervision of student services. None of the private rural agencies used graduate students and one occasionally had a varying number of undergraduates. The public agencies as a rule did not take on student nurses.

With the increasing demands on every efficient public health nursing agency in the country, with the present impossibility, indeed, of meeting the most urgent needs, persons other than nurses should obviously be employed for whatever services they can properly perform. Clerical workers and business managers in offices, clinics, and welfare stations; trained attendants, nutrition workers, social workers and housekeepers in the homes; assistants of different kinds in the schools; volunteers everywhere—these are some of the allies and colleagues of the public health nurse employed by public health nursing organizations.

Clerical Workers: Record Keeping

It would appear a mere matter of course that nurses should be freed from all clerical work which can be delegated to others. In large organizations, public and private, an adequate clerical force is essential to success. Owing chiefly to lack of funds, but due in part also to bad management and failure to appreciate the waste of nurses' time involved, clerical workers of good grade are rarely provided in sufficient numbers. Cumbersome and antiquated systems of record keeping are tolerated, which require often 2 hours or even more of the nurse's 7- or 8-hour day. Small wonder if among nurses giving such excessive time to records the chief business of visiting the homes is found to be rushed and infrequent.

Clerical work must, however, necessarily be involved in record keeping. The keeping of adequate records is admittedly one of the tests of good public health nursing. Both to check up the work and as an incentive for the individual nurse showing her comparative daily, weekly, monthly, and yearly accomplishment, a simple but accurate system of record keeping is a *sine qua non*. In determining the policies of a nursing bureau or association, such as the distribution of visits among acute, chronic, and maternity cases, the proper number of visits per day and per patient, and many other technical points, current and trustworthy figures and facts are no less indispensable. Indeed, adequate record keeping by public health nursing agencies is contributing materially to the whole field of vital statistics.

For an admirable discussion of the value and best methods of record keeping the reader is referred to a series of articles by Dr. Louis I. Dublin, Statistician of the Metropolitan Life Insurance Company.[46]

Use of Trained Attendants, "Practical" Nurses, etc.

In a subsequent chapter on private duty nursing we shall discuss the use of trained attendants; that is, persons who have had training or experience sufficient to enable them in minor illness, in chronic or convalescent cases, and in maternity care to take over or supplement the work of the more highly trained nurse. With the present personnel it is manifestly impossible for public health nurses to cover the field. As we show later, an essential part of the public health nurse's work consists in enlisting the services of other members of the family, or of relatives, friends, and neighbors, and teaching them how to assist and give care between her visits. There remain many cases in

[46] Records of Public Health Nursing and Their Service in Case Work, Administration, and Research. Louis I. Dublin, Ph.D., Statistician, Metropolitan Life Insurance Company, New York, 1922. (Reprinted from The Public Health Nurse.)

which none of these alternatives in the way of assistance are available, or in which some more experienced person is needed. Various efforts have been made by nursing organizations regularly to employ less highly skilled workers to give simple nursing care.

The difficulties which have in the past beset these efforts has been the lack of any standards in the training or capacities of these workers; the almost uniform tendency for them, after a short period, to drop their work under guidance of the association and to assume responsibilities in the care of the sick for which they are not fitted, charging in emergencies prices which are often equal to or even higher than those charged by the fully trained nurse.

With these difficulties we deal in our subsequent discussion of the nursing aide or attendant, and we consider the only practicable method of protecting the public and standardizing the training of a less highly skilled class of workers through a system of licensing similar to that which has long been effective in other professions and trades.

Size of Staff

IN RURAL AGENCIES: PRIVATE AND PUBLIC

The size as well as the organization of the staff of a public health nursing agency naturally varies in accordance with the size and character of the agency. Of the 7 privately administered rural organizations included in this study, 5 had only one nurse, who comprised the entire staff in all but one instance. In this case the nurse, a woman of exceptional initiative and experience, undertook to train "practical" nurses to work under her direction. Several of these women were actively associated with her work. She had also a list of those who had completed her course on whom she could call in emergencies. The 2 remaining private rural agencies served one or two small towns in addition to the more dispersed population of the countryside. They employed, respectively, 2 and 3 graduate nurses in addition to a supervisor.

The public rural agencies were of a somewhat different character from the private ones and therefore had a larger personnel. Of these 4 agencies only 2 gave bedside care; one of them, a county tuberculosis committee, had but one nurse, and the other, doing general work in a county surrounding a large city, had a staff of 3 nurses and a supervisor, besides having from time to time a few students from a public health nursing course. The other 2 public rural agencies were state nursing bureaus engaged in supervisory or demonstration work; one of these had a force of 7 nurses, the other a force of 15 nurses.

IN URBAN AGENCIES: PRIVATE AND PUBLIC

The urban agencies had for the most part larger staffs than the rural organizations. Among the 17 privately controlled city organizations, the largest number of nurses employed by any one agency at the time of our inquiry was 119, exclusive of the supervisory student and clerical staff. The next largest number was 90. Four agencies had 50 or more on their staffs; half had more than 27. Only 5 had less than 10 staff nurses.

Among the publicly supported urban agencies the staffs were even larger, ranging from 20 to 308. The next largest number employed was 174. Of the 9 public urban agencies reporting, half had more than 56 nurses on their staffs.

REQUIREMENTS FOR STAFF CANDIDATES

HOSPITAL TRAINING

As we have seen, the hospital-trained nurse was taken over as field agent first for district nursing, and later for public health nursing in its different forms. Various causes have made it necessary, however, to set certain standards in the employment of these staff nurses.

In the first place, with the rapid multiplication of hospital training schools, many of them are, as we shall see in Part B, schools in name only. They have neither clinical nor teaching facilities to give students adequate experience or instruction. In the effort to standardize the training, and to give the public the same protection in engaging a nurse which it has in selecting other persons legally licensed to practise such as physicians, or dentists, or pharmacists, etc., most states have enacted laws defining certain minimum requirements for state registration as R. N. (registered nurse). Persons without training and without state registration, passing themselves off as trained nurses, cannot legally use this title.

Public health agencies have availed themselves of the protection afforded by state registration, and usually require that candidates be graduate nurses, registered in the state in which the agency is carrying on its work. Some organizations do not require registration, but do require graduation from a hospital training school. All agencies, public and private, urban and rural, put first in their list of requirements that candidates be either graduate nurses or registered nurses or both. Some organizations go further and make certain specifications about the type of clinical training required. Out of 36 agencies reporting on their requirements for staff nurses, 12 have accepted the standard of one of the professional public health nursing associations, most often that of the National Organization for Public Health Nursing. This standard requires a 2-years' course of training in a hospital having a daily average of at least 30 patients, including work in obstetrical, medical, surgical, men's, women's, and children's services. Two more organizations, in addition to the 12 above mentioned, require training courses of 3 years but without the other conditions of the National Organization for Public Health Nursing standard.

SPECIAL TRAINING IN PUBLIC HEALTH NURSING

Only 10 of the 34 agencies reporting required special training in public health nursing. Of these, 3 required completion of some course in public health nursing in addition to hospital training, 1 demanded previous experience in the public health nursing field, and the remaining 6 required either experience or a course in the special branch of nursing. A few of the organizations specified that the course be at least four months long, but the majority made no definite requirements as to the length of either training or experience.

One agency included in this study preferred to train its own workers, and in fact went so far as to refuse to take nurses who had had any previous experience with a public health nursing agency. This was an organization with a very high standard for its work: workers coming to them from other less efficient agencies had so much to unlearn that their previous experience proved a handicap rather than an asset.

In view of the recent establishment of special courses of training in public health nursing and the comparatively small number of nurses who have yet received such training, it is hardly surprising that completion of such a course has not been made prerequisite to employment. A significant departure has recently been initiated in the state of California where special training in public health nursing is now mandatory by law for employment in the state public health nursing service.

Some publicly supported agencies require civil service examination. Of the 12 reporting on this point, 3 demanded it, while the remaining 9 made their appointments without formal examination, provided their other requirements were met.

WORKING CONDITIONS

SALARIES OF STAFF NURSES

In view of the need of increasing fivefold the number of public health nurses now in the field, the conditions of work in this new profession for women are of considerable importance. What are the material inducements for girls and women of fine calibre to enter upon this career, which admittedly requires physical strength as well as the necessary personal and professional qualifications?

Many organizations have set a definite scale with a minimum initial salary and a fixed upper limit beyond which no staff nurse can pass, no matter how long she remains in that capacity in the agency. Some have no minimum and maximum but pay all members of the staff at the same rate, regardless of experience or length of service. Still others have no set salary scale.

Of the 31 organizations reporting salaries paid to staff nurses, half were paying a minimum salary of less than $101.67 per month and a maximum salary of less than $120.45 per month. The minimum salary paid to staff nurses ranged from $65 monthly in a small southern city and $70 in a New England rural district to $125 in several country agencies having only one nurse, in which the minimum was also the maximum. The maximum salaries ranged from $75 monthly (in the same rural organization which had a minimum of $70) to $140, in one large city association, and $150 in a small town agency which employed but one nurse.

In Rural and Urban Agencies

The median [47] salary in the rural agencies studied, was higher than in the urban. It should be remembered in this connection

---

[47] When all amounts are ranged in order of magnitude, the median is the middle amount.

that the rural agencies of our group had, for the most part, only one nurse who carried on the work single-handed, performing various functions usually assigned to different members of larger staffs. Moreover, this one person may have organized the work when it first started, and had frequently had a long tenure of office, her salary increasing gradually. In one small town, for instance, the nurse had advanced from $65 per month to $130 in the course of six years. The salary scales of city and country agencies are thus not strictly comparable.

In Public and Private Agencies

It is interesting to note that the salaries paid in the public and private city agencies studied are on about the same level. Two organizations, one public and one private, located in two of the largest eastern cities, offered no incentive to their staff nurses in possible advances over the initial salary. In both, the minimum beginning salary was also the maximum, and unless a staff nurse was promoted to the position of supervisor she had no prospect of an advance in salary no matter how long her period of service with the organization. This fixed salary in the public agency was $91.67 a month and in the private agency $100 a month. Some of the agencies had a definite scale for advancing salaries, but in the majority increases were made irregularly or in a haphazard fashion.

The salary figures used in this report were obtained in the winter of 1919-1920. Some organizations, notably two large private city agencies, have in the interval raised their salaries. On the other hand, the salaries of clerical and industrial workers, are lower today than they were two years ago, when even the average mediocre stenographer was receiving about $1,200 a year and an able girl could easily earn in such work $1,500 to $1,800 or more. The salaries of public health nurses compare favorably with the salaries of teachers in the public schools, though teachers have, it is true, been notoriously underpaid.

SALARIES OF SUPERVISORS

The salaries paid to the supervising staff did not greatly exceed those paid to the rank and file of the nurses. The lowest salary paid to a supervisor was $85 a month, the initial salary

for the supervisor in a small rural society. The highest was
$175 monthly, the maximum salary for supervisors in two large
private city organizations. Half the agencies included paid a
beginning salary to their supervisors of less than $120 a month
and a maximum salary of less than $133.33. A third of the
agencies paid maximum salaries to their supervisors of $150
a month or more.

VACATIONS WITH PAY

Of 31 organizations reporting on this point:

    10 gave a vacation with pay of 2 weeks,
     1 gave a vacation with pay of 3 weeks,
    18 gave a vacation with pay of 1 month,
     2 school nursing organizations allowed the entire summer
       vacation of the school year.

WORKING HOURS

The work of the public health nurse involves so much walking, so much stair-climbing, so much actual physical exertion,
besides the strain on her sympathies and the constant effort involved in continually meeting people, teaching them, and attempting to persuade them into doing a variety of things for
which they may have little inclination, that her working day
must perforce be a fairly short one. In the organizations
covered in this study, the vast majority had a working day for
their staff of from 7 to 8 hours. In a 7-hour working day
the nurse comes on duty at 9 o'clock in the morning and continues until 5 o'clock in the afternoon, taking as a rule an hour
off for lunch in the middle of the day.

Of 34 organizations reporting:

    8 had a 7-hour working day,
    1 had a 7¼-hour working day,
    9 had a 7½-hour working day,
    8 had an 8-hour working day.

Of those organizations which exceeded eight hours:

    3 had an 8½-hour working day,
    1 had a 9-hour working day,
    1 had customarily an 11-hour working day.

Two others laid no claim to any fixed schedule and reported their hours as "irregular," while, on the other hand, one baby hygiene association claimed as short a working day as 6 hours.

OVERTIME

In many cases, however, nurses stay on after the day's work to finish writing up records; or emergencies arise which demand overtime from the staff. Overtime in the organizations reporting was irregular and dependent on emergent situations which may arise. At certain seasons of the year, as in the winter when there is more sickness, overtime is apt to be more prevalent than at other times. Some agencies have considerably more overtime than others. Those which conduct a maternity service are apt to have calls at all hours, and for this reason often organize their staff so as to have a special detail of nurses for this particular work, whose time can be adjusted to the demands of the service. This plan is followed frequently even in agencies which otherwise have a generalized staff.

SUNDAY WORK

Most organizations, especially the majority that provide bed-side care, find it necessary to provide a certain amount of the most essential service on Sundays. Various schemes have been devised to make this Sunday service possible with the least possible demand on the staff. A number of organizations have a regular schedule whereby each nurse on the staff expects to be called for Sunday work at some definite interval. The length of this interval varied from 2 to 9 weeks. One rural organization in which the superintendent rarely allowed herself a day of rest arranged for her assistants to have alternate Sundays off, and in a large city association each member of the staff was expected to give a half day every other Sunday. Other agencies called for Sunday duty every 3 weeks, once a month, every 5 weeks, every 6 weeks, or every 9 weeks. Still others had no regular arrangement, but required Sunday service, some of them "irregularly but frequently," some "not very often," and some "in emergencies." More than four-fifths of the organizations arranged for a Saturday half-holiday throughout the year.

SUPERVISION OF THE WORK

For the success of public health nursing, supervision of the right order is a prime requisite. It is essential not only for planning the work of the staff and co-ordinating their activities, but as a stimulus and guide for the individual nurse both in her function of teaching the principles of health and in giving bedside care.

Adequate supervision involves the actual accompaniment of nurses on their home visiting. The more experienced supervisor or director brings to the nurse's aid, especially in non-acute cases where changes are slow from visit to visit, a fresh point of view, a greater ability to see new angles of old cases. Good supervision is thus in a sense the crux of public health nursing.

In organizations large enough to have both superintendent and supervisors, the direct oversight of the work of the nurses is in the hands of the supervisors. Procedures naturally vary in different agencies, but under the best system the supervisors assign the work, hold daily individual conferences with the nurses, give advice on especially difficult problems, accompany the nurses regularly in their home visits, etc. The supervisor is thus the field executive, seeking to develop, in democratic relations, the initiative and imagination of the nurses under her direction. She is responsible for reports on the work of each nurse, regular inspection of their bags, group meetings of the staff, etc.

NUMBER OF NURSES PER SUPERVISOR

Of the 37 organizations included in this section, 29 had staffs of more than one nurse and therefore required some type of supervision. The number of supervisors in each agency varied with the size or resources or standards of the organization. As a rule under the system of "generalized" nursing, more supervisors are needed than in a "specialized" agency, to direct and keep the balance between the claims of the different nursing specialties. One organization with a generalized staff of 78 nurses had one group of 10 supervisors, each responsible for the work of a district, and another group of 7, each responsible for supervision of a single specialty. On the other hand, an agency with a specialized staff of 40 nurses had 6 supervisors.

This is an extreme example of variation between different agencies, but even among those with the same type of staff organization the number of nurses per supervisor varied considerably. The number of nurses per supervisor differs also in the various districts of one organization or in the different specialties covered.

Of the 23 organizations reporting on the proportion of nurses to supervisors:

> 9 organizations had a minimum of less than 5 nurses to a supervisor;
> 7 organizations had from 5 to 10 nurses to a supervisor;
> 2 organizations had from 10 to 15 nurses to a supervisor;
> 5 organizations had 15 or more nurses to a supervisor.

Twenty-four agencies reported on the maximum number of nurses per supervisor, and of these:

> 3 agencies had a maximum of less than 5 nurses to a supervisor;
> 4 agencies had a maximum of from 5 to 10 nurses to a supervisor;
> 9 agencies had a maximum of from 10 to 15 nurses to a supervisor;
> 8 agencies had a maximum of 15 or more nurses to a supervisor.

Half the group showed a minimum of less than 7 nurses to 1 supervisor, and a maximum of less than 13. These figures well indicate the diversity in the assignment of nurses to supervisors even within the same organization.

ACCOMPANYING STAFF NURSES IN HOME VISITING

In 22 of the 29 organizations reporting which had a supervising staff, the supervisor regularly accompanied staff nurses in their home visits; in two others it was the custom to do so only occasionally. For the supervisor to visit in the homes without the nurse was a less general practice. Yet in as many as 16 organizations she did so regularly. In 3 agencies supervisors never visited in the homes unless accompanied by the district nurse.

EFFICIENCY RECORDS

In 9 agencies of the 29 in question, the supervisors kept formal records of the efficiency of each nurse's work. Where such records were not kept, judgment of the individual nurse was based on her reports of cases, on observation of her work in the field, and on personal conferences, but there was no current record available on the progress and development of the work.

WRITTEN INSTRUCTIONS

The larger agencies frequently have small printed manuals containing instructions which are given to the staff nurses when they begin work with the organization. Many of the smaller agencies have printed or typewritten directions which are given to their workers. Of 34 associations reporting, 22 gave some sort of printed or written instructions to their staff for guidance, while the remaining 12 relied on verbal directions. Eight of the 12, it may be noted, were agencies with one nurse each, and hence naturally had not worked out formal regulations.

REPORTING AT HEADQUARTERS

A part of the nurse's daily routine is regular reporting at headquarters. In large organizations with many subdivisions or districts, nurses usually report at the district office; in small organizations, as a rule, there is but one office where all the staff reports regularly. With but few exceptions nurses are expected to report at least once daily. This is usually the first thing in the morning when the nurse stops at her office to get her bag and either to receive her day's assignment or to work out her day's program herself, according to the degree of responsibility allowed her under the prevailing method of supervision.

Of 26 organizations reporting in which there was a supervisory staff, 11 required their nurses to report once a day.[48] Of the remaining 15, 5 required that the staff report twice daily in person; 3, that they report three times daily; 3, that they report once in person in the morning and once at noon by telephone in order to get emergency calls which might have come in during the interval; and the remaining 4 required either a weekly reporting only, or had no definitely stipulated time, leaving it to the nurse's discretion. Two of this last group were state nursing agencies whose staff was scattered throughout the state and could not be held to any fixed schedule.

Even when not required to report more than once daily, nurses frequently drop in at the lunch hour to get new calls or to talk over troublesome cases with the supervisor or other members of the staff, and then stop in at the end of the day to write up records and leave the bag. In a number of agencies the nurses lunched together informally at headquarters; and these

* In one of these, reporting by telephone rather than in person was allowable.

luncheons were found by our investigators to be fruitful to the nurses and to promote good fellowship among them.

Meetings of the entire staff are held at more or less regular intervals, varying in different agencies. The majority hold these conferences either weekly or monthly, more inclining toward the weekly plan than to the monthly. In the organizations in which the staff was regularly assembled for conference, the director of the agency usually issued the call for the meeting and presided.[49] The entire field staff attended these meetings and usually the supervising staff as well. A few agencies did not have their supervisors attend because separate conferences were held for them with the director, but for the most part the supervisors joined the general meeting regardless of whether they had special meetings or not. In some agencies members of the association's executive committee or of the nursing committee attended, and in one or two public bureaus the deputy health commissioner responsible for the nursing bureau of the department came to staff meetings. Usually the general problems of the organization were discussed, but special questions and cases were also brought up, and sometimes arrangements were made for an outside lecturer to address the staff on some health subject.

Besides the regular staff meetings, 14 organizations had case conferences held at regular and frequent intervals, and 2 others held them irregularly. These were more informal meetings designed especially for thrashing out particular problems arising in specific cases, and sometimes were held jointly with social workers who were working on the same cases. The staff nurses in a number of agencies also attended meetings of other organizations, to keep them abreast of current issues and modern methods in their field of work.

6. Successes and Failures

We have now given in our first four sections a general survey of the field of public health nursing. In Section 5 we have

---

[*] Where the staff included also an associate director she occasionally conducted the meeting, and in one instance the supervisors were assigned to this duty.

outlined the most important facts in the organization and administration of public health nursing agencies, to show the background of the nurse's activities.   In order now to fulfil our primary purpose and make clear the kind of training needed for successful public health nursing in the United States, we have next to trace further the causes of the success or failure of the nurses in their various functions and relations as observed in the field.

A ROUGH CLASSIFICATION OF 147 NURSES

In order to supplement our detailed case study and description of individual nurses, we have attempted roughly to classify, according to their degree of success or failure the 164 persons observed or interviewed in the course of our study.   For various reasons 17 persons had to be omitted in this rough classification,[50] leaving 147 nurses whose work could be fairly appraised.

Obviously, it is difficult to set any rigid standards of performance in such a general appraisal, or strictly to grade individuals in work in which so many varying factors must enter. However, with the information at our disposal gained from discriminating observation of each nurse in the field, we have based our judgment on five essential elements in the work of each: her personality, teaching ability, nursing technique, and social understanding, together with the organization of the work; and we believe that, in spite of the limitations of any such informal rating, these elements have afforded a fair basis for conclusions.

Of the 147 nurses in question, broadly speaking,

69 were successful,
42 were average,
36 were unsuccessful or below average.

VARYING DEGREES OF SUCCESS AND FAILURE

Of the 69 nurses counted as successful, 26 were of outstanding excellence in personality, training, and in the results achieved; 43 were well above the average, though not of the very first rank.

Of the 36 at the other end of the scale, 16 were unmistakable

---

* Ten nurses were not observed in the field but only met in conference, so that there is not sufficient basis of information on which to gauge the excellence of their work.   Seven other persons, not nurses, were either employed by public health nursing organizations as social workers, etc., or were doing some form of public health work, such as dental hygiene, etc. Twenty-four industrial nurses are not included in this classification.

failures, some of them totally unfitted by character for any
kind of nursing work, others without any grasp or even understanding of the special field of public health nursing. The 42
rated as average were doing work not discreditable but more
or less routine or humdrum.

THE HANDICAP OF POOR ORGANIZATION

The direct influence of the organization of the work on the
success or failure of the individual nurse is brought out in this
informal classification.   For more than one-quarter of all the
nurses ranked average or below might have made a different
showing had they not been handicapped by poor policy or management in the agencies in which they were employed.   These
nurses were either so overworked or so inadequately supervised
or so limited by their agencies' policies that those of good native
ability fell short of success and those of mediocre ability were
completely unsuccessful.

In undertaking now to analyse further the success or failure
of the nurses accompanied in their work in the course of this
investigation, it is important to bear in mind several general
considerations.   Public health nursing is, as we have seen, a
new form of an ancient service.   This new profession for women
is only in process of development: its possibilities are almost
day by day being further explored and demonstrated, as the
old curative functions of nursing, like those of medicine, are
supplemented by the new stress on hygiene and prevention of
disease.

All education for public health work, medical as well as
nursing, is of very recent date, and itself in process of development, almost of definition.   It has therefore been a matter of
necessity, not of choice, that many nurses have learned only
by trial and error in the field, that they have, as one eminent
public health nurse says of herself, "struggled into this new
profession of public health nursing with no preparation other
than that afforded by a hospital training school." [51]   The justice,
therefore, of criticising the nurse for the various lacks and
failures which we are about to describe and for which her lack
of special training is in many cases responsible, might be open

[51] Public Health Nursing and Industrial Hygiene. Mary Beard, R.N.,
Director, Instructive District Nursing Association, Boston.   Journal of
Industrial Hygiene, July, 1919.   Page 195.

to question, if it were designed merely to appraise the performance of different individuals. But in the interest of an objective statement, to contribute towards further standardizing the function of the public health nurse and deducing the objectives of training, examples of failure are clearly as illuminating as examples of success. We have accordingly given about equal weight to each.

Teaching Ability: Examples of Failure

In turning next to concrete examples, we take up first the ability to teach. The final measure of the nurse's success is indubitably her ability not only to make her message clear, but to do it so persuasively or with such skill in teaching, that the desired measures will not only be understood but put into practice.

As in all teaching, the active participation of the person taught is a condition of success. Indeed, the ability to call forth the participation of others, to give free play to their individualities, is a test of success not only in the schoolroom but in most human relationships. For the nurse, this capacity of obtaining an active response, a free give-and-take in her intercourse with people, instead of trying to impose *ex cathedra* instructions is peculiarly important, since her sphere of influence is to include persons of the most diverse sorts, adults and children, men and women, and since, moreover, in many situations she will feel herself taught by the fortitude and patience she encounters rather than being herself the teacher.

The failures in teaching which we encountered may be roughly ascribed to two main causes. The causes are:

1. A lack of appreciation on the part of the nurse of her rôle as health teacher and of the preventive measures to be taught.
2. A lack of knowledge on the part of the nurse of methods of teaching, or a lack of sufficiently definite information as to what should be taught.

From among many examples, we may choose a few to illustrate these main causes of failure.

A PARODY OF PUBLIC HEALTH NURSING

We have already described the successful instruction of Miss O., an efficient nurse under a municipal department in a large cosmopolitan city (see page 74).   In contrast to her, Miss W., another nurse in the same department, gave what may well be called a parody of public health nursing, an example of complete failure which unfortunately might be duplicated in other cities.   This nurse, like the successful Miss O., also spent her mornings in the baby station and her afternoons in home visiting.   But where the first nurse paid 5 visits during the afternoon in homes showing, by the care with which feedings were prepared, etc., unmistakable evidences of her intelligent teaching, the second nurse paid 12 visits, so hurried, so inconsequential, that our investigator comments immediately afterwards:

"The calls were made with such rapidity that I cannot remember all of them or their details.   Many of them were on top floors of tenements and it was rather disconcerting after having climbed up seven flights of stairs to turn about in less than one minute and walk right down again."

In the first home visited, the anæmic young Jewish mother, delivered less than three weeks before, complained of pain in her chest and around her heart.

"Nurse put her fingers on patient's pulse for a moment— then pronounced patient O. K.   Did not look at baby or ask regarding his condition.   Asked regarding husband's continued unemployment and sympathised with mother because of unpaid rent.   Her sympathy was of no constructive value, however, for her only advice was, 'Poor thing, poor dear! Well, do the best you can.   Good-bye.'"

Obviously from any point of view these so-called "home visits" of one or two minutes apiece were a mere farce, or parody of public health nursing.   That they should be tolerated by a large city health department is evidence of the total lack of adequate supervision in the field.[52]   Such a performance is not only dishonest on the part of the nurse and patently valueless for baby welfare, but worse, it often leads to a deserved contempt on the part of the mothers for all health work.

But even when the nurse pays an honest visit she may fail as

[52] It is perhaps worthy of note that the superiors of this nurse were so totally unaware of the futility of her performance that she was rated as a good exemplar of the department's activities.   This department chanced to be the only one visited twice, in order to substantiate certain facts, in the course of our investigation.   After the lapse of eight or nine months, Miss W., the nurse in question, was assigned to our second field agent, a public health nurse, as she had been assigned to our first who was not a nurse.   Precisely the same comments were made by both observers.

entirely for lack of appreciation of her rôle of instructor and for lack of knowledge of preventive measures.

NO APPRECIATION OF HEALTH TEACHING

Thus, for instance, in an environment far removed from the large eastern city just mentioned, in a small mining town of wretched aspect, the failure in teaching of another nurse was observed by another of our investigators. Through one of the most crowded streets of this town runs an open sewer partly clogged with sewage. On each side of the sewer is a narrow roadway and sidewalk and rows of houses in which the foreign families live. The object of the nurse's visit to one of these homes was to look after a 10-year-old girl whose sore throat she had noticed at school the previous day. Owing to the prevalence of diphtheria, she was calling to see the child's condition.

Here was a woman who, in our agent's opinion, was inspired by "zeal, sincerity, and one hundred per cent faithfulness," who even "takes a certain grim pleasure in hardships, such as making a difficult call in bad zero weather." She averages in her scattered territory between trolley and railroad trips, six miles a day of walking.

Yet, says our agent, in spite of these assets the nurse "has no glimmering notion of real preventive work or of social problems." She has little skill in securing information because her questions are awkwardly worded and chiefly—a criticism not infrequently made of other nurses—because she seldom listens to a reply, being herself an incessant talker. She has no skill in leading up to a question or asking it indirectly. She has never had any public health training, has never read anything on the subject, and does not even know the names of other types of public health nursing or other social work. Small wonder that in the day's visits, beginning with the 10-year-old girl, our agent failed to find any evidence of health teaching or preventive work, even though, through her ministrations in sickness, the nurse undoubtedly had won a "very great influence over her people."

In the case of suspected diphtheria the child was called in from an adjoining bedroom which was not inspected.

"The nurse asked question after question, without waiting for an answer. Such directions as she gave were so jumbled, that I failed to get out of them all one single thing she had told the child to do, while the child herself stood staring at her, mute and showing no evidence of understanding. None of the other four children were examined in any way. Quite as a threat, and one which I am sure the mother failed to understand, the nurse said: 'If you don't look out, you'll all have diphtheria.' "

The same failure to give any clear directions or even to grasp the situation was shown in her other visits. In stopping to see some infectious skin cases, for instance, the nurse and our agent found a small boy under the care of a doctor, with what was called a "bad liver."

"Her inquiries all seemed pointless," is the comment on this visit. "Not a single definite helpful suggestion was made. . . . The family were Russians, extremely hospitable and courteous. They seemed eager to learn. Yet even their own questions were not clearly answered."

NO KNOWLEDGE OF PREVENTIVE MEASURES

The lack of definite knowledge as to what should be taught may be illustrated also by a midwestern county nurse, working among a mixed population of native American mountaineers and foreigners, chiefly Italians and immigrants from the old Austria-Hungary. This nurse had been placed in positions of responsibility in her hospital training, first as charge nurse during her last eight months, and then as assistant superintendent of the hospital. Her only "preparation" for the public health work into which she had drifted consisted in reading her predecessor's reports and three books loaned to her by the state supervising nurse, "one about public health nursing, one about school nursing, and one about something else,—I've forgotten what," as she described them to our field agent. With such a background it was scarcely surprising that she should have been found sure of herself only in her relation to the little local hospital and in her actual nursing in the homes. Of her attempts to instruct, we may quote the following:

"Visit 9. Elderly patient, living in fairly good surroundings, with daughter's devoted care. Diagnosis: cirrhosis of liver, 'leakage of heart,' and suspected TB., although three sputum tests had been negative. Forced feeding advised for TB. condition, although liver condition makes food distasteful, especially milk and eggs, which nurse urged patient to eat in quantity. Much time spent in advising re TB. precautions, etc., but information was given indefinitely, and absent-mindedly, and very much at random.

"Visit 11. Family of several small children, Italians; parents and all felt honor of nurse's call. Four-month-old twins; nurse had previously advised re diet, and insisted upon calling doctor. Twins had improved. Nurse had called perhaps eight or ten times. Feeding was reviewed, without any demonstration, and both nurse and mother laughed when they failed to understand each other about anything so important as proportions, quantities, and frequency of feedings. It seemed worse than futile. As in every other call made, nurse seemed to lack definite available information with which to advise. Constantly she made use of 'Let me see—' and would close her eyes with a certain affectation of eyes and smile. Her suggestions were so hazy, that I, listening sympathetically and interestedly, was never once clear as to what her advice really was."

NO KNOWLEDGE OF TEACHING METHODS

In these cases, the failure of the nurse was as much due to her own inaccuracy and lack of definite knowledge of what should be taught as to her inability to teach. In other instances the nurse may herself be precise and painstaking, but may entirely fail to appreciate the need of explicit directions and explanation of procedures which are totally new to an ignorant though well-disposed lay person. Thus, for instance, another infant welfare nurse was accompanied by one of our investigators in a southern city to an 8-months-old baby whose ears had been lanced at a dispensary.

"The mother was told to remove the cotton from the child's ears," says our agent; "if the cotton was soaked she was to wash the baby's ears three times a day with syringe, if not, once a day would be enough. She was told to use boric acid, but was not asked whether she knew what an ear syringe was like, nor told how often to use it in each ear, whether water should be warm or cold, what amount of boric acid to use, what care to take after cleaning ear out."

Less immediately serious, but from the point of view of preventive work equally unsuccessful, was the performance of another child welfare nurse accompanied by one of our field

agents in a large midwestern city. The first visit was paid to
an intelligent Russian couple. Their only child was about 7
months old, and the object of the call was to follow up the child's
feeding and to teach the mother how to cook farina. The
"demonstration" is thus described by our agent:

"The nurse measured the farina, boiled and measured the
water and stirred the farina until it was thoroughly cooked.
Meanwhile the mother bustled about her work, not even
noticing what the nurse was doing although both of them
were chatting vigorously and intimately. Before the call
was over, quite as an afterthought, the nurse reminded the
mother to measure the farina with level, not heaped, table-
spoons, and gave purely verbal instructions, quite disasso-
ciated from any actual teaching. Apparently all she had
accomplished was cooking the day's cereal!"

A similar call was next paid to another fairly comfortable
home. Here the nurse was supposed to be teaching the mother
how to make up a formula for the 2-months-old baby, who cried
a great deal at night. The same futility characterized the instructions given.

"The mother," says our field agent again, "was quite in-
attentive during the making-up of the formula by the nurse
who in a well-equipped kitchen, worked daintily and prettily.
Frequently, with her back toward mother, she would say,
'You see——,' but there was no actual demonstration. Only
part of the 24-hour formula was made up, and nurse and
mother argued pleasantly, as they differed over proportions,
etc. Each insisted that doctor had given a different formula.
Then followed a pointless conversation as to causes of colic
in babies. Numerous possibilities suggested by each as to
why baby cried so much at night. No suggestions made as
to better ways of caring for baby. Mother seemed a very
heedless sort of person, and argumentative. Nurse appeared
to exercise no sort of professional advantage over her."

IGNORANCE OF EMERGENCY MEASURES

Perhaps the most serious instance of failure to teach encountered in the course of our study was that of another child
welfare nurse who was not only deficient in teaching ability but
also ignorant of the emergency measures which her clinical
training should have taught her.

This nurse was called by a neighbor to a baby in convulsions. Our field agent, herself an accomplished public health nurse, accompanied her and thus describes the visit:

"Nine-months-old baby registered at station as feeding case. Baby was just out of second convulsion on our arrival. Mother terrified. Nurse embarrassed—did not know how to proceed. Took temperature—found normal. On my suggestion examined stool. Found every indication of intestinal disturbance. Baby appeared to be suffering from cramps. Nurse advised: 'If convulsions return put baby in mustard bath. I don't know the proportions but I think it's a tablespoon to a quart of water.' It did not occur to her to warn mother against danger of burning baby from too strong a solution until I reminded her as casually as possible. Her further directions were: 'Cut the baby's diet in half for 24 hours, then if he's all right put him back on full diet.' Baby should have been put on barley water *only* for 24 hours and not returned to full diet for several days. I tried to get her to 'phone the family physician for orders to give a normal salt enema (nurse said standing orders do not include this but I learned that they do) but she did not feel it of sufficient importance. Baby was white and dazed and likely to go into another convulsion at any moment yet nurse permitted mother to dress him completely, pinning and buttoning everything securely.

"Two days later Miss S. told me that at 2 p.m. of the day of our visit the baby went into a convulsion—had had sixteen during the p.m. Two doctors were in attendance. They pronounced it feeding upset and intestinal disturbance. Miss T., the supervisor, heard her report this to me but she made no inquiries regarding her procedure."

EXAMPLES OF SUCCESS IN TEACHING

We have already shown concrete instances of good teaching in our general survey of public health nursing. Some further examples of clear cut and effective instruction, in contrast with the deficiencies above described will serve to emphasize elements needed in the training of the public health nurse.

CLEAR CUT QUESTIONS AND EXPLANATIONS

In a rural district on the Atlantic coast a visiting nurse association has been formed covering three townships. Seventeen villages and the intervening country are included in these townships. On the coast a large number of the people make their living by fishing. In the villages there are many small businesses, such as groceries, garages, carpenter and plumber shops, etc. The people in the country are poor but have a lucrative source of income during part of the year from the summer boarders. "This seasonal occupation furnishes practically the entire support of many families," says our investigator. The association provides three automobiles for the use of its nurses. Because of the large territory to be covered the number of visits paid per day is comparatively small, averaging six. The nurses of this association were found combining bedside care with teaching of unusual excellence.

"Without exception all the families visited displayed great confidence in her," says our agent of one of these nurses. "Her methods of teaching were far superior to those of nurses in general. Her questions brought out the facts. Her directions were given in a simple, clear cut fashion which admitted of no confusion. She always asked the patient or care-taker before leaving what was to be done. Their replies showed that they had understood her instructions."

Thus in one family living in a poor house in the open country, the nurse's questions elicited from the mother all the facts as to her own and the month-old baby's habits respecting food, regularity of feeding, fresh air, exercise, hours of sleep, etc. It was learned that the baby was fed whenever she woke. Thereupon the nurse not only instructed the mother as to the value of regularity and reassured her as to the baby's going to sleep again after feeding, but worked out a detailed feeding schedule which should not conflict with the mother's many other duties.

The nurse's questions had likewise shown that the mother was so rushed in the mornings to get breakfast for her husband and her two little boys that she often went without eating herself. She was impressed with the need, for the baby's welfare, of sitting down with her family to eat a regular meal, and specific changes in the diet were advised by the nurse, on learning that she was in the habit of taking all manner of laxatives. The nurse showed her practical insight by not only urging the mother to encourage her little boys to wait on the table, but herself securing from them an enthusiastic response by offering to help make, on the following Saturday, a wooden shelter for the baby to sleep out of doors.

That the clear cut and definite instructions of this nurse were not only understood but acted upon was proved in various other visits during the day. In visiting a prenatal patient, for instance, the nurse's questions showed that the woman was taking no out-door exercise, eating very little and entirely improper food because she would never, to her husband's indignation, wear her false teeth and could not chew without them. The nurse took much time to explain why such a way of living was foolish and what the mother must do to have a healthy child and avoid difficulty for herself. On learning further that the woman was having serious symptoms and intended to get a patent medicine recommended by a neighbor for kidney trouble, the nurse persuaded her that she was "throwing her money away." She insisted that the physician engaged for this confinement be called in. "The woman seemed loath to have him," says our investigator, "but finally agreed to have the nurse arrange for his call the next day."

This nurse, it is clearly apparent, had the teaching instinct. She had her information well in hand, but more than that, she knew how to arouse the right motive for action in the person she was advising.

Another excellent example of teaching in a somewhat similar situation was seen in visiting a prenatal patient, with an infant welfare nurse in a large western city. In this instance a dose of a cough mixture used by the entire family was to be given to the year-old baby. The grandmother who was visiting, insisted that having had eleven children, eight of whom had died, she was as competent as a doctor to prescribe for "mere teething and a little cold."

"The nurse," says our field agent, "to my surprise did not begin to attack use of the cough mixture. Instead she advised liquid diet, plenty of water, orange juice, sleep and quiet, the baby being much handled by the fond relatives. She advised the pregnant woman as to her own condition and allayed her fears as to premature delivery. Loquacious grandmother considerably controlled by nurse's quiet dignity and definiteness of questioning.

"Just as call ended the nurse picked up the patent cough mixture and said almost casually that she would hardly use that for a year-old baby. It might not hurt a mature man or woman. She recognized the mixture as an expensive medicine, she said, but suggested investing an equal amount for a doctor's visit. . . . She would be glad to help them carry out any new directions he might give.—Promised to come the next day."

TEACHING IN COMMUNICABLE DISEASES

Another example of resourceful questioning to get the facts was seen in a visit with a visiting nurse giving general care and instruction in a far western city.

"Our last visit," reports our agent, "was to a newly reported tuberculosis case. It proved to be a young girl of 22 who had had the disease four years before, . . . and spent a year in a sanitarium. She was taking excellent care of herself, running a very slight temperature but with no cough. Miss M. was very clever in getting information indirectly. For instance, when she wanted to find out whether there had been any previous tuberculosis in the family, she looked at the mother, a buxom woman and said: 'Well, you certainly don't look as if you had ever had any such trouble,' to which the mother replied: 'No, but I did just a little, when I was about her age.' This naturally led to inquiries about the rest of the family.

"In offering pamphlets on some phases of the disease Miss M. got their interest and consent to read them by saying ingenuously: 'You probably know most of these things, but I know you are interested in reading about your disease, and you just *might* find something new or different from what you have learned before.'

"The visit was very well done," concludes our investigator, herself in this instance a public health nurse of high standing. "It was social but professional and took perhaps 20 minutes."

Again, in a very different environment, in a congested district of a large city in the Middle West, where housing conditions were very bad—several frame houses being built on each lot, four or five families living in each house—well-conducted instruction was observed by one of our agents. The purpose of the call was to take cultures for release of a diphtheria patient. This work, performed by the board of health nurses in other parts of the city, was in one district given over to nurses working under the supervision of an admirably directed school of public health nursing. These nurses combine general bedside care and instructive work. In the visit in question, the family was found breaking the quarantine rules in allowing a child that had been released from quarantine to play with an "unreleased contact." Without being disagreeable, the nurse made the family understand unmistakably that quarantine would be extended if they did not strictly observe the rules. Her manner of speaking, in our agent's opinion, did not endanger their friendship; she gained added respect. The care which the nurse herself used in taking the release culture, putting on mask and paper apron which she had left on her last visit, made a deep impression on the family.

Before going into the room where the convalescent diphtheria patient was in bed, the nurse gave care and instruction to other members of the family, examining a little boy who was supposed to have a fever, inquiring into the progress of the mother's asthma, and recommending some changes in the little sister's diet.

"When she left the home," says our agent, "she most assuredly had the good-will of the entire family. This nurse has a friendly pleasing manner in approaching her patient. Their cordial way of welcoming her indicates the regard in which she is held. She can be firm in a kindly, intelligent way. Her work is carefully planned before entering her district in the morning and she is careful to read the family record before going in."

She had had considerable experience in public health nursing, after a short time in private duty, and was completing her special training.

RELATION TO RELATIVES AND FRIENDS

The success or failure of the public health nurse often depends on her relation to, and use of, the relatives and friends of the patient or person whom she is advising. For it must be constantly borne in mind that the nurse's responsibility does not end with her visit. Her success is conditioned by the skill and foresight with which she makes provision, during the hour or less of her visit, for the remaining 23 hours of the day. In cases of sickness, the care or at least the oversight of the patient must be deputed to relative or neighbor; in cases needing advice and instruction, co-operation and friendly relations are scarcely less necessary to secure, if the nurse's instruction is not to be counteracted or undone during her absence.

The increasing hold which the visiting nurses are year by year obtaining on the interest and confidence of the families in their neighborhoods is clearly shown by some figures published by a leading nursing organization, giving the sources of their calls.[53] In the four years between 1916 and 1920 the calls from families rose from 16.9 per cent of the total calls to 26.6 per cent, or from 6,803 to 10,707 calls.

"This certainly evidences," says the report, "the growing appreciation of the family of the value of nursing care, which is the first and a most important step in their realization of the part such oversight plays in the prevention of disease."

To illustrate the nurse's success or failure in this phase of her work, we may show how in various instances she gained the confidence and assistance of the husband or failed to do so.

Too often, owing to the father's absence from home during the daytime, he is seldom or never seen by the nurse. Yet without the consent and co-operation of the wage-earner and head of the household, especially in families of foreign birth, the mother's efforts to change such matters as diet or other living habits of herself or the children may go for naught. In special instances the husband must be seen at his work-place, or by a special visit to the home in the evening. To enlist his interest in the family's health problems is obviously to double the chances of successful teaching. When not himself sick it is naturally in connection with maternity care for his wife that he is most often and most readily accessible to new ideas.

THE EDUCATION OF AN ITALIAN HUSBAND

An excellent example of the active backing which may be obtained from a husband genuinely awake to preventive measures was shown in accompanying a visiting nurse in a large midwestern city, where she came in contact with many different nationalities. In an Italian home the nurse had been giving prenatal care. The mother had promised, but without much assurance, to have a physician for her confinement. On the nurse's stopping in to make inquiries, it appeared that the baby had been born three days before, a midwife having opportunely "happened to be just across the street" when needed, making a last maternity call on the patient's sister.

[53] The Henry St. Nurse, May, 1921. Page 7.

"We were ushered into the mother's room by the proud father," reports our field agent. "He first shook hands with the nurse declaring in English: 'You nurses do much good.' The baby was shown, encased in regular Italian fashion, standing almost upright against numerous pillows. The mother was also sitting quite erect, beside the baby. The nurse examined the baby first, asking permission before she unwrapped him, later suggesting that he be allowed to lie flat,—so! so!"

But it was upon the nurse's offering the mother some suggestions and urging her to lie flat, that the husband burst out affectionately:

" 'What did I tell you? When I want you to be like an American woman you know so much! Now, hear the nurse's advice.' Then to the nurse: 'That damn woman of mine has seven children and she ain't got no more sense than the one that's three days old. I ain't a woman, but I know more about a woman than she does. She feels good, so she wants to get up the second day. I tell her, it ain't how she feels the second day, I care. It's how she feels next year, and in ten years. . . . She says she feels young and healthy and strong. That's good. It is for her to stay so.' Again he damned her," adds our appreciative observer, "but added with a laugh that because she had given him such a fine boy, he couldn't beat her as she lay in bed! There was no question about his sincerity in wanting to be 'like an American husband,' as he said."

There was no question, either, of his having benefited from the nurse's prenatal teaching on the need of rest and care. It was he who asked the midwife to "put the drops in," as his wife explained on seeing the nurse's examination of the baby's eyes. Both parents welcomed the nurse's offer to call regularly and watch the baby's progress.

OTHER EXAMPLES OF ASSISTANCE

In a smaller western town, it was a Polish husband whom the visiting nurse had taught to prepare for her postnatal visits, to have supplies and hot water ready, to assist in bathing his wife, and to go for whatever might be lacking, from a paper of safety pins to a new flannel night gown, both of which articles he ran out to purchase on the bitterly cold day of our agent's visit, warming the night gown before it was offered to his wife.

In a flat fertile prairie county, where few foreigners lived, and where there was neither great wealth nor real destitution among the farmer population, it was a husband of native American stock who read the prenatal pamphlets of the Children's Bureau loaned to his wife by the nurse; who "was interested as much as she in having her do whatever was best for herself and the baby," such as changing the usual heavy meal at night to a light supper, etc. Here another young farmer insisted on paying $10 for the nurse's care at confinement and $2 each for subsequent postnatal visits at which he had been present and assisted. On the nurse's remonstrance against such rates his proud satisfaction could not contain itself. "Don't you know it's worth more than money to have the girl so well—and say, ain't the boy a dandy?"

So might instances be multiplied of the nurse's success in educating, and utilizing the services of, others than husbands, of grandmothers, and other relatives and neighbors. One of these, with some experience in practical nursing, we found utilized in the laborious work of giving treatment every fifteen minutes to a baby with gonorrheal infection of the eyes. This was in a city where the nurse could call several times during the first day to satisfy herself of the woman's reliability.

FAILURE TO UTILIZE THE ASSISTANCE OF OTHERS

But unfortunately in other instances the nurse showed neither native insight nor resourcefulness in enlisting the co-operation of others, nor had her training taught her how to do so. One flagrant example was encountered of actual abuse and bullying of an unfortunate Polish husband by a nurse who resented his well-meant efforts to care for his wife and new-born baby before her arrival.

He had himself delivered his wife at night, the doctor having arrived just too late; he had washed all the clothes, etc., from the delivery, so that the children "would see nothing which they shouldn't;" and after waiting for the nurse had himself washed the baby in the morning. It was for this and the danger of infecting the cord and eyes that she violently harangued him and threatened never to come again.

"I wish," says our indignant observer of this nurse, "that I could have had for this report the probable remarks of this

decent, fairly intelligent family after our departure; their
resentment was apparent; their courtesy and probably some
sense of obligation kept them still."

This nurse, though in her own way a conscientious and hard
worker, was obviously unfit by temperament or character to be
entrusted with the care and direction of other people's lives.
The innate coarseness shown in the course of her work should
have debarred her from being allowed to complete training in
any well-supervised school of nursing.

Other types of failure in utilizing the services of others were
also encountered in our study. One of the simplest but most
ordinary misconceptions was illustrated in a city on the Pacific
coast, in a home of exceptionally good standards. Here a daughter of 17 years was to give care to her sick mother between the
nurse's visits. But no effort was made to show her how to
turn the patient in bed or arrange her pillows, or give her assistance so as to cause her least pain. The daughter watched
everything the nurse did, anxious to learn, but the nurse made
no effort to teach or encourage her.

Another striking failure to utilize the services of a member
of the family—in this case the mother of a bedridden girl of
16 suspected of tuberculosis and running daily high temperature—was seen in a midwestern city. The nurse, accompanied
by our investigator in this instance, was a student in a public
health nursing course, in charge of her own district. Neither
the patient nor her mother had been successfully taught the
necessary preventive measures; the window was closed, the
patient held the unprotected bedclothes up to her lips and no bag
for paper napkins was in sight. How little the nurse appreciated
the need of active participation on the part of those whom she
was attempting to teach, was shown by her failure even to take
the mother into her confidence. A note had been left by the
doctor asking to have the girl removed to a sanatorium from
her present hopeless surroundings:

"The nurse did not discuss note with the mother but discussed it later with me," says the observer, herself one of
our nurse investigators. . . . "I felt that the mother should
have been taken at once into the confidence of the nurse
regarding her plans. The mother needed reassuring—needed
to have things explained to her. This nurse conformed out-
wardly with the general technique of public health nursing.
She knew her patients and all about their troubles; she knew

what resources to call upon for their relief. She seemed to have her instructions fairly well in hand. But there was evident one fundamental weakness: a lack of appreciation of the patient's and the family's side of things."

This tendency to see in the patient only a subject for nursing not only indicates a lack of constructive imagination and sympathy on the part of the nurse, but leads to the complete failure in teaching which this case illustrates. In the incident described, the nurse was a student who might still be taught to take a broader and more adequate view of her opportunities.

The Barriers of Language and Racial Customs

In dealing as she constantly must do with persons of various nationalities, the public health nurse, to be successful, should be equipped with at least some knowledge of their various backgrounds, characteristics, and prejudices. For a full and sympathetic study of public health work among immigrants, the reader is referred to a recent volume in the Americanization Series of the Carnegie Foundation.[54] Mr. Davis here points out the obvious difficulty of the nurse in making good contacts from ignorance of foreign languages, and her more fundamental difficulty from ignorance of the immigrant's point of view. The use of interpreters, either children or adults, is obviously necessary in many cases. Foreign language literature to distribute for instruction has its obvious uses. Some personal knowledge of the immigrant's home language is invaluable for the nurse, even if it is enough only to "build a bridge between the newcomer and the American." This is likely to be supplemented by a subsequent growth of vocabulary in the daily work.

Even more important than language to the health worker, if she is to win her way, is some appreciation of the background of the new-comer, and of the various traditions as to the common human experiences of birth, marriage, and death, which have been handed down from generation to generation, and still dominate at times the sons and daughters of a later transplanted era.

Traditions about women in pregnancy, about the care of babies, about fresh air and bathing and unfamiliar foods, all call for tolerance and wise teachings on the part of the nurse.

[54] Immigrant Health and the Community. Michael M. Davis, Jr., Director, Boston Dispensary. Harper & Brothers, New York, 1921.

Accordingly, as part of her course in social problems, it is important that the nurse should have some instruction in these various racial characteristics and myths.

Group conferences with leaders of different races and with persons who have first-hand acquaintance with them, have proved to inform and modify profoundly the nurse's whole attitude towards a given group of immigrants.

In our investigation various examples of success in dealing with these immigrant traditions and prejudices were observed. To leave the baby of Jewish parents unbathed on the day of circumcision; to leave the new-born baby of Mexican parents clad only in cord dressing and miniature "sombrero" of flannel; to leave the Italian baby tightly swaddled until the opportune moment comes for urging it to be unwrapped!—these are examples of wise yielding on the part of the nurse to traditions which are not permanently harmful, gaining her friends instead of arousing resentment. On the other hand, we encountered also the nurse who shouts at the non-English speaking immigrant to make her meaning clear; the nurse who "would not demean herself" by accepting hospitality from the foreign-born; the nurse who expresses her unfavorable views of all foreigners and all foreign ways in the presence of those who speak and understand English, etc.

RELATION TO PHYSICIANS

The efficiency of the public health nurse's work must be in large part conditioned by her relation to the physicians with whom she comes in contact, such as those to whom she persuades people to go for remedial services, etc., and those under whose direction she gives bedside nursing care.

It should be clear from our various narratives of the nurse's activities, that far from interfering with the doctor's practice, those activities necessarily increase it. The true prevention, as we have seen, means primarily correcting defects or weaknesses *in time*, before it is too late for cure; and in proportion as the nurse has been educated up to and applies this newer view of prevention, she brings to the physician defects, weaknesses, and suspicious symptoms of which he has usually had no knowledge and to which he would have no access in the majority of cases until actual sickness developed.

Where physicians are awake to the overwhelming needs of

prevention, they have welcomed and aided in developing public health nursing; where they have been uneducated to this great issue or have feared jeopardy to their own practice or authority, they have failed to co-operate with public health nursing or have offered obstacles to it.

So, for instance, in two rural communities visited in the course of our study, not far distant from one another, the medical support accorded to public health nursing showed the most marked and informing contrast. In one of these communities, a well-organized and well-supported visiting nurse association had in the course of a few years succeeded in so well demonstrating the value of preventive as well as curative nursing that the six physicians practising in the township were all actively co-operating with the association. An excellent beginning had been made in preventive work in the schools, in prenatal and tuberculosis instruction, etc.

In the other community, practically nothing was being done in the way of prevention. Of the six physicians practising in this township not one had any vision of preventive medicine. Two of them in conversation justified themselves by insisting that their people would gladly pay to be cured in sickness but would not listen to any advice as to how to keep well. The nurse, in this instance but a few months out of the training school, with no experience of public health nursing, and no efficient organization to back her, was striving, overworked and discouraged, merely to supply the necessary bedside care. Two of her predecessors had broken down in health, owing probably to the unfavorable conditions of work. In this organization undoubtedly only an experienced public health nurse with constructive ability, could demonstrate to the community, which is practically all American-born and with little actual poverty, what preventive nursing means, and thus in time educate it to meet its obligations in the way of health and to support preventive as well as curative efforts.

It is obviously necessary that in rendering bedside care the ordinary professional ethics between doctor and nurse should prevail, according to which the doctor and not the nurse is recognized as in charge of the case and responsible for it. But in the new functions which have devolved upon the public health nurse—in teaching prevention of disease, in discovering suspicious symptoms in the homes, schools, and work-places of a community, and in arousing community interest in public health measures—a wide range of opportunities has been opened up, unknown to the nurse in private duty, in which necessarily the ordinary rules of professional etiquette do not apply.

How strict and rigid these rules have in the past been is shown in a standard volume on public health nursing written only a few years ago by a leading public health nurse. According to the enumeration:

"She (the public health nurse) should not diagnose, should not prescribe, should not recommend a particular doctor or change of doctors, should not suggest a hospital to a patient without the concurrence of the doctor, and should never criticise, by word or unspoken action, any member of the medical profession."

But when the nurse has been made responsible for finding any suspicious symptoms in the course of her work, and persuading people to avail themselves of medical and surgical and obstetrical and dental care, to mention no other specialties, when she usually refuses to give nursing care unless a physician is called in, it is obviously often her duty to recommend medical or hospital treatment of some kind, and it may sometimes be very difficult, in the interest of the patient, to avoid indicating the special direction in which treatment should be sought.

Moreover, to the lay observer, unable to agree that a nurse in entering her profession must resign her conscience as well as her common sense, as strict observance of these rules would require, the comments of an enlightened physician are welcome:

"These rules," says Dr. Burnham in his handbook on the community health problem, "appear to me too severe and I believe that in time they may be modified so that a nurse will not be compelled to serve under a physician who is palpably ignorant or dangerously careless. In such cases the nurse should report to her immediate superior who, if she is experienced and resourceful, can usually find a way out of the difficulty." [55]

With tact and a command of the facts, in various instances in the course of our investigation, nurses were found able to protect their patients and the community from lapses in preventive care on the part of the physician, without arousing his resentment and without infringing on the domain of the physician.

[55] The Community Health Problem. Athel Campbell Burnham, M.D. Macmillan, New York, 1920. Page 43.

RELATION TO SOCIAL WORK AND SOCIAL AGENCIES

From the preceding examples of success and failure it is evident that in making her contacts and grasping a family situation, the public health nurse needs also some knowledge of social case work. Without some instruction in modern methods of social diagnosis and treatment she is often hampered if not baffled.

In so far as social case work means making better adjustments between individuals and their social environment, the nurse must obviously use case work methods.[56] She, too, by her teaching, her planning with the family the solution of their health problems, her efforts to aid her patients and those whom she visits to establish habits of hygiene, aims at accomplishing the "socially useful adjustments" for individual persons which is the essence of social case work.

How far the nurse enters into the more intensive social case work of the professional social workers, that is, in Miss Richmond's analysis, the development of personality through a better adjustment between individuals and their social environment, is a matter of degree. In teaching a mother, for example, in the care of her baby such seemingly simple matters as the need for regularity in feeding and sleeping, the development of the mother's own self-control, patience, and a certain degree of resourcefulness is an almost inevitable corollary. In teaching a tuberculous patient, or one threatened with tuberculosis, the right prophylaxis, the development of spiritual qualities, of patience, fortitude, and unselfishness, is often as striking as physical improvement.

In practice it is often difficult to draw a distinction between the adjustment of the health problems and the social problems of the family, since at so many points health and social relations touch and react upon one another. Yet it should be clearly understood that the nurse is not a social worker in the professional sense. By a wise tradition she is herself debarred except in exceptional cases from giving material relief. She must, however, for successful work, be acquainted with the social problems underlying physical disability or illness and must know the social agencies with whom she is constantly to co-operate and on whom she can call.

---

[56] What is Social Case Work? Mary E. Richmond. Russell Sage Foundation, New York, 1922.

This general rule, obviously, often cannot apply in rural districts. Where there are no social or relief agencies, the nurse working alone must be not only supervisor and staff nurse in one, but social worker also, as best she may. The need of some social training is therefore indispensable, especially for those intending to devote themselves to rural public health nursing.

The tradition that nurses should not themselves give relief is based on the correct principle that health work should not be regarded in the same category with the giving of material assistance, and that the nurse is not fitted to undertake, and should not be distracted from her own functions to undertake, to relieve the social and economic needs of the family.

EXAMPLES OF FAILURE

It is perhaps scarcely surprising, in view of the limited number of public health nurses who have had the advantage of special training, how many combine with excellent nursing technique and even with teaching ability ignorance of the most rudimentary principles of family rehabilitation.

That a nurse engaged in work of outstanding excellence in a crowded city district, combining bedside care and instruction with unusual success, should herself pay, during many weeks, for milk for a certain baby rather than "subject the family to the associated charity inquisition"; that she should send to the associated charities, without inquiry into the family resources or the possible assistance of relatives, a $16-bill for special shoes and brace for an orthopedic patient; that she should justify her procedure by insisting that "most people are good and we don't investigate our friends;" show how easily a worker highly skilled in her own field may undermine family responsibilities and do harm in the very act of physical rehabilitation.

Nor is Miss C., the nurse in question, exceptional. In another city a nurse was visited who was, on the one hand, sending in to the associated charities a request for daily delivery of ice for a sick baby and for clothing for the other children, while, on the other hand, she was encouraging the baby's family of father, mother, and six children, to buy a house by installments. A school nurse saw nothing undesirable in, and indeed herself suggested, the exhibition on a concert platform of a little cripple, for whose benefit—to enable her to buy an artificial leg—the concert had been arranged.

Another nurse was accompanied on a maternity visit to a woman with whose living arrangements and plans for the future the nurse was, on her third visit to the home, totally unacquainted. She knew that the woman had been deserted by her husband and lived with her son who worked and a daughter of 11 who was at school. But she did not even know how the woman was being fed.

EXAMPLES OF SUCCESS

In contrast to these flagrant failures, nurses were met who exercised wide discrimination in bringing family maladjustment to the care of the right social agencies and in obtaining relief.

Thus, for instance, through the aid of the Catholic priest, a nurse working in a southern county interested an important resident, herself an invalid confined to her chair, in the problems of poverty in the community. Through this invalid, the nurse was assured layettes if necessary, clothing and other relief, and a small fund for medical prescriptions. Of even greater aid was the committee appointed to confer with the nurse and adjust social problems.

"Good nursing and good teaching and good social work," is the comment of one of our agents on the living arrangements made by this nurse for a colored man in the last stages of tuberculosis. Because institutional care could be secured only in the county jail or insane asylum, the nurse was caring for this patient at home. She had successfully taught him how to use and burn paper napkins and sputum cups, etc. An old uncle gave care between the nurse's visits. The house was kept clean by a colored woman living next door, herself pregnant and under the nurse's care.

Another admirable example of co-operation and shared responsibility between nurse and social worker may be quoted from the small western city of B. in which extremes of comfort and poverty meet. A woman whose husband had left her for another wife came several years ago to live in this town. Here her second child was born. She was both hopeless and helpless, ignorant and slatternly, with no sense of responsibility for her children. Through her maternity care, Miss N., the nurse in question, became this woman's confidant and adviser. She secured for her the assistance of the united charities, which provided generously both material relief and the friendliness which she bitterly needed. Work was also found for her in a day nursery where she could be with her children. Now the assistance of the charitable society is no longer needed.

On the day of our visit her two boys were sick with influenza. Miss N. gave directions for their care and offered to send in supplies from a neighboring grocery store. But she accepted the woman's money to pay for the groceries. In spite of frequent backsliding and changes of work, the steady improvement of this woman in keeping up her home and educating her children is in Miss N.'s own words "the greatest gratification of her nursing service in B."

FAILURE ON THE PART OF SOCIAL WORKERS

It is also important to bear in mind that in many instances of antagonism between nurses and social workers the fault lies with the social agency. Nurses are often justified in resenting the failure to give emergency relief at the moment when it is really needed. Obviously, in matters of health the timeliness of the relief may be all-in-all. Nurses are justified in resenting stereotyped and formal methods of dealing with human needs such as too often characterize the work of social agencies without vision or real understanding. Nurses may justly criticise the failure of social workers to observe elementary health precautions in dealing with families referred to them.

So, in one instance, the serious health problems of a family consisting of a young widow and four children were not only ignored, but their chances of improving jeopardized by the incredible neglect of a social worker from the united charities which was paying the rent. The rooms in which the mother and children were living had been secured by this worker. The husband had died of tuberculosis; the young widow had developed disturbing symptoms and on the nurse's recommendation was about to have a medical examination. The two younger children looked anæmic; the baby had rickets.

On attempting to teach the mother how to ventilate the cold damp rooms the nurse's dismay may be imagined on finding that not a single window could be raised, every one being stuck fast with paint. The damp walls and exposed location of the rooms and the tight closed windows were indeed such a menace to health that the nurse, though fearing that the united charities' worker would "be peeved at having the nurse call them to her attention," felt obliged to do so.

It is clear that only mutual patience and tolerance on the part of both nurses and social workers can overcome antagonisms due primarily to the failures of the unenlightened in both groups. That this antagonism is happily yielding to a better understanding, on the part of each, of the other's work and contribution, was well illustrated by a conference between these two groups of workers attended by one of our observers. It was decided that under a working agreement all cases needing hospital care should be at once reported to the visiting nurse association, since that association was best fitted to prevent duplication and handle the cases. Emergent relief was to be given by the associated charities to acutely sick patients on the nurse's recommendation, without waiting for investigation of the family, which was to be postponed until after the acute emergency had passed. The visiting nurse association, on the other hand, agreed that relief work should be entirely in the hands of the associated charities.

Up to this point we have illustrated, from instances seen in the field, successes and failures in certain salient features of the public health nurse's work; namely, in teaching, in her relations with families and neighbors, with physicians and with social agencies.

We have reserved for our final discussion the most important questions of organization of the work, previously referred to in this report; that is, the relative merits of combining or of separating curative and preventive nursing; and the relative merits of the system of "generalized" nursing, wherein one nurse gives all nursing care and instruction in a given area, as contrasted with the "specialized" system, wherein the nurse devotes herself to one field of nursing only, irrespective of geographical areas, and usually to instructive work only, in her own field.

Clearly these issues, while matters of organization, necessarily and intimately affect the success or failure of the individual nurse, and as necessarily dictate the kind of training which she should have as an adequate preparation for the work.

Relative Merits of Instructive Nursing and Bedside Nursing Combined with Instruction

The relative merits of purely instructive nursing, and bedside nursing combined with instruction as given under the generalized system, are hotly contested issues in public health nursing.

Advocates of the entire separation of curative and preventive nursing assert with some justice that when they are combined, the bedside care of disease constantly interferes with the apparently less urgent claims of instruction; that nursing in sickness is "of necessity emergency work," and that emergencies tend to take precedence over the systematic routine of preventive nursing such as the prenatal, instruction in infant welfare, tuberculosis, etc.

Most advocates of instructive nursing go further and assert that nurses cannot successfully combine instruction in the various specialties; that to do good work they must be restricted to the single field which they may elect.

WEAKNESSES IN GENERALIZED NURSING

It is indeed true, as illustrated in various visiting nurse associations giving bedside care, and it should be admitted at the outset, that the weakness of generalized nursing often lies in its too great emphasis on curative work alone to the detriment of the preventive. The necessary supervision of well babies, for instance, may suffer, when pneumonia is unusually prevalent. Yet to admit this weakness is not therefore to deny the theoretical and practical benefits of the generalized system. The possible over-emphasis on curative work is in our opinion a failure of administration, not of principle. It is the result of attempting in the generalized system to cover too large a territory with an inadequate force or without the proper supervision by specialists which is admittedly indispensable to keep true the balance between the various kinds of service rendered. To do good tuberculosis work in generalized nursing, for instance, the specialist in tuberculosis is needed to supervise the technique and general adequacy of the work and to clarify its special problems; the nurse who has specialized in child welfare is needed to supervise and direct the child welfare activities, etc.

But even admitting that the curative work of the generalized agency may tend at times, unless carefully guarded against, to overbalance the instruction, nevertheless in our opinion the advantages of the system far outweigh its possible weaknesses. The bedside care it offers and its stress on a local unit of work for each nurse are, in our opinion, irreplaceable assets, opening doors to the nurse at which she knocks in vain with instruction only.

WEAKNESSES IN INSTRUCTIVE NURSING ALONE

It is often asserted by opponents of instructive nursing alone that its inferiority to the generalized system lies in the fact that it renders no actual service and offers only words of counsel for aid. This contention is not in our opinion borne out by the facts. The competent instructive nurse through her demonstrations of baby care, her preparation and teaching of milk formulæ, her prenatal advice, her examination of persons suffering from communicable disease,—all instructive functions,—does perform a genuine service, "practical and educational," as its advocates claim.[57] It is inaccurate as well as unfair to underrate these functions as merely verbal aid. In our opinion the inadequacy of instructive nursing alone arises from a far more fundamental, a far deeper cause, deep-seated in our common human nature. Its failure is a failure in psychology.

What is, indeed, the fundamental problem in all public health work, in all the great educational movements of our time, summed up in Wells's phrase as "the race between education and catastrophe?"

CAPITAL IMPORTANCE OF THE CONTACT

The essence of this problem is plainly the approach to the individual, the contact. How, among the vastly increased conflict of motives, interests, and objectives in man's modern life, shall we obtain for a given idea that degree of attention which is needed to give it some degree of permanence and to release its dynamic power? How shall we combat for a given object not only mental inertia—the natural human inclination to think only when we must—but also the active opposition of natural human prejudices in favor of our own way of life, however mistaken? "To approach a well man or woman with excellently intended hygienic advice is a difficult proposition," says the Carnegie Foundation study of public health work among the foreign-born, already quoted.[58] The report then touches with sureness on the cardinal point which has emerged from our studies.

"It is a sound principle, borne out again and again by this study of the foreign-born, that curative medicine provides an

---

[57] U. S. Department of Labor, Children's Bureau. Publication No. 60, 1919. Standards of Child Welfare. Discussion. S. Josephine Baker, M.D. Page 210.

[58] Davis, op. cit. Page 418.

approach to preventive. Our goal is to teach people how not to get sick, 'how to be healthy and well.' But we generally find that the best way to get this instruction accepted and put into practice by the recipient is to give it when the recipient or some member of his family is sick or threatened with sickness."

Or when a relative or neighbor has been sick or threatened with sickness, we would add, for the testimony of relative or neighbor, of one with the same racial or neighborhood prejudices, appears to be equally effective. Again and again in our study, as in the special study of the foreign-born, this principle that curative care provides an approach to the preventive has been illustrated. Gratitude for relief in suffering, or for the relief of those who are dear to them, is a potent motive in opening the minds as well as the hearts of men.

The Vantage Ground of Generalized Nursing

This, then, is the fundamental lesson which, starting with no preconceptions and no brief for any system of nursing, our field study has brought home to us. This is, in our opinion, the strength of generalized nursing, combining bedside care and instruction as against instruction alone, that it offers a natural, an unforced approach to the individual and the family, because it is itself sought. It works with, instead of against, deep in-grained instincts of normal adult life.

This is, again, in our opinion, the great asset for preventive health work of the nurse, that she stands in the minds of the ignorant as well as of the better informed, for a person who has at her command a training in the treatment of disease which at any emergency is indispensable; a person who through her clinical experience can give bedside care at need and is thereby entitled to a hearing from those to whom she has ministered in sickness or to whose family or friends she has ministered.

The instructive work of the generalized nurse starts from this vantage ground. Her concern for the health of the entire family further reinforces this initial advantage. Each member of the family whom she can aid by nursing care and advice adds to the sum of her influence. With the instructive nurse, on the contrary, each member of the family whom she must refer to another nurse for nursing care or for instruction in a different specialty, detracts from her influence.

THE HANDICAPS OF POVERTY

It must, moreover, constantly be borne in mind that among wage-earners and persons of inadequate means, all the psychological difficulties of re-education and of inculcating new habits are immeasurably increased by the sheer physical difficulties of conforming to hygiene. Overcrowding, bad housing, long hours of industrial work, poor food, a poor grade of milk, above all inadequate wages—these things which are the mere commonplaces of tenement life, and corresponding handicaps in rural life, all combine to make of good hygiene at all times a far more difficult and precarious goal than it is among the well-to-do. Often the counsels of hygiene appear a mere mockery to those without material means of carrying them out.

All the greater must be the influence of the teacher of health to arouse the motives of self-preservation and self-interest, love of family, altruistic scruples against scattering infection, pride in the neighborhood or community, etc., which may ultimately assist in the formation of new habits, if the physical difficulties are not overwhelming.

On this point, from her experience in the field, the director of the Bureau of Public Health Nursing of the American Red Cross bears effective witness:

"We seem to think," says Miss Fox, "that our American people are most anxious for advice. I do not think public health nurses would agree with that point of view. American people think they know how to run their own affairs pretty well, and are not anxious to be told by some one else how to do it. But when the nurse who comes into the home and nurses them when they are sick, and does something for them when there is suffering, tells them what they ought to do, they are going to take her advice, because it is . . . counsel from a person who has helped them out in time of need.

"We have all gone into homes and tried to tell mothers about the care of the family, and when we have gone back we have found that we had not made much impression. They have said politely, 'Yes,' but they did not do what we told them to do. It is the person who has been there repeatedly, who has done something for them, and who has dropped these little kernels of advice as she went along in casual remarks, who really gets the thing over to the family. This may not seem to be preventive medicine, but in this way the nurse may work a revolution in the home which she could not possibly bring about in any other way." [59]

Instructive and Generalized Work under Official Agencies

The opinion is sometimes expressed that generalized nursing, however desirable for privately endowed societies, should not be undertaken by official health agencies, and that these should confine their activities to educational functions and not engage in the curative. If this contention were strictly enforced, even well-baby campaigns and prenatal nursing, which have grown to be important departments of municipal and state health work, might be questioned as encroachments upon curative functions. While it is undoubtedly true that curative nursing under official auspices is often viewed askance, yet such activities are in fact being carried on in rural communities and even in some municipalities. Bedside care when needed, for instance, in tuberculosis, is accepted as part of the program of public health nursing under public control. It is not unreasonable to expect that the undoubted difficulties of combining nursing in sickness with preventive educational measures now deemed more appropriate for official health agencies, may be ultimately overcome.

Some Contrasting Results of Generalized and Specialized Nursing

In the course of our investigation, the advantages for preventive work of generalized nursing as opposed to specialized were repeatedly and unmistakably demonstrated. Some concrete instances may serve to show the causes of the difference. Thus, to quote a single diverting example, in a certain family visited, the nurse, who had given prenatal care to the mother and was now caring for the baby in sickness and health, became, as our agent states, a "health authority" for a member of the family with very different health problems. This was the unmarried uncle, who chanced to be the baby's adoring godfather, and who, in spite of the differences of sex and need, accepted the nurse's rules of hygiene for himself purely owing to the success of her prenatal and baby care!

* U. S. Department of Labor, Children's Bureau. Publication No. 60, 1919. Standards of Child Welfare. Discussion. Elizabeth Fox. Page 209.

It is also abundantly evident that all possible reinforcements which generalized nursing may offer are urgently needed by the nurse to make her persuasions effective in the face of poverty and need. It is often her difficult task to persuade people to spend money on remedial medical or surgical services for ills or weaknesses whose bad effects they are not themselves able to gauge and may not believe in. The Boston Instructive District Nursing Association reports for instance that of 177 cases of correctable defects entailing such possibly serious consequences as hypertrophied tonsils and adenoids, rickets, defective teeth, defective vision, malnutrition, etc., 49 per cent refused, even after an average of six visits each, to take any action. In 51 per cent of the cases, however, remedial action was taken.

On the other hand, the ill-effects for the specialized nurse of having to depute to another nurse functions performed by one individual under the generalized system was well illustrated in visiting a certain southern city. Here there were four agencies employing visiting nurses.

"In general in C.," says our investigator, in this instance herself an experienced social worker, "there always seemed to be some other agency to do the work, no matter what nurse I went around with—visiting nurse association, child welfare, board of health, or infant hygiene. This was not so much that the nurses lacked training as that the work had become so highly organized and specialized that every family seemed to need ten visitors to cover the particular problems of that family."

For instance, in one home visited by our agent in this city there was a baby suffering from ophthalmia neonatorum. A board of health nurse had first been called in upon learning that nursing care was needed. She referred the case to the visiting nurse society. The nurse from this organization, on finding that care was needed for a baby, referred the case to the infant welfare society. The call being received on Labor Day, a holiday, and not being marked urgent, was laid over a day. The properly designated nurse after the lapse of two days found the mother, though willing to follow directions, wholly uninformed of the necessary measures to be taken or even of the nature of the disease. She was washing both eyes with the same cloth, and was naturally ignorant of the dangers of infection.

Thus it took three visits by nurses from three different organizations to take elementary precautions in the care of the baby's eyes and to teach the mother how to do so. Even after the infant welfare nurse was giving daily care, the duplication of visits continued. For the board of health nurse returned to learn whether the baby had been taken to a dispensary for treatment and managed by altercation still further to arouse the mother's resentment.

Obviously some of this duplication might have been avoided by ordinary intelligence in reporting and referring cases. Advocates of specialization are apt to minimize the duplication of work by different specialist nursing organizations, and assert that there is little evidence to prove that it results in the entrance of various nurses into the home. The obvious reply to this contention is that if under the specialized system there is little duplication, there should be a great deal. For the absence in a given home of other nurses than the nurse giving a special type of care usually means that other physical disabilities are unrecognized and neglected.

SOME DISADVANTAGES OF SPECIALIZATION

An even worse example of unintelligent specialization than the instance of three nurses visiting the baby with infected eyes was encountered in accompanying a tuberculosis nurse in a crowded Italian quarter of another city. A visit was paid to a little Italian boy of 7 years with a tuberculous cervical gland. This the tuberculosis nurse dressed carefully and with excellent technique. But she did not touch an extensive infected area on the child's scalp. When questioned about this by our field agent, she replied that

"she was not supposed to attend to the scalp since her work was in the tuberculosis department of her association and an infant welfare nurse was attending to it."

She had no idea when or how often the other nurse called though it was clear that an ointment had recently been applied.

A more ridiculous extreme of specialization could not easily be imagined, yet it was not exceptional in this nurse's performance. In visiting with her another Italian home, where the mother was an arrested case, our agent found several children at home. The youngest child, of 6 months, was in swaddling clothes; the next one, of 22 months, was engaged in taking coffee from a nursing bottle which had just been prepared for her by an older sister.

"When about to leave," says our observer, a public health nurse, "I was unable to restrain myself from talking to the mother about the advantages of taking babies to the welfare station (where I knew swaddling would be discouraged) and also mentioning the unsuitability of coffee. A visiting neighbor on seeing my interest in the baby, went and got hers, 2 months old, also swaddled. She was rather apologetic about swaddling. On being told that I should take that baby if he were mine, to the baby station to show him off because he was so good-looking, she said she thought she would when it stopped raining. A good baby conference could have been worked up with those two mothers then and there. But the nurse made no suggestions whatever, since she was doing tuberculosis work!"

One organization, which was engaged in changing its nurses from the specialized to the generalized system, offered an unusual opportunity for comparing the effectiveness of the two types of work, some districts being still specialized while others had been changed.

It is of some interest to note that the investigator reporting was in this instance another public health nurse, herself trained and experienced in specialized nursing, who had in the course of our investigation been converted to generalized work by the greater excellence of the results observed. Of the association's specialist work she says:

"The loss through specialization manifests itself in several ways. First, the multiplicity of departmental details which each supervisor must administer. . . . Each supervisor evidently gets in touch with social agencies for the families under her jurisdiction; she must make her separate contacts with hospitals and other resources; in many ways she must exactly duplicate the work some other supervisor is doing for her department for the same district, if not for the same families. Second . . . the loss in the nurses' time and usefulness in covering all of a district in a specialized way, instead of part of a district in a generalized way. In going about with the specialized nurses I noted we spent from twenty to thirty minutes and frequently longer, walking from one case to another. With the general nurse little time was lost between cases.

"The instructions of the generalized nurse, even in tuberculosis and child welfare cases, seemed to be better rounded and more practical, for with her knowledge of the family needs and neighborhood resources she knew how best to make them fit in."

One of the salient features in the change from specialized to generalized nursing in the association mentioned above has been precisely the saving of time emphasized by our investigator. In the generalized district one-sixth of the total number of nurses are doing one-fifth of the work, and the bitterest opponents of the change, including the specialist supervisors, have become satisfied by the operation of the new system.

DEMONSTRATION OF SPECIAL NEEDS BY SPECIALIST ORGANIZATIONS

It is true that valuable demonstrations of special phases of nursing care have been made by organizations specially devoted to one object, such as many tuberculosis societies. Indeed, the generalized system of nursing could not have developed if such demonstrations of special nursing had not first been made and certain standards of performance set by such specialist organizations. It may still, in various instances, be desirable to continue such demonstrations.

TENDENCY TOWARDS GREATER INCLUSIVENESS IN SPECIALIZED NURSING

Moreover, in contrast to the extreme examples of unintelligent specialization encountered, we may note in some specialized nursing a distinct tendency towards a greater inclusiveness. We have already referred to the prenatal work inaugurated in the interest of the baby's health and safety by various infant welfare societies. Some tuberculosis societies give prenatal care, when needed. Even those persons most impressed by the value of specialized nursing in affording intensive application to one subject, incline to generalize so far, for instance, as to give over to one nurse all phases of child welfare from the unborn child up to school life.[60]

How indeed should it be otherwise? The increasing stress on prevention carries back and ever further back the starting point, the point of departure, for nursing care and instruction. It is being increasingly recognized that the inadequacy of much prevention work, such as that done, for instance, in the schools, is due to the fact that it has been too long postponed. *Too late* is

*Public Health Nursing. Mary S. Gardner, R.N. Macmillan, New York, 1918. Page 255.

nature's answer to remedies attempted in adult life for defects or weaknesses which should have been corrected in childhood or youth. Too late, even in school life, are remedies which should have been undertaken between the ages of two and five years. Too late, even in those early years, are remedies for defects which should have been corrected in infancy, or which prenatal care should have wholly prevented.

It is not, therefore, only by its immediate benefits to the mother in confinement that the effectiveness of prenatal care must be measured, but, as a leading public health physician points out, by "the number of babies who die in the early months of life from congenital defects and diseases and the number who survive in good health." And again of infant care:

"Efforts for the care of babies cannot be measured by consideration of the infant death-rate alone. . . . The reduction in the death-rate under five years of age is the only sure index of the worth of the care given under one year of age." [61]

Thus the measure of success achieved in any one period of child life is most truly shown by its subsequent effects. In this large view of child welfare, the child is "father to the man" indeed, and any break is to be deplored in the continuity of nursing care throughout these various periods.

From such an extension of nursing in the "specialty" of child welfare it is not far to the general family care, which is the goal of generalized nursing. For the child is pre-eminently a member of a family and the tuberculosis of the father, or any other illness in any other member of the family, inevitably affects its environment, and must be guarded against. The "specialties" of child welfare and tuberculosis thus inevitably meet and overlap in family care.

From the educational point of view which has guided our investigation, this enlargement of public health nursing into general family care is of profound significance. With the family as her unit of care, the nurse must evidently have a training which shall enable her to recognize and to gauge the importance of any symptoms she may encounter in the family, whether she refers some to another specialized nurse or, as seems to us sounder in both theory and practice, herself takes the necessary curative or preventive measures. In either case the condition of success is that she should be trained to *know the symptoms*.

[61] Cleveland Hospital and Health Survey, Part III. A Program for Child Health. S. Josephine Baker, M.D. 1920. Page 319.

The Unit of Population Served

We have said that the tendency, in generalized nursing, to allow preventive work to be overbalanced by curative must be constantly guarded against. It is clear that this can be effected only by the limitation of the nurse's area and unit of population. It is generally held that a nurse giving generalized service cannot successfully serve more than 2,000 persons. In the remarkable "block nursing" which is one of the latest contributions of the Henry Street nursing service to the development of public health work in the United States, experiments are being tried in various parts of a cosmopolitan city among various nationalities having various standards of living and comfort, to provide nursing care and instruction to all families in the block. The public schools, clinics of various kinds, special classes, and demonstrations—all are utilized in the effort to teach health and heal the sick. The outcome of these experiments appears to show that for successful work the nurse should probably not be assigned to a larger unit than a population of 1,500 persons.

The Future Outlook

Clearly, under present conditions, it is impossible to reach or even to approximate the desirable unit of population per nurse. To provide public health nurses enough, in a short time, to reach any such proportion is beyond human possibilities. Nor, if they were available, would there be sufficient funds in the community to support them nor, even more important, sufficient expert direction to supervise them. It must be frankly recognized that today, no more than in the past, can all the sick be succored nor all those taught the elements of health and hygiene who need it. Today we have more knowledge than ever before of the extent of the need; but by no fiat or short cut can those long existing needs immediately be met.

So far as concerns public health nurses, needed in numbers not only in the United States, but through the world, the best hope, in our opinion, lies in no short-sighted efforts to turn out large numbers quickly, but in deeper and more fundamental considerations.

Indubitably, the three years' hospital training which is all that most public health nurses have had to prepare them is a totally inadequate preparation for this field; the balance of this report is devoted chiefly to a consideration of the changes needed to provide more and better trained nurses.

But behind all changes in methods of education, we must look for that democratic understanding and appreciation of public health nursing which alone can give adequate support to the nurse's work and can give backing against the vested rights of the hospital to the needed changes in education. In our opinion, to organize the work on the best possible basis, to demonstrate its remarkable possibilities in whatever way local conditions approve, but so as to make the most complete demonstration possible with the existing personnel, is the best way to secure growing democratic appreciation and support. Every able demonstration even in a limited area furthers it; every failure serves to delay or alienate it.

To make the most of its present personnel the public health nursing bureau of the National Red Cross thus wisely begins county work, if only one nurse is available, with school nursing which is almost universally demanded. In her home visiting, this school nurse demonstrates as much of care in tuberculosis, of infant and child welfare, of bedside nursing in sickness as she can compass. Part of the school work is thus necessarily delayed; several years may elapse in covering the county. But meantime, in an intensive way the fuller possibilities of public health nursing have been made clear to the community; support for additional nurses usually follows. Chief of all, a sound foundation has been laid for the public recognition of public health nursing and enthusiasm for its results has been engendered which will do more than any short cut methods to enlist new workers and to support, financially and morally, the fundamental reorganization of nursing education which is the ultimate condition of success in public health nursing.

Educational Implications

Of the facts assembled in the preceding chapters, the educational implications are unmistakable. From our study of the concrete functions of public health nursing as observed in the field, from the results achieved even under unfavorable conditions, with a personnel inadequate in numbers and training, we may justly deduce the kind of training which is indicated to accomplish even better results in the future.

At the outset it is plain that, in both success and failure, the personality of the nurse plays a very large part. Tact, insight, a feeling heart, a quick mental grasp of persons and situations, dignity, persuasiveness—these things come by grace of nature. Yet in other professions too, among teachers, doctors, clergymen, those pre-eminently the essence of whose work lies in their personal contacts, personality plays a commanding if not determining part. It has, however, yet to be suggested that in these professions the personal powers are not to be supplemented or guided by training.

So far as concerns the public health nurse our analysis of the facts indicates clearly, in our opinion, the kind of training with which she should be equipped, however well endowed by nature, and with which those less well endowed should be enabled to achieve a considerable measure of success. We postpone to a later chapter the detailed discussion of this training for public health nursing. Here it suffices to state the general conclusions to which we have been impelled.

NEED OF CLINICAL TRAINING

It is worthy of note that the conclusions derived from our study of nurses and of the problems towards the solution of which their efforts were directed, were effectually reinforced by observation of the attempted teaching of health and hygiene by certain persons other than nurses. These examples were in a sense negative testimony; showing by salient omissions, the lack of adequate preparation in these workers.

During the war the shortage of nurses led to serious consideration of the desirability of establishing courses, much shorter and more limited in scope than those for preparing nurses, to train lay persons as "health visitors" of a purely instructive and specialist type, for dealing with single needs such as child welfare, tuberculosis, etc. In Europe the dearth of qualified nurses has led to the establishment of such courses, the results of which are variously viewed.

The teaching of habits of health and hygiene in schools and in homes by lay persons trained at one experimental course in this country, and observed in the course of our investigation, could admit of but one view: its essential incompetence and lack of authority, reaching back unmistakably to a lack of adequate clinical experience.

For the general family health work towards which the best public health nursing in the United States is tending—alike for the generalized and the specialized, the curative and the preventive—a sound clinical training is plainly dictated as the first requisite, the *sine qua non.* For the functions which distinguish the public health nurse from all other workers who are contributing in their several capacities to the manifold varieties of public health work, a sound clinical training is indispensable and basic.

In our subsequent discussion of the hospital schools of nursing and the invaluable clinical experience which they offer in wards and dispensaries, we emphasize the need of a radical change in training to provide for all student nurses a new stress on methods of prevention as well as cure, and that minimum of social interpretation of disease which is indispensable in modern health movements.

To aid in obtaining nurses in greater numbers and better trained for public health nursing, we recommend higher entrance requirements, better teaching, a reduction in the length of the undergraduate hospital course, above all, the endowment of nursing education, as all other conceivable education has been endowed.

NEED OF SPECIAL PUBLIC HEALTH TRAINING

We have already pointed out that the nurse who comes from her hospital training unawakened to the medico-social problems which underlie physical disability and sickness cannot, however well trained in bedside care, do effective health teaching.

It is abundantly evident that however good her clinical training, however accurate her knowledge of disease and even of prevention, she is at a grave disadvantage, if not totally at a loss, without a thorough grounding in the principles of teaching and in the principles of social case work. Without the first, her own personal nursing services may be totally inadequate to effect a cure or to improve injurious conditions; without the second, her work with families is necessarily halting and uncertain.

LENGTH OF TRAINING

The basic clinical course which in our opinion must be the groundwork of the public health nurse's work is discussed in detail in the chapter on the hospital training school. This course must be sufficiently long to cover the services essential for the demands of public health work, and to equip a nurse so that she shall be safe to send out into the community. These services in our opinion can be adequately covered in two hospital years, following a preliminary four-months' period of instruction.

The special public health training should in our opinion be given at the completion of the basic clinical course. The necessary subjects can in our opinion be covered in an academic year of eight to nine months. The public health training can thus be completed within three years.

7. Industrial Nursing

We have reserved for separate brief discussion a type of public health nursing which has been one of the latest to develop and which is as yet one of the least standardized, yet whose potentialities in effective service equal if they do not exceed the types of work which we have been considering in schools, clinics, and general visiting nursing. This recent form of public health nursing, as yet one may say practically in the making, is industrial nursing; that is, the nursing care and instruction of industrial workers, in connection with their employment, at or centering at their places of employment. Here obviously in mere numbers alone without going afield to render service the industrial nurse shares with the industrial physician rich possibilities for preventive work. According to the census of 1920 a substantial proportion of our entire nation, 13 million men and women spend their working days congregated in manufacture and mechanical pursuits, and another million and a quarter as salespersons in stores. Clearly, if industrial medicine and nursing were organized on the proper scale, and had the personnel adequate to reach these individuals effectively for the care of their health, for protection against occupational hazards and diseases, and for the teaching of good hygienic habits, the health of the nation would soon be appreciably affected.

Scope of a Brief Survey

In the course of our investigation into industrial nursing, 27 different industrial and mercantile establishments were visited. These establishments were situated in or near two prominent industrial cities, one in the Middle West and one on the Atlantic Coast. The industries represented were the following:

Manufacturing
    Metals and metal products 8
    Food and food products 6
    Textiles 3
    Clothing 2
    Shipbuilding 1
    Scientific instruments 1

Mercantile
    Department stores 4
    Mail order house 1
Transportation
    Telephone exchange 1
          Total 27

The size of the labor force in these establishments—ranging
from 277 to 10,000 workers—shows the magnitude of their health
problems. All but three establishments had 500 workers or
more; nearly three quarters had each at least 1,000 workers.
Industrial nursing began and has hitherto centered largely in
the first aid room. With the rapid growth of workmen's compensation and the increasing attention given to the care and
prevention of industrial injuries, the demand has grown for the
nurse in industry and from the first aid room her work has
developed in many directions.

Our survey of industrial conditions in Cleveland showed that
there were in 1920-1921 in that great industrial center 7 full-time
industrial physicians and 104 industrial and mercantile nurses.
The 27 plants studied in our industrial inquiry employed 51
nurses; only 4 employed a full-time physician. In 19 of the plants
one or more part-time physicians were engaged for varying
periods of time. In some instances they spent from one to four
hours per day at the works, in others a day or several hours twice
a week; in still others they did not come regularly but were called
at need. In the remaining 4 establishments no regular provision
for physicians' attendance was made; neighboring doctors were
called. In addition to these arrangements for medical care,
13 plants also had specialists—oculists, chiropodists, and dentists—who came regularly to examine and treat employees.

TYPES OF WORK

The fact that so large a proportion of nurses are working in
industrial establishments with part-time physicians who visit
plants only a few hours per day or per week is highly significant
of the nurse's great and varied responsibilities and opportunities.
Obviously, no hard and fast rules can apply to the activities of
the industrial nurse. They vary necessarily with the size and
management of plants, the organization of the medical department, the calibre of doctors and nurses. Industrial nursing has
developed even more markedly than other branches of public
health nursing empirically, at haphazard and may be observed

today in various stages of development from the single nurse in one plant combining in her own person not only nursing but welfare work, safety and personnel work, to the large group of supervising and staff nurses and attendants in another plant under a well-organized medical department.

In the best type of industrial nursing, surgical work in the first-aid room is chiefly an introduction to the nurse's subsequent more extended activities in preventing disease and disability, in getting the workers under proper medical care, and actively forwarding their health. Because her contacts arise for the most part in the first-aid room or dispensary, because the workers themselves in the first instance seek her there for assistance in need, great or small, from a cinder in the eye to temporary indisposition or serious injury, she shares the same vantage-ground as that of the generalized nurse on which we have laid stress, the advantage, namely, of combining, or at least having the possibility of combining, curative and preventive care.

Of the 27 plants covered in our special inquiry, 14 employed one nurse, one plant running on the 3-shift system employed three nurses and the remaining 12 had each a supervising nurse with a staff of from one to four nurses. The varied activities of these nurses are summed up in the following table:

TABLE 3

TYPES OF SERVICE RENDERED BY NURSES IN 27 PLANTS

Type of Service	Yes	No	Does Not Apply	Not Reporting
First-Aid Room......	27	..	..	..
Employment Dept.:				
Physical Exam. ...	8	17	2	..
Other Service	20	7	..	..
Plant Conditions:				
Sanitation	15	12	..	..
Labor Laws: Aid				
in Enforcing ...	14	13	..	..
Welfare Work:				
Rest Room	9	9	9	..
Lunch Room	3	22	2	..
Recreation	5	21	..	1
Safety Work	14	13	..	..
Health Education ..	22	5	..	..
Home Visiting	18	9	..	..
Bedside Care	13	13	..	1
Absentees	10	17	..	..
Relief	5	17	2	3
Other	10	17	..	..

First-Aid Work and Its Development

As we have already noted the primary work of the nurse for which she is usually engaged is in the first-aid or hospital room. Here employees come for treatment or advice, here the nurse has regular office hours and keeps records, from here her other activities usually radiate. In following up in the plant employees who do not return as directed for treatment, in developing contacts made in the first-aid room, the nurse obtains her foothold both in the factory and in the confidence of her patients.

But many nurses, either through pressure of first aid, through lack of vision on their own part or through the restrictions of physician or management spend practically all their time in the dispensary and become in fact little more than surgical assistants as ignorant of plant conditions or of the lives of the employees whom they are to influence as though they were permanent fixtures of the first-aid room, mere agents for binding up wounds or dispensing pill or bottle. To three girls in succession complaining of headache did one nurse visited give out aspirin tablets without further word of inquiry or advice; three times in the course of one day did another bind up cuts received by workmen at the same machine. In this instance indeed the nurse was prevented by the management itself from seeking out the causes of injury as she was forbidden to leave the dispensary.

Few industrial nurses were encountered who could say with one highly qualified nurse that to every patient seen by her she sought to teach something about proper habits of living. Yet in this instance, the nurse's interest in instructing each individual with whom she came in contact had not narrowed but extended her conception of her duties. She it was who gradually persuaded her firm to engage a full-time physician; she it was who acquainted herself with all processes in the factory, who "kept her eye on all places likely to show bad effects of the work on employees" and obtained permission to speak to the assembled workers in any department before the noon hour on desirable methods of preventing possible injury. Thus in one department in which raw silk was handled, infection of cuts and scratches previously frequent was eliminated by the nurse's success in enlisting the men's interest in these small injuries and in having them immediately treated with iodine by the foreman.

Contrasting examples of success and failure on the **part of** the nurse in following up injurious processes in the plant were shown in two factories manufacturing biscuits and crackers. The most common injury in these factories was abrasion of the finger tips. The girls who pick up crackers, etc., from canvas tables on which they are emptied from the conveyors break the skin of the finger tips almost daily. In one plant employing 1,500 women the nurse estimated that many thousand treatments were given during the year for this cause. She had provided adhesive strips at each table so that girls might bind up their finger tips before the skin was broken but had not succeeded in having them used and apparently accepted the present situation as unavoidable. In the second plant employing about 6,000 women the nurse had persuaded workers at the canvas tables to bind up their fingers before they were hurt. But better than this, alternation of work, by transferring girls from standing to sitting positions during part of the day and thus shortening their periods of work at the canvas tables, had automatically reduced the exposure to injury.

EXCESSIVE MEDICATION

Many nurses, as we have already indicated, rely upon giving drugs for such common ailments as indigestion, constipation, and headache instead of seeking to teach hygienic habits of living. This custom of giving sedatives and medication, without individual or standing orders of the physician, is not only contrary to principles of preventive medicine but often in direct violation of the state medical practice acts and should be abandoned.

WORK WITH EMPLOYMENT DEPARTMENTS

One of the most important functions of the industrial nurse is assisting with the medical examination of applicants. The increasing use of such examinations in the interest of placing workers at tasks for which they are fitted instead of indiscriminate hiring is one of the most promising steps in the program of industrial efficiency. The nurse in many instances might and often does examine workers for communicable eye and skin diseases, varicose veins, flat-foot, etc. In some instances she trespasses upon medical practice and is found making heart and chest examinations which she is not fitted to perform. Undoubtedly, in the medical examination she should act as the

assistant to the physician who may delegate to her certain parts
of the routine.

On the other hand, the transfer of workers physically unfit
for certain operation to work better suited to their physiques is
a genuine health measure which the nurse may well recommend
to the management. Not only are good workers thus retained,
labor turnover reduced, and production increased, but equally
important, good-will is engendered between men and management.
The nurse has substantially contributed towards improving the
human relations which lie to a far greater extent than is ordinarily recognized, at the basis of successful production.

Examples of transfers successfully conducted by industrial
nurses in the plants visited were the removal of men with hernia
or fracture in a foundry to suitable light work; transfer of men
suffering from chronic indigestion or bronchial affection in a
huge baking establishment to outdoor jobs; change of girls who
developed hysterical symptoms at speeded textile machinery to
the clerical department; removal of girls affected by dermatitis
from a process involving handling of sugar, etc. In one instance
the nurse discovered that a girl stitcher in a corset factory,
diagnosed by both family and company physician as having
appendicitis and diagnosed at a leading city hospital as having
ovarian trouble, was in fact suffering from constant use of her
right leg at a stitching machine. After transfer to "attachment
sewing" which required only finger work, she gradually ceased
to suffer any pain and was thus spared an unnecessary operation.

SANITATION, SAFETY WORK, AND WELFARE WORK

The nurse's share in the sanitary, safety, and welfare work of
plants obviously depends almost altogether on their size and
organization. In small establishments she is often the only
worker whose function it is to care for plant conditions such as
ventilation and cleanliness as well as for the reporting of accidents, for the lunchroom, the restroom, and the social welfare of
employees. While she clearly is not an expert along all these
lines, she can do much to improve plant housekeeping. Where
she combines so many functions, however, health work proper
must often inevitably suffer.

AN EXAMPLE OF GOOD SAFETY WORK

Because she is often responsible for all the accident records
on which compensation claims are based, the nurse in many in-

stances makes a special point of following up accidents in the plant. While she is obviously not equipped to do safety work in its technical sense, which properly falls within the province of the safety or production departments of plants, she may render valuable service in bringing the facts to the attention of the management or in using her influence with employees to utilize safety appliances, etc.

Thus, for instance, in a large sugar refinery employing about 3,000 men and women, the nurse has posted above her desk a chart of the entire plant with the name of each department written on it, together with a list of the foremen in each department, and the numbers of the workmen under him.

"When she first took the work," writes our field agent, "she insisted upon seeing the whole plant and understanding the entire process. She said: 'I wanted to know when a man said he was a mixer just what he did and where.' Through the chart she has become further acquainted with the organization of the industry. If an employee comes as a victim of an accident, she questions him closely regarding the cause, and if she cannot understand, she goes with the employee to the scene of the accident and sees for herself. The preliminary report of the accident is made out by the nurse. She feels great responsibility about getting accurate information on account of the compensation department, and also because she thinks it her duty to know how accidents happen."

With a few questions, on the day of our agent's visit, this nurse got a complete account of an accident from a man severely injured by a hit in the groin, and then carefully read her account to him, asking him to correct her if she had made a mistake.

LACK OF RECORDS

It has seemed worth while to describe this nurse's activities somewhat in detail, both because of her unusual intelligence and ability and also by way of contrast with the slipshod methods and deplorable absence of records in many industrial nursing departments. The lack of records and statistics these departments indeed share with the medical departments. In many cases neither management nor physician encourages or indeed takes any interest in the nurse's reports, yet as we have already noted in general public health nursing, without reports and records the nurse cannot gauge her own progress or prove her points to her superiors. An accurate system of record keeping is indispensable for good work, showing so far as possible the relation of nursing care to such matters as compensation claims, accident statistics, illness, and absence of employees.

Obviously with the elaboration of personnel work, especially in large plants, with the employment of safety and sanitary engineers to deal with these technical functions, the nurse's share in them naturally lessens. The relation of the nurse with other departments dealing with plant conditions and the welfare of employees remains in most instances to be successfully worked out and in our special inquiry the loss to efficiency from lack of co-operation between nurse and social worker or sanitary or safety engineer, was clearly evident. In other cases the nurse worked harmoniously with these other specialists, without duplication of effort or loss of good-will.

HOME VISITING

Considerable difference of opinion exists as to the desirability and the value of home visiting by industrial nurses. Undoubtedly a knowledge of the home conditions of employees is essential to advising them in matters of health. Such information the tactful and competent nurse can obtain through her confidential relations with those for whom she cares at the plant. Visits to the homes of those who are reported sick should undoubtedly be a function of the industrial nurse, to make sure that even though she cannot herself give bedside care, adequate attendance is being furnished by a member of the family or by the visiting nurse association or other appropriate agency.

Often indeed the health and industrial productivity of workers is vitally affected by the illness of another member of the family and the nurse's aid in remedying home conditions is as effective as in caring for the employee himself. Not infrequently impaired strength and decreased efficiency on the part of men workers has been traced by the nurse to anxiety and loss of sleep incident to the arrival of a new baby, without adequate medical or nursing care for the wife, a lack which in more than one case known to the writer the nurse has made good by recourse to hospital or visiting nurses.

We have already referred to the work of a prominent visiting nurse association in contracting with the employees' mutual benefit association of a large plant to give care to its members.

Many visiting nurse associations render services to employees of industrial establishments either by contract with the firm or with the employees' association or in individual cases, as called by the industrial nurse. For this reason, because she should know in various contingencies what social agencies to call on, a knowledge of community resources should be part of the equipment of the industrial nurse, as of any other type of public health nurse. She may, indeed, find it necessary herself to make good nursing facilities which are lacking in her community. Thus one industrial nurse of unusual insight and experience in public health nursing, in one small town without a nursing association, gave prenatal care and advice to wives of employees as well as to women in the employ of her company, averaging 26 per month, and also devoted one afternoon each week to conferences on baby care.

FOLLOWING UP ABSENTEES

Unfortunately it is not to care for the sick or advise on health matters that most industrial nurses are employed in home visiting, but to inquire into causes of absence of employees, and to urge the return of delinquents. This service which may well be performed by lay assistants, is not medical care or supervision, but connotes espionage for the company and can scarcely fail to detract from the employees' confidence in, and respect for the nurse.

EDUCATION IN HYGIENIC HABITS

While the majority of firms studied, 22 out of 27, reported that their nursing service included education of workers, and several nurses stated that they considered such education their most important function, in fact as we have already intimated, not many of them either appreciated or made the most of opportunities for preventive teaching.

Often the nurse's reluctance or inability to speak to a group prevented her from utilizing valuable opportunities for pointing a moral or enlisting the workers' co-operation. In 6 of the 27 plants studied, classes in hygiene were held; in 5, posters were used, especially in time of epidemic, pointing out various precautions for the preservation of health. In other factories occasional speakers were invited to discuss health problems; in 1, the plant doctor gave talks from time to time. Or again, in some places bulletins on the care of health and hygiene were published, or government pamphlets and literature distributed. One nurse had "health hints" inserted in the weekly pay envelope.

Undoubtedly all such group and graphic methods of education should be carried much further than they yet have been in industrial establishments, relating the advice given to what is naturally one of the workers' foremost needs, that is, the preservation of his working capacity. Here is a motive which may rightly be invoked, not as a mere brutal necessity for the good of the business, a plea quickly resented by self-respecting workers, but in the interest of the individual as well as the common welfare. The desire to preserve his working capacity, if rightly aroused, may therefore aid in dissipating the inertia natural to most human beings with regard to changing established habits of living, especially when such changes are rendered more difficult by inadequate means.

Above and beyond all group methods of education, however, the nurse's daily and hourly opportunities of influencing those to whom she renders service differentiates her in the factory and store, just as in the school, clinic, or home, from other social agents. It is her nursing care and supervision which is at once her best claim to a hearing and the actual basis of her best teaching.

TRAINING FOR INDUSTRIAL NURSING

While nurses in industrial work as in other specialities have achieved success through their own initiative and persistence, yet the lack of special training for this special field has been a grave handicap for the most capable and has often nullified the efforts of the less capable. No less indispensable for the industrial nurse than for other public health nurses—for the detection of disease, incipient and acute, for educational as well as curative work—is the preparation which we have already outlined for all public health nursing. This should consist of a basic hospital course of 2 years and 4 months, followed by sound training in public health nursing, with special emphasis and time devoted to training in industrial conditions.

For lack of such preparation and because they have come into industry direct from the hospital or from private duty, immature and inexperienced, many industrial nurses fail in the educational possibilities before them. It is perhaps more remarkable that many without special training succeed and have left a mark not only on the special plants with which they have been connected but on the whole progress of industrial hygiene. On this point an unusually just and generous-minded industrial physician has expressed himself unequivocally:

"The progress of industrial hygiene," writes Dr. Wade Wright, "has been due in large measure to the contributions of industrial nurses. The truth of this may be readily evidenced if one endeavors to withdraw from the fabric of industrial organizations the threads representative of the services, the influences, and the personalities of able industrial nurses." [62]

This is high praise from a man himself in the forefront of industrial medicine and research. In order, now, to enable more nurses to win the praise accorded to the few, in order to initiate more able nurses into the special problems, needs, and possibilities of industrial work, additional postgraduate teaching in industrial nursing is urgently needed. A course offering unusual opportunities has been given, for instance, at the Boston School of Public Health Nursing whose students were admitted to the courses on industrial hygiene of the Harvard Medical School and to the Industrial Clinic of the Massachusetts General Hospital.

USE OF LAY WORKERS

In many plants the functions of the industrial nurse are undertaken by persons other than graduate nurses, by "practical" nurses, who may or may not have had any training or experience, or by persons who have merely had some "first aid" lessons. Undoubtedly, just as in other fields, the "practical" nurse of good native ability may, through prolonged experience, render valued and valuable services. It is also true that the employment of lay workers or of persons with less training than that of the graduate nurse may wisely be carried further than it has yet been in industrial plants. Clerical assistants are urgently needed in the nurse's office; nursing aides or attendants may well be employed under competent direction in the dispensary; lay messengers should be used for tracing absentees.

We believe, however, that such special aides should in general be subsidiary to the fully qualified nurse. From our study of the successes and failures of these nurses in industry it is evi-

*Cleveland Hospital and Health Survey. Part VII. Industrial Medical Practice. Dr. Wade Wright. Page 529.

dent that their functions are too important, too fraught with potential benefits to the whole trend of industry, in its human
relations no less than in matters of efficiency, to entrust them
to persons without the requisite equipment. No more than in
any other field of nursing, we must conclude, is there a short
cut to efficient preparation. In justice to the nurse herself in
view of her prospective responsibilities, in justice to those whose
welfare is entrusted to her, in justice above all to the community
which pays in deteriorated manhood and womanhood for the
unrepaired injuries of industry, the industrial nurse needs a sound
and rounded training.

"How can we get the employee to take an interest in
and to look after his own health?" asks another able industrial physician. "There is only one way, and that is almost
exclusively by education. . . . The greatest and most enduring
effort is not by any short cut or wholesale method. It is
through personal contact established by a good medical department enjoying the confidence of employees, by the daily
advice of the doctors and nurses to the individual patients
given when they are in receptive mood. . . . No short cuts—
a lot of work and personal confidence are necessary." [63]

* The Art, Not the Science, of Industrial Medicine. C. C. Burlingame,
M.D. South Manchester, Conn. Journal of Industrial Hygiene, February,
1921. Page 372.

II. THE NURSE IN PRIVATE DUTY

Her Function

We turn next to consider private duty nursing, that is, the continuous care of one patient.

As we have seen in Chapter I, the nursing of today is only the modern form of an ancient service: tending the sick has been an immemorial function of women. But at the beginning of the nineteenth century this ancient tradition of service had sunk into ignominy and decay. Florence Nightingale's supreme service lay in this, that in the course of a few short years she transfigured the whole status of nursing, and the Sairey Gamps, dishevelled and tipsy, vanished or seemed to vanish before the white cap and gown, the professional skill and resource of the modern era.

From the latter half of the nineteenth century on, it is not too much to say that trained nursing in sickness has been accepted as one of the assets of civilized life. In the cities of the United States, at any rate, recourse to the trained nurse in any emergency has been one of the signs and tokens of our national prosperity.

Undoubtedly the center and focus of the nurse's work in private duty is the actual bedside care of the sick. With the slowly growing medical emphasis on prevention of disease, she may have the opportunity as well of teaching hygiene to the individuals to whom she gives nursing care and to the members of their families. This is notably true of obstetrical nursing. Teaching a mother something of baby care is for the private duty nurse as for the visiting public health nurse the natural corollary of maternity care.

But unlike the public health nurse, the nurse in private duty does not seek out in the community her patients or those to whom she is to give instruction in the rules of health and hygiene. She does not have the opportunity of continuously seeing these patients and their families and friends over a long period of time, sometimes for years, and thus establishing friendly relations on the basis of a long acquaintance. The private duty

nurse comes and goes. She takes a given case usually on the
call of the physician. Not often does she continue her professional relation with her patient on completion of the case.
Broadly speaking, her function is the bedside care of sickness,
and it is for this that her education must be designed and discussed.

In entering upon this discussion we enter on one of the most
hotly contested controversies in the medical field. On the one
hand, we have the extreme view expressed by many physicians
that for bedside care the present nurse is "overtrained;" that
her charges are so exorbitant as to be prohibitive for all but the
very rich; that the nurse is merely the doctor's "extended hands;"
hence, that any biddable girl can be quickly trained to obtain
the necessary deftness and skill to carry out his orders. It is of
course true that a leading element in the medical profession
does not share these views.

On the other hand, there has undoubtedly been a great reluctance if not a refusal on the part of many nurses to admit the
need of persons less highly trained than themselves for any bedside care of sickness. This reluctance, in many instances, is
based on the fear that in advocating the services of any persons
of a lesser degree of skill and ability than the graduate nurse's,
abuses of all sorts will inevitably follow. How far these fears
are justified we must presently discuss in detail. There is no
doubt that nurses have in the main failed to gauge fully the
size of the problem, that is, the really large numbers of subsidiary workers who are urgently needed throughout the United
States. Yet it is only just to add that such efforts as have been
made to clarify the present situation with regard to the training
of a subsidiary group, have been due to the initiative of members of the nursing profession.

It is clear that before the extreme views on the part of physicians and nurses can be reconciled or modified, or an intelligent
inquiry be made into the objectives of training for bedside care
of sickness, we must first define what is meant by the term and
what is needed in such bedside care.

DIFFERENTIATION OF CARE ACCORDING TO SERIOUSNESS OF SICKNESS

Certainly, a distinction must be made, not as to the financial
status of the patient, but as to the nature and degree of serious-

ness of the sickness in question. To treat as one problem the nursing of a pneumonia or diphtheria or cardiac patient and the nursing of one confined to bed with some mild affection, or a chronic or convalescent bed case is merely to confuse the issues.

Let us then first consider the care of acute disease. In such cases—whether cared for at home or in the hospital, whether rich or poor, irrespective of the means or race of the patient,—it is evident that the nurse's function is a highly responsible one.

She must be equipped to deal promptly, in the doctor's absence, with emergencies of all sorts; to observe and record symptoms of all sorts, often obscure enough, the basis of the doctor's diagnosis and treatment; she must be able to give nursing treatments ordered by the doctor which often require a high degree of skill and judgment; she must know, from hour to hour, how to further what is often the sole condition of cure, that is, nourishment of the patient and the conservation of his strength. The difference between good and bad nursing, between nursing which has been carried to a high degree of professional ability and mere rule-of-thumb attendance, is reflected in the mortality statistics of countries where scientific medicine exists but where modern nursing is unknown. Only recently, mortality in the influenza epidemic varied largely with the provision and competence of nursing service. Again, the condition of patients before Florence Nightingale's day shows in how far modern nursing has reinforced scientific medicine and has itself contributed to alleviating the world's suffering.

In our subsequent discussion of the hospital schools of nursing we analyse the methods of training in vogue today, good, bad, and indifferent, and seek by concrete illustration to show the effects of these varying methods. We outline the minimum requirements needed, in our opinion, to fit nurses for the responsible care of acute disease. These requirements include the educational preparation of the student before entrance; the hospital services in which she must be trained; the classroom instruction which must accompany and interpret her practical ward experience.

PROTECTION OF THE PUBLIC THROUGH NURSE REGISTRATION LAWS

We have already referred to the fact that, in the efforts to standardize the training of nurses and to give the public the same protection in engaging the services of a nurse which it now has in selecting other persons legally licensed to practise, such as physicians, pharmacists, dentists, etc., most states have enacted laws defining certain minimum requirements in courses leading to a diploma of R. N. (registered nurse). To carry out the provisions of these acts, state boards of examination and registration are usually provided in the law. Persons who are not registered cannot legally use this title.

In engaging a nurse, therefore, the public has some legal guarantee as to the training and professional equipment of the person to whom the sick are entrusted. In our subsequent study of the hospital schools of nursing we point out how deficient the guarantee of the R. N. still is, and how it may cover gross inequalities in equipment. With the present wide discrepancies in the scope and competence of instruction, the public, seemingly protected by the guarantee of the R. N., may still obtain for the care of the sick, under that title, graduates of schools totally lacking in some essentials of training such as experience with children, or with tuberculosis, etc. The plan proposed in a later chapter recommending minimum requirements for a basic course is designed to carry further the standardization of the R. N. with a view to its more genuinely guaranteeing to the public the product of a rounded and well-balanced educational program.

THE NEED OF A SUBSIDIARY GROUP

Before entering more at length into the scope and need of a fully trained registered nurse, let us next consider the cases in which persons of less training and ability are able to give routine care. There can be no doubt in any unprejudiced mind that in the long list of minor illnesses which keep patients in bed, during convalescence, including after-care in maternity, and in chronic cases, the superior skill, judgment, and initiative of the graduate nurse are unnecessary. Her abilities so bitterly needed for acute disease are wasted. Yet without some person who can provide some nursing care, such as giving baths in bed and other simple nursing treatments, taking temperature and pulse, preparing the patient's food and keeping him comfortable in bed, minor illnesses may readily develop into acute, serious relapses occur in convalescence, and chronic cases suffer hardship.

RESULTS OF A BRIEF SURVEY

In the effort to obtain some concrete information as to the waste of graduate nurses on cases for which they are not needed, an inquiry was directed during the course of this investigation to a selected group of physicians and nurses. From them, it was felt, some authentic information might be obtained as to the extent of such unnecessary employment. Physicians and nurses genuinely interested in the problem from their own practical experience should be able to gauge the degree of nursing skill required on given cases.

But to obtain any current and detailed information from persons as hard pressed as busy physicians and nurses proved a difficult undertaking. Since concrete facts rather than general off-hand opinions were desired it was soon found that either appropriate records of cases must be kept during a specific period of time or information must be based on existing personal records.

After some experimenting, it proved best to make out a record form for the nurses whose co-operation was secured in this inquiry; they were asked to keep a record card for each case nursed during a sample period of three months, giving information on the following points:

Diagnosis of the case.

Whether it was nursed at home or in a hospital.

Dates of going on and of leaving case, with amount earned.

Whether the case could have been adequately cared for without the full-time services of a graduate nurse.

Four hundred and fifty separate cases were reported on by the 118 nurses who kept records during three months.[64] Two

---

[64] Names and addresses of nurses were secured through the courtesy of registrars and superintendents of nurses of representative hospital training schools in nine states: Connecticut, Iowa, Maryland, Massachusetts, Missouri, New York, Pennsylvania, Texas, Wisconsin. The 450 cases were distributed approximately as follows:

Per Centage	Locality
28	New York City
20	St. Louis and other cities in Missouri
12	Connecticut
10	Philadelphia
10	Rural-suburban areas in Massachusetts, Connecticut, and New York
10	Other states
5	Boston
5	Milwaukee
100	

hundred and five nurses were personally interviewed to explain the object of this inquiry and enlist their interest. One hundred of these responded by keeping records of their cases. One hundred and twenty-seven additional nurses were reached by letter; of these, eighteen kept a continuous record. From the replies, interesting data were acquired on various allied and contested points, such as the annual earnings of the graduate nurse, length of annual employment, duration of employment, etc.

UNNECESSARY EMPLOYMENT

The average length of time reported on by the nurses was about three months. During this period each nurse had on the average nearly four cases. Of the 118 nurses reporting, no less than 79, or almost two-thirds, considered themselves unnecessarily employed in one or more cases. The large number of nurses so expressing themselves is of special significance because the period studied was relatively short and fell in the winter months when the shortage of nurses is usually thought to be much greater than in summer. Moreover, the basis of selection used in securing names of nurses for the study was such as to eliminate those interested in holding easy jobs, and included only those with a genuine professional interest in their work.

The average nurse spent one-quarter of her employed time on cases which in her opinion might have been carried by less expert care, and the entire group of 118 nurses wasted over 2,000 days or 25 per cent of the total days reported on such cases.

KINDS OF SICKNESS CARED FOR

Three-quarters of the 450 cases reported on were acute. Nearly half the patients were surgical, one-third were medical, one-tenth were obstetrical, with a relatively small proportion of nervous and mental cases, communicable diseases, and children's diseases. A little over two-fifths of the cases (183) were nursed at home; three-fifths (266) in a hospital.[65]

WASTE OF NURSES IN VARIOUS TYPES OF SICKNESS

The waste of graduate nurses is most significant in connection with the type of sickness cared for. Geographical distinctions were found less important. Naturally this waste is greatest among chronic cases, rising to nearly 50 per cent of such cases.

[65] One case was cared for in a doctor's office.

In acute cases the proportion of those not needing a graduate nurse was slightly less than one-third.

It is important to note that of the total cases (149) in which the graduate nurse might have been dispensed with, 83, or 56 per cent, could have done without her altogether, while 66, or 44 per cent, could have dispensed with her only in convalescence. Many patients, that is, could well be cared for by persons less skilled than the fully trained nurse after a brief period of expert service. Among the cases studied this was most often true of obstetrical patients. The tendency to keep graduates unnecessarily in convalescence was slightly greater among surgical than among medical cases. The highest proportion of cases employing graduates unnecessarily and for the entire duration of the cases was found in the care of children and of mental and nervous diseases. The highest proportion needing a nurse throughout was, naturally, in the care of communicable disease.

These cases of unnecessary employment are often of long duration; our returns included some lasting from year to year, the patients refusing to release nurses even temporarily for service in epidemics. Nurses so employed are as completely lost to the community as though disabled or imprisoned. Their names cease to appear on their hospital registrar's lists, they are no longer on call, have no longer varied experience to keep them in touch with the developments of their profession or of medical science, and eventually deteriorate to the stage where a case needing real nursing care would find them completely at a loss.

The group of nurses studied, it must be remembered, were a picked group chosen for their serious interest in their work. Among the general run of private duty nurses, the number of those willing to exchange the great possibilities of the profession for a sinecure would not improbably be larger.

While this study was too brief and circumscribed to be of statistical value, nevertheless it offers some evidence, from one angle of approach, as to the need for persons of less expert equipment than the graduate nurse. It is disinterested if limited evidence, since the nurses reporting themselves unnecessarily employed would by the elimination of such engagements probably add to their excessive annual period of unemployment, already amounting, during the three busy winter months, to one-quarter of the total employed time.

The average of one unnecessary case out of three among the 450 cases studied, consuming one-quarter of the average nurse's time, is certainly, as we have indicated, exceeded among the general run of private duty nurses.

EARNINGS OF THE PRIVATE DUTY NURSE

To the often-made claim of exorbitance on the part of the private duty nurse the statistics obtained in this study give no support. There is no doubt that, in emergencies, conscienceless registered nurses, like other profiteers, have made the most of their advantages and have driven hard bargains. But a profession cannot be indicted for individual cases of profiteering and, as a matter of fact, during influenza epidemics untrained and ignorant "practical" nurses have in authentic cases asked and obtained higher prices than graduate registered nurses. .

It is often thought that, since the private duty nurse usually receives meals and a place to sleep while on duty, she is practically exempt from any living expenses except for her clothing. Her high rates of pay are therefore supposed to be pure profit with few if any necessary expenditures. But this popular assumption is not borne out by the facts and does grave injustice to a class of workers whose excessive periods of unemployment have never been sufficiently recognized as justification for fairly high rates of pay.

SEASONAL UNEMPLOYMENT

Nursing, as is too often forgotten, is in strict truth a seasonal occupation. Markedly during the fall and summer, somewhat less in the spring, sickness decreases. Thus, for instance, during the mild fall and early winter of 1921-1922 as late as Christmas time, private duty nurses were idle and waiting at their registries for work,—in one instance, known to the writer, to the extent of one hundred at a time. The incidence of a light epidemic of influenza quickly absorbed them all and again brought on a shortage. For such seasonal irregularities of employment there seems to be no cure. No more than in industry can there be a floating reserve large enough to cover the peak of employment. Even with the present personnel, which is insufficient in epidemics, unemployment during certain seasons is a regularly recurring phenomenon. Nor do there appear to be any kindred occupations to which private duty nurses could apply themselves during the scarcity of work, except vacation work in hospitals or work on the permanent graduate nursing staff of hospitals. But the time of need within the institution may well coincide with the private nurse's period of maximum employment. Rates must therefore of necessity take into account periods of unemployment unknown to women in kindred occupations such as teachers, social workers, etc.

We have already referred to the fact that of 118 nurses keeping records during the three busy winter months, the average nurse spent about a week each month waiting for cases or in recovering from illness. For a quarter of her total employed time, that is,—even at the peak of employment during the three busy winter months,—she was out of work. Moreover, these figures understate the extent of unemployment even at this season, since nurses who were long unable to secure work ceased to report cases and were thus dropped from our records.

Furthermore, the unemployment shown by our statistics during three months of an average winter would be much increased during the seasons when work necessarily slackens. The necessity of supporting herself entirely from three months up to possibly six months in the year makes serious inroads into the private duty nurse's earnings.

LIVING EXPENSES

It must also be borne in mind that even when the nurse receives meals and a place to sleep while on duty, she invariably keeps four walls which she can call her own. There she must keep her belongings since there is room for only the barest necessities on duty. There she must retire for rest and sleep and such social life as her occasional return allows. The cost of keeping up such a little home throughout the year, as well as the cost of living during unemployment, must be counted in considering the income of the private duty nurse.

During the winter of 1920-1921, when this inquiry was made, rates of pay varied in different cities. The rate reported was $7 per day for 24 hours' duty and $6 for 12 hours in New York; $6 and $5 in Boston, and some cities in Missouri, Wisconsin, etc. In Connecticut $5 and $4 were reported, rarely $6. The average monthly earnings of the 118 nurses studied, allowing for the amount of unemployment reported, was $120. But, as we have pointed out, this income cannot be counted on for the year.

It must, finally, be recognized that private nursing is not in itself a career with a future. Earnings do not increase with experience. There seems, on the contrary, to be a tendency to

regard the private duty nurse as obsolete or worn out after a
length of service which in other professions would find a woman
at the height of her earning capacity. The need, consequently,
of saving for old age or incapacity must be more seriously considered than in other professions.

OPINIONS OF 52 PHYSICIANS

In the opinion of the 52 physicians in private practice interviewed on the question of a subsidiary nursing group, the need
of a larger proportion of persons of less training and ability
than the fully trained nurse was clearly indicated. Physicians
representing practices both among the wealthy and among persons of small means were interviewed.[66]   But our inquiry among
this small selected group of physicians in various cities was not
sufficiently rewarding to warrant extending it more widely. Even
by consulting their charge books, definite statements as to the
degree of nursing skill needed on their cases were difficult to
obtain; the general opinions of the physicians on the subject
exhibited all shades of difference, varying from that of the doctor
who considers untrained assistants and midwives as "a menace to
the community" to the views of those who would accept a six-
months' training course for nurses, "the rest to be picked up
under the doctor's direction."

Grouping the statements of 48 physicians who were willing
roughly to estimate the amount of necessary and unnecessary
employment of graduate nurses on their cases during a recent
period of time (usually a month), it appears that about one-
fifth (10) reported no unnecessary employment of graduate
nurses; at the other end of the scale about one-fifth (10) estimated that on practically all their cases, that is, on 75 per cent
or more, graduate nurses were unnecessarily employed. A little
more than one-fifth (11) estimated unnecessary employment
on less than 25 per cent of their cases, and the remainder (17)
estimated such employment to amount to between 25 per cent
and 50 per cent of their cases.

As a matter of fact, among 40 of the physicians questioned
on this point, all but a few employed persons of less training,
such as so-called "practical" nurses, attendants, former mid-

---

[66] Physicians were seen in Philadelphia, New York, in rural-suburban
places near these two cities, and in Detroit.   Half (26) had medical
practices, about a third (16) surgical and obstetrical, about a tenth (11)
were children's specialists, and the rest (4) were neurologists.

wives, etc. Commenting on their experience with these workers, the physicians were about evenly divided between those who considered them entirely satisfactory, "as good as a graduate nurse," and those who considered them unsatisfactory or satisfactory only with certain qualifications such as the following: "Satisfactory, if the doctor shows them everything." "Some really do good work, though their ideas of asepsis would make one's hair stand on end. Wish they could have asepsis training," etc.

Our inquiry to physicians and nurses thus added to our information only a consensus of opinion that bedside attendants less expert than graduate nurses are needed, in numbers estimated at from one-quarter of the total number of bedside nurses to a very high proportion.

Moreover, these estimates do not take into account the scope of the subsidiary group of workers in the two other fields of nursing, institutional and public health. We have in our first chapter on public health nursing pointed out the insistent recurring need, for cases in which the necessary assistance cannot be given by relatives or neighbors, of having some person to call on for continuous bedside care under supervision of the visiting nurse in the intervals between her daily or twice or thrice daily calls.

In our subsequent study of the hospital we show the possibility of much needed economy in the disposition of student nurses' time by employing trained attendants on the wards for the minor duties of daily care, such as in well-ordered hospitals are performed on the male wards by orderlies. The numbers of subsidiary workers needed must therefore take into account these extensions of the field.

THE NUMBER OF TRAINED AND UNTRAINED NURSES IN THE UNITED STATES

According to the census of 1920, there were in the United States 300,000 nurses, male and female. Of these about half were trained registered nurses, whose number showed the phenomenal increase during the decade of 83 per cent (from 82,327 in 1910 to 149,128 in 1920). Some 11,000 of this group are engaged in public health nursing, approximately the same number in hospitals and other institutions, leaving over 120,000 in private duty. How many of this number have dropped out of nursing either through marriage, death, or change into other professions is unknown. An effort made in the course of this study to learn by questionnaire from a sample group of 10,000 graduate nurses their present occupation or whether they had retired from nursing, proved unsuccessful.

According to the census figures, there is thus one trained registered nurse to 700 persons, for the country as a whole. If we add to the 149,128 trained registered nurses the 54,953 student nurses in hospitals and the 151,996 attendants, etc., below the grade of the registered nurse, we obtain the ratio of one nurse trained or untrained to every 294 well persons, the country over. Evidently, then, the problem of caring adequately for the sick is a problem of distribution and of financial need rather than of actual numbers. It is a problem also of training and standardizing the status of the subsidiary nursing group which we are next to consider.

The Standardization of a Subsidiary Group

To urge training for this group is not thereby to create any new type of nursing service. The subsidiary worker is already here in numbers practically equal to the graduate nurses. Of the 276,000 women nurses recorded by the census of 1920, 44 per cent were of the lesser grade of ability and training, known variously as practical nurses, undergraduate nurses, attendants and the like. They range in calibre from women who through native endowment and practical experience have become really proficient in routine care, to those who approximate to the old type of Sairey Gamp, preying on the public under the generic name of nurse, at prices not much less than those asked by the professional trained nurse.

What constructive efforts, we may ask, are being made to stimulate girls and women of good calibre to enlist in the ranks of licensed or trained attendants or whatever designation is used for sickroom service less highly qualified than the graduate nurse's? Let us examine the present situation. Various attempts have been made in the United States to provide short training courses and attract candidates for such work. Measured by the number of girls and women of good address graduated or at present in training, these efforts, it must be conceded, have hitherto had only a very small degree of success.

We do not include in this connection short courses which are intended only for instruction in personal hygiene and home care of the sick by members of their families. Such are the courses of lessons given under the auspices of the American Red Cross to high school girls, to mothers, and to groups of women throughout the country. Over 2,000 nurses are engaged in this service. These lessons are not intended to prepare girls and women to take care of serious disease but to give them some training in the household nursing of which almost every woman is sure at some time to have need, and of which modern life has left most girls as ignorant as though it consisted of secret rites and mysteries. How to make a bed properly, how to protect mattress and bedding, how to do simple cookery and serve a meal appetizingly, to make morning and evening toilet in bed, the rudiments of baby care—knowledge of these things would go far to lessen the need for paid assistance in chronic and mild sickness, and enable families to some extent to help themselves in times of emergency.

A much advertised so-called 8-weeks' course given free by the Chicago Board of Health (except for a $5.00 "diploma") has during the past few years attracted some thousands of girls and women. The course has consisted of 24 lectures on nursing subjects lasting 1½ to 2 hours each, and might be of genuine value in informing a large if totally heterogeneous body of women of some of the essentials of home care. But unfortunately, by registering for nursing service those who have had approximately 48 hours' lectures, and by sending them out to nurse the sick for hire, this course, instead of contributing to intelligent home care, puts a premium on fraud and incompetence. Persons who have completed this 48-hours' course, posing as nurses, have asked and received the same $35 weekly fee as the graduate nurse.

SHORT COURSES FOR TRAINED ATTENDANCE

Totally different in content and design are such short courses as those conducted by various local Young Women's Christian Associations, the course given in Boston by the Household Nursing Association, and those promoted in various parts of the country by the Bureau for the Home Care of the Sick, with offices in Boston, under the Thomas Thompson Trust. Of these courses we may briefly describe two, as examples of the best types of short training now being carried on.

The New York Young Women's Christian Association has, for instance, during the past 12 years conducted a course in practical nursing designed to fit girls and women "to care for convalescent patients and to give valuable aid to doctors and to trained nurses." Emphasis is thus laid in the announcement of the course on the scope of training. It has consisted of 11 weeks' daily lectures and demonstrations, with some experience of hospital work for a limited number. Each student is required to practise until proficient in the practical procedure taught. Since 1921, in compliance with the New York state law setting certain minimum requirements for persons desiring to obtain a state license for employment as "trained attendants," the course has supplied 6 months' practical training in a hospital for candidates desiring to register under that title.   Similar courses are offered by the Young Women's Christian Association in Brooklyn, which has also arranged a 6-months' hospital affiliation, and in other places.

In Boston, the Household Nursing Association was incorporated in 1912 and opened a registry to provide household nursing by persons less highly trained than graduate nurses, who should work under the supervision of graduate nurses. This household nursing includes housework and help in the home such as is necessary for the welfare of the patient, but does not include heavy cleaning, scrubbing, or laundry work. After five years the difficulty of gauging the competence or experience of the attendants led in April, 1918, to the establishment of a course of training. This 7-months' course consists of 6 weeks' household training in residence at the headquarters of the school, 4 months' training at either of two small general hospitals with which affiliations have been made outside of Boston, and 6 weeks' maternity training at either one of two maternity hospitals. After completion of 7 months, the attendants are sent out on cases under supervision of the Association for an additional 6 months, the diploma not being awarded until the 13 months are completed.

The hospital training offered in this course, as observed by us at one of the small general hospitals mentioned, is admirably fitted to give the attendants experience in simple routine nursing while at the same time safeguarding the patients by a generous provision of graduate nurses. The hospital, having approximately 50 beds, with additions now building to double its capacity, is maintained by a private corporation. It has no training school for nurses. On the day of our visit there were 15 attendants in training and 18 graduate nurses including the supervisory staff. There is a special instructor of the attendants.

During the first 3 months on cases under supervision, the attendant is supposed to receive $17 per week; after graduation, $22 per week. Families having these attendants are asked $1 per week supervision fee.

The Boston Household Nursing Association was modelled on the Mutual Aid Association of Brattleboro, Vermont, established in 1907 under the Thomas Thompson Trust. This latter association was formed to furnish standardized household nursing under graduate nurse supervision, and within a few years opened its training course. A few other experimental demonstrations, some of them since discontinued, have been carried out under the Bureau for the Home Care of the Sick mentioned above, at Lynn, Massachusetts, Rhinebeck, New York, Milwaukee, etc.

GENERAL CHARACTERISTICS OF THE COURSES

Undoubtedly these short courses have many excellent features. They have wisely sought to enlist two classes of applicants,— girls whose lack of preliminary schooling prevents their entering a hospital training school for nurses, and older women who have passed the age for entering training. The emphasis on helping in the household which usually includes general oversight of children though not the care of babies, is invaluable, especially when the mother of a family is obliged to stay in bed. The supervision of the attendants in training who are sent out to give bedside care during the second six months of the course, appears to be satisfactory as judged by our field agents, who accompanied graduate nurse supervisors both in Boston and in Brattleboro.

TENDENCY TO DISPERSE AFTER GRADUATION

But the question which at once arises concerns the work and scope of the attendants after graduation. Here we touch on the crux of secondary or subsidiary nursing as it is sometimes called, that is, the irresponsibility of the unlicensed sickroom attendant, under whatever name she is known.

Between 1918 and 1921 the Boston Household Nursing course admitted about 150 applicants. About 50 completed the course, of whom approximately half remained on the registry. The Brattleboro course between 1917 and 1920 had about 30 graduates, of whom 19 remained on the registry varying lengths of time. Thus the number of girls and women attracted to these courses is not only so small as to be almost negligible but the proportion remaining under supervision is even more significant.

Similar figures are available from the Detroit Home Nursing Bureau organized in 1913 to furnish similar household nursing care, but with no training course. Of the 440 women who have been on the directory during 7 years ending December, 1920, about a half (209) stayed on the average 3½ months; another quarter (117) averaged a little over 6 months; only a handful (43) remained between 2 and 7 years.

It appears unmistakable that the graduates of the short courses, as well as attendants placed through registries, tend soon to leave the registries and to practise independently under whatever name and at whatever price they may choose. The whole object of preparing and placing a subsidiary or secondary group of nurse assistants is defeated. Thus, for instance, in its annual report for the year 1919, the Boston Household Nursing Association says that its work has been greatly restricted owing to the fact that many of the attendants left the registry during the epidemic of influenza. "Only a few have returned," says the report, "as they are able to get much higher wages by working independently."

This was the experience also of the Visiting Nurse Association of Cleveland with the trained attendants whom the Association made a determined effort during three years to employ. High hopes were entertained of having by the engagement of these subsidiary workers met the problem of giving continuous bedside care when needed, under supervision of the graduate visiting nurse. But in this instance also the tendency of the attendants to leave the Association, to accept nursing calls on their own initiative, and to assume responsibilities for which they had neither training nor experience, led to the abandonment of the attendant service.

The practice of commercial employment agencies in sending out to nurse the sick, especially at times of widespread sickness, persons without any qualifications even as to personal character aside from any proficiency, is too well-known to need comment.

With the unquestioned tendency of newly trained subsidiary workers to disperse after graduation and the impossibility of gauging the competence or training of those already working independently, we are forced to query what procedure shall be advocated to fill the unquestionable need for bedside attendants in large numbers, while safeguarding on the one hand the patients whose lives and comfort may be jeopardized by incompetence, and safeguarding on the other hand the hard-won status and guarantee of the R. N.

PRIMARY NEED OF LICENSING

The answer seems unmistakable. For different grades of need, different grades of service should be provided. To safeguard the distinctions between these different grades of service no new device needs be invented. The same system should be possible which has proved successful in guaranteeing the designation R. N. and in guaranteeing certain standards in other professions and trades; that is, legal recognition and license to practise under a given designation, with penalties for fraudulent use of the title.

From the present chaos of irresponsible workers,—among whom the public is unable to distinguish the ignorant or the dishonest from those genuinely able to provide routine nursing care,—it should not be impossible to evolve a system whereby those now competent to give such care may be certified as capable by some legally constituted body and the way be opened to obtaining a sufficiently large group of new candidates for training each year.

A beginning has already been made in this direction in five states, New York, Missouri, Michigan, California, and Maryland, where bedside attendants as well as registered nurses may be legally licensed to practise. In these states, with the exception of Maryland, the title of "attendant" guarantees to the public that the person so designated has met certain minimum requirements.

Under the New York law enacted in 1920 a candidate must be over 19 years of age and have a grammar school education or its equivalent, and must be a graduate of a nine-months' course approved by the educational authorities of the state. As in all nurse registration laws, a period was provided before the law went into effect during which applicants might be licensed on satisfactory evidence as to their qualifications. Approximately 400 attendants were licensed under this proviso.

During 1922 similar legislation was enacted in both Michigan and Maryland.[67] In California, under an earlier law, a year's hospital training is required.

In Missouri the movement has gone further and contains a feature of first importance which should be followed in all legislation on this subject. That is, under the law enacted in 1921, in the five cities· of the state having each more than 30,000 inhabitants, no person may engage in the care of the sick as an attendant for hire unless licensed by the state board of nurse examiners, after a specified course of training. Age and educational requirements for candidates are the same as in New York. . Between July, 1921, and February, 1922, approximately 1,545 attendants were licensed under the proviso allowing licensing on satisfactory evidence, before the law went into effect. An additional 1,000 attendants were licensed outside these five cities on mere certification by a practising physician that such persons are "competent or qualified to engage in caring for the sick," which is all that the law requires in second class towns.

We are driven to the conclusion that before training or seeking to enlist additional numbers of girls and women, the first imperative need, the crux, the sole safeguard of a subsidiary group, is to include in state licensing laws subsidiary nursing attendants as well as graduate registered nurses. In no other way can the sick be protected so that they may know by the title of the sickroom attendant what grade of service they are receiving, and subsidiary nursing be given its own distinctive character, status, and name.

THE PLACE OF SUBSIDIARY SERVICE IN A PROGRAM OF NURSING EDUCATION

Without a more distinctive character, status, and name than it has had in the past, subsidiary nursing by persons less highly trained than the registered nurse seems destined to remain in its present condition of irresponsibility and chaos, unsatisfactory alike to doctors, nurses, and the public, in effect an incentive to fraud. For the temptation to the so-called practical or household nurse or attendant to pass herself off as a fully qualified registered nurse, since she has no recognized standing of her own,

* For criticism of the name "practical nurse" incorporated in the Maryland act, see page 179 of this Report.

is almost irresistible. Let a recognized and honorable status
and name be accorded her, with penalties for those who use
the title illegally, and it may well prove possible to develop
among these subsidiary groups a more professional attitude
towards their work, a recognition of the functions they can
safely undertake and of the code of ethics which it has been
one of the shining achievements of the nursing profession to
enunciate and live by.

In seeking to give to the subsidiary nursing group a more
definite status and dignity than has hitherto pertained to them,
a factor whose importance has for the most part been ignored
is the designation or name by which they are known. The
name "trained attendant" commonly used is, it is not too much
to say, almost uniformly disliked and resented by those whom
it is intended to designate.

The importance of the name of the subsidiary worker is often
brushed aside in discussion, and held to be of little, if any,
significance. But much may be in a name, from the psychological point of view so germane to our present discussion, and
if the term hinders instead of helping the standardization of
function for which we aim, if it actually acts as a deterrent to
women and girls of good address from entering these subsidiary
ranks, then the designation is actually a factor of real
significance.

In a personal experience of many years with members of the
subsidiary nursing group, the writer has never known one will-
ingly to use the name "attendant," and such is the testimony
of most of those who have taken part in training this group.
Even those who appreciate most fully their own limitations and
have no desire to assume responsibilities beyond their powers,
resent the name and feel a right, by virtue of their ever-so-
small share in nursing service, to some designation which shall
indicate that service.

This deep-seated desire might, in the opinion of the writer,
be capitalized for good, instead of being allowed to continue
among attendants as a sense of wrong, a real incentive to falsely
representing themselves as fully trained nurses. The term
"practical nurse" in common use for the subsidiary worker has
this grave disadvantage that it marks a false distinction between the subsidiary worker and the registered nurse who is
no less practical, though trained for different ends. The term
"nursing aide" or "nursing attendant" (licensed as N. A.) would

be a better designation and would meet the need of sharply differentiating the two groups, while giving the subsidiary worker a name in which she might take a legitimate pride.

Education of the Public

The fear is often expressed that even with the safeguard of a licensing act, the work of the subsidiary group will not be limited to non-acute cases and that they will seek to undertake functions beyond their abilities. Nor is this fear groundless. There is no doubt that whether or not the subsidiary group is standardized and recognized by law, a supremely difficult period of transition lies ahead. The only safety lies in the education of the public. The success of the licensing system is absolutely contingent upon the education of the public as to the differentiation of function between the two licensed groups. In this education physicians as well as graduate nurses and the state authorities supervising nursing schools must be enlisted, so that the public shall be entirely clear as to the type of service offered.

That the superior qualifications of the fully trained graduate nurse will in her own sphere hold their own, there can in the long run be no doubt. The financial inducement to employ the less expert worker will not be overwhelming. Again with the precariousness of employment in private duty, her rates of pay must be such as to provide a decent standard of living. About $25 per week is the usual charge as against $35 per week for the graduate nurse.

As we have seen, to advocate a new training for this group is not to advocate the creation of any new grade or type of worker but to urge the establishment of standards for a class already numerically large but entirely heterogeneous and irresponsible. Training by small centers and associations needing special endowment which send their students to hospitals for short periods will not in our opinion suffice to solve the problem.

We postpone until after our study of hospital training schools suggestions for training and a curriculum for the nursing aide. Here it suffices to reiterate with all possible emphasis, our opinion that no program of nursing education, however well framed, however well devised to supply the graduate nurse personnel can succeed, if it fails to take into account the parallel need of educating a subsidiary group for nursing attendance which shall be more satisfactory to physicians and to the sick

themselves than any group existing today. We cannot blind
our eyes to the wholly subordinate and inadequate place which
such training has in the past held and still holds in plans for
nursing education. We cannot, if we would, blind our eyes
to the actual need for such attendance, on a large scale, for
the types of illness and disability which we have defined.

In rural districts and even in small country towns the problems of attending sickness are even more sharply accentuated
than in the cities. The dearth of country doctors leaves the
sick peculiarly destitute of care. In country districts the private duty nurse has practically never been known, except for
single individuals occasionally imported for special cases. Even
in the small state of Connecticut, almost all parts of which are
comparatively accessible, a search for private duty nurses made
outside of cities during this investigation was practically un-
rewarded. Nor is it likely that in such communities private
duty nurses could make a living the year round.

Here it is that the increased number of public health nurses
entering rural work offers the best hope for the future. The
scope and interest of rural public health nursing, its increasingly
recognized status, and the career it offers to women who combine with love of nursing some executive abilities and a taste
for adventure, seems to assure a steady increase in personnel.
But for continuous bedside care, when needed, in rural districts
as in the city, the services of the public health nurse must be
supplemented. In the past, country people have had to depend
for any bedside care chiefly on relatives or neighbors, who may
or may not have had some practical experience in nursing. To
make available for them the services of the subsidiary group
under supervision of the public health nurse, would undoubtedly
tend to lessen the hardships of sickness in the country.

THE OUTLOOK FOR PERSONS OF MODERATE MEANS

It is often asserted that while the wealthy can afford to pay
any price for the best nursing, and the poor have recourse to
the free wards of the hospital and to free visiting nursing, persons of moderate income who are unwilling to accept charity,
have least access in sickness to nursing care, and it is for them
that the subsidiary group is proposed.

It is undoubtedly true that families of moderate means are
unable to afford for long the expense of the full time graduate

nurse. Yet to suggest any material reduction in her rates of pay does not, in view of her early superannuation, appear to be justifiable.

Furthermore, that a subsidiary nursing group alone can in any sense solve the problem of nursing the sick of moderate means in their homes, as has been the too sanguine expectation of some of the protagonists of the short courses, seems to us idle to expect. To differentiate between grades of nursing skill, not according to the degree of seriousness of the disease in question, but by the financial standing of the patient, seems to us thoroughly mischievous. It is a truism that acute disease is none the less acute among persons of small or no means than among the wealthy.

We have in our discussion of public health nursing pointed out the increasing number of pay patients on the rolls of the visiting nurse associations, indicating increasing recourse to the visiting nurse service, on the part of persons other than the very poor. This increasing use of the daily or twice or thrice daily visits of the visiting nurse in serious disease foreshadows indubitably the most promising ultimate solution of the nursing problem in homes of moderate income; it foreshadows, that is to say, a community solution, the development of community programs for the care of disease and the promotion of health.

COMMUNITY HEALTH PROGRAMS

Insurance schemes for providing bedside nursing as well as medical care are only in their infancy. The Missouri Valley Industrial Hospital at Kansas City, for instance, proposes to offer medical, nursing, and hospital care to participating members at one dollar per month paid three months in advance. The institution is beginning by taking in only large groups with the proviso that the central organization of the group shall collect the money and turn it over to the institution.[68] Medical and nursing care is to be given either at home or in the hospital as proves necessary. Another promising attempt now being initiated in New York City proposes to provide maternity care, hourly bedside nursing, and even instructive household supervision at a cost of only $6.00 per year, on a basis of 5,000 participating members. The success of this effort at group insurance it is too early to predict.

* Hornby's Hospital Magazine. Kansas City, Mo. January, 1922. Page 35.

While for individual nurses the precariousness of "hourly" nursing requires the setting of a rate too high to be of any substantial benefit to families of moderate means, group organization might with a fair return to the participating nurses provide nursing by the hour or half-day at markedly lower rates.

Whatever the system inaugurated for continuous home care of the sick, in minor disabilities and convalescent and chronic cases the services of the subsidiary nursing group will remain appropriate and urgently needed.

USE OF HOSPITALS FOR ACUTE DISEASE

In community health programs, the increased use of the hospital for acute disease seems assured, at any rate for adults. For children, the remarkable results achieved by medical and nursing care in the home, even under adverse conditions of poverty and overcrowding, have inclined some child specialists to set such home care above hospitalization for children. For adults, however, among persons of moderate means as well as among the wealthy, use of the hospital for surgery and in confinements has within less than a generation developed to an extraordinary degree, and only less so for medical cases. More and more the use of hospitals for acute disease seems destined to be an inherent part of the community care of health.

Such increased hospitalization is not incompatible with a shorter average stay in the hospital per patient, especially for surgical cases. The extra-mural after-care of surgical patients by doctor and nurse, successfully inaugurated at some hospitals, obviously means lessened expense both for patient and institution.

III. THE NURSE IN INSTITUTIONS

1. The Graduate Nursing Staff

In the interest of deducing a desirable training for the nurse in her several fields of work, we have aimed in Part A to discuss her function and calibre as observed in action; and in Part B to gauge, in the light of this survey, the effectiveness of the current and projected methods of training.

There is one large and important group of nurses, those, namely, on the permanent graduate nursing staff of hospitals and other institutions, to whose function we give no separate analysis, as it consists primarily of the duties of bedside care, which we have already outlined in relation both to the public health and to the private duty nurse. The work of the graduate nursing staff in hospitals must inevitably be influenced to some extent by the fact that it is performed in an institution and not in a private home; yet in its basic requirements such bedside care in no way differs from other bedside care and therefore needs no separate treatment.

2. Instructors and Administrators

The study of the function of the nurse as instructor and administrator in schools of nursing is postponed to Part B. For obviously her duty in these capacities is of necessity touched upon again and again in the discussion of the training school, and can therefore best be summed up at the conclusion, in connection with a study of the existing facilities for the training of nurse teachers and administrators.

PART B

TRAINING OF THE NURSE

IV. THE HOSPITAL SCHOOL OF NURSING [1]

1. Present Status of the Training School

In the preceding chapters we have sought to study the function and performance of the nurse in her various fields of service and have been impelled to the conclusion that for all forms of nursing a basic clinical training is necessary. This basic clinical training we are next to consider in detail, and for this purpose we must turn away from the homes and schools and factories which we have been considering, to the hospitals and hospital training schools in which, during the last fifty years, nurses have received their education.

Our studies of the nurse in action have thrown into relief some of the strong and some of the weak features of that training: its prime asset in teaching the symptoms and care of disease, without which the teacher of health is fatally handicapped; its weakness in failing to give due weight to the prevention of disease broadly conceived, and in failing owing to a variety of causes to meet the greatly increased demand for applicants of high calibre.

To gauge more accurately the causes of both success and failure, to estimate what changes are needed to supply larger numbers of graduates, better equipped to meet far-spread needs, we must next analyse in detail the educational resources of the hospital, which alone can provide the indispensable clinical opportunities.

SCOPE AND METHOD OF THE INVESTIGATION

On January 1, 1921, there were in the United States approximately 1,800 schools of nursing, having a total of 55,000 students and graduating each year approximately 15,000 nurses. According to the Biennial Survey of Education in the United States

---

[1] The investigation upon which this report is based was made in the years 1919-1921. Notable improvements have been made since that time in a number of the training schools studied, and many others are under consideration.

for 1919-1920, made by the Federal Bureau of Education,[2] the rapid rate of increase during the last 20 years is shown by the following figures:

Years	Number of Schools
1899-1900	432
1904-1905	862
1909-1910	1,129
1914-1915	1,509
1919-1920	1,755

During the same span of time the increase in the number of students was from 11,164 to 54,953.

In order to reduce to manageable proportions an inquiry into the training given in so large a number of schools, including all the factors which affect the life of the students during three years' residence, it was manifestly necessary to limit our field. An intensive study of a small number of schools would, it was concluded, be more enlightening than an attempt to cover a large number briefly. Indeed, the nature of the inquiry, which was not statistical, but aimed to evaluate the quality of the education given, required our studies to be intensive.

In choosing the training schools to be studied, differences in the type and size of the hospital with which the school was connected were, for our purposes, the most important factors. We chose therefore for scrutiny training schools maintained by hospitals publicly and privately supported, by hospitals large and small, general and special. We included also training schools connected with hospitals but independently organized. The different types of hospitals all involve corresponding differences in the schools of nursing maintained by them and illustrate the varieties of training given.

Again, within the hospital, among the innumerable questions of hospital management, it was essential to focus our inquiry on those factors which are related to the education of the student nurses. To gauge the kind of teaching given, it was obviously necessary to learn as much of the organization and administration of the hospital as determines the conduct of the training school.

In the first place the scope of the school's activities depends on the financial and educational policy, or lack of policy, of

[2] U. S. Department of the Interior, Bureau of Education. Bulletin No. 51, 1921. Statistics of Nurse Training Schools, 1919-1920. Page 2. (Advance Sheets from the Biennial Survey of Education in the United States, 1918-1920.)

the hospital. Hence these primary factors were necessarily included in our inquiry. The training is clearly conditioned also by the clinical facilities available, hence a knowledge of the clinical details was essential, such as the kind of ward used for training; the type and activity of the services, acute and chronic; the number of beds; the ratio of students to patients, to supervisors, and to graduate nurses; and similar closely related data. Within the training school, the educational requirements for entrance, the curriculum, the methods and equipment for teaching, the hours of duty by day and by night, the living conditions and social relations of the students, were among the important question at issue.

The Committee was fortunate in obtaining, for this portion of its study, nurse investigators of high standing who had themselves been teachers or administrators in training schools, and who were thus able to judge the performance of students and the technical problems of management. In addition, it was thought desirable to compare the instruction of the nurses with teaching in other educational institutions of similar grade. For this purpose most of the training schools studied were visited also by field agents of the Committee who were teachers of science and who could gauge the calibre of the lectures, quizzes, and laboratory work.

Our field agents generally lived in the nurses' home of the school and always accompanied students on duty to see all phases of their training. Every facility for observation and for conference with students and staff was afforded in each hospital visited.

Basis of the Investigation:
Hospital Training Schools Covered

The facts on which this report is based were thus obtained for the most part by personal inspections. Twenty-three schools were intensively studied. Four affiliating schools offering maternity training were more briefly inspected. Two schools maintained by tuberculosis hospitals were studied for the special training given, but are not included in the general statistics. It should be noted that throughout this report the term "private hospital" is used to designate a hospital supported by private funds as distinguished from one supported by state or municipal funds.

Type of Hospital	No. of Hospitals	Bed Capacity	Students Enrolled
Municipal	4	2,700-750	685
Large private	10	750-150	1,254
Small private	5	150- 50	154
Special *	2	160-135	126
University	2	850-190	187
All Schools	23		2,406

* Includes one children's and one women's hospital.

To determine the exact disposition of the students' time, a special study was made of· the daily assignments during three years' training of about 250 students in these schools. The personal histories of about 2,000 students and 200 teachers and supervisors in the schools were obtained and analysed.

In addition to these intensive studies, the records of a newly completed and unpublished survey of 80 schools of nursing in two western states were kindly put at our disposal. Reports on 5 schools maintained by state hospitals for the insane and 5 schools connected with psychiatric institutions in various parts of the country were also made accessible to us.[8]

Finally, our findings were supplemented by examination of about 200 students' records from approximately one hundred different schools of nursing,[4] by study of the literature of nursing education, and by informal conferences of the writer with physicians, superintendents of hospitals and of training schools, students, graduate nurses, and dietitians. Approximately two and one-half years have been spent in making this study.

INCLUSION OF THE BEST SCHOOLS IN THE GROUP STUDIED

At the outset of this report it should be clearly stated that the 23 schools of nursing intensively studied, while including examples of superior and inferior types of training, are not as a group representative of the great majority of training schools throughout the country, or of the average training given, as indicated by the Biennial Survey of Education in the United States for 1918-1920, already quoted.

In the group of schools intensively studied, a disproportionate

[8] Through the courtesy of the National Committee for Mental Hygiene.
[4] Through the courtesy of Teachers College, Columbia University, in allowing access to records of all students in the classes graduating 1919 and 1920, who had received their hospital training within ten years preceding date of graduation.

number of the best schools was deliberately included. In our general findings therefore as to the calibre of training, students, and equipment, the better schools in many particulars outweigh the inferior ones. Thus, the average hours of duty in the schools visited are shorter than in the great majority of schools; the clinical and teaching facilities are better; the students are somewhat older and better prepared than in the general run. Taking the country as a whole, for instance, of all training schools maintained by general hospitals almost 40 per cent (36.2 per cent) are connected with hospitals of less than 50 beds. In this study schools having access to less than 50 beds have been omitted as by general consent in many cases unfit, and always needing extensive affiliations in clinical or educational opportunities, for training nurses.[5]

Wherever information was at hand, we have indicated how and to what extent our general findings diverge from and are superior to the data relevant to the great majority of schools of nursing. Moreover, and more important, all the illustrations of principles and procedures, all the concrete examples with which the writer has sought in every case to illuminate the discussion, are drawn alike from the best and the worst schools and thus give due weight to the inferior as well as the superior practices.

For our inclusion of a disproportionate number of the best institutions, the reason is obvious. The weaknesses and failures found too abundantly true of these, are obviously even more true of the inferior schools. Moreover, the intention of this study looks towards the future. It is not in order to convict the training schools and hospitals of error that the facts have been sought and analysed, but to show what has been accomplished under the present system and the possibilities of the future. While inferior schools point the worst failures and the chief obstacles in the way of education and the recruiting of students, it is on the pattern of the better schools that the future must be modelled. To include a larger proportion of the better schools was therefore more fertile and more in conformity with our purpose than to insist upon an even balance of all grades.

[5] Compare rulings of the Red Cross, Bureau of Public Health Nursing, and the National Organization of Public Health Nursing, excluding respectively graduates of training schools connected with hospitals of less than 50 beds or having less than a daily average of 30 patients.

Florence Nightingale and Nursing Education

Before entering upon our study it may be enlightening briefly to recall the genesis of nurse training and the gradual evolution of its educational status which is in progress today.

We have already referred to the signal achievement of Florence Nightingale in practically founding the modern secular profession of nursing and building up from the best sources which existed in her day, a new system of hospital training. We do not here digress into the history of this unique figure of the nineteenth century, whose extraordinary record and command of such diverse matters as vital statistics, hospital construction and administration, poor relief and housing, as well as nursing, is accessible in recent illuminating studies.[*]

Certain antecedents of hospital training for nurses it is valuable, however, in the interest of a better understanding, to recall. Nursing, as we have already pointed out, dates from far back of the Christian era, as a natural exercise of the maternal instincts of women. During the middle ages it became a function of religious orders, and with that persistence of accepted ideas and conventions which marks all human affairs, there survive to this alien day, as ideals deemed appropriate to nursing, the monastic ideals of asceticism, self-abnegation, and obedience to authority.

To these monastic influences there must be added further the influence of the military model which it was natural that the first hospital training schools should adopt, following as they did so closely upon Florence Nightingale's Crimean episode and her reorganization of the army medical service.

These monastic and military traditions have, until very recently, dominated to an extraordinary degree not only the actual working of the schools of nursing but our habitual thinking about them. It has been an accepted tradition that the nurse in training should yield to her superiors an obedience which transcends even that of the good soldier, for it has no court of appeal; and that she should be governed by a sole dedication to duty which is derived from the earlier religious devotion of votaries.

But in a modern world and with the entrance into the training schools of young women actuated by the same mixed motives

[*] The Life of Florence Nightingale. Sir Edward Cook. Macmillan, London, 1913.
Eminent Victorians. Lytton Strachey. Putnam, New York, 1918.

which animate their contemporaries in other pursuits, these traditions are bound to be modified. In this report we describe the process of modification which is today going on and which is inevitably a cause of profound unrest in the training schools.

For the student of nursing education it is significant to note that the first school for nurses, to whose endowment at St. Thomas's Hospital Miss Nightingale devoted the national gift presented her after the Crimean war, was established not to furnish nursing service for the hospital but solely for the education of nurses. The school had a separate economic foundation, distinct from the hospital. Lectures, class work, and practical work under supervision were provided for the students, who were destined to go out from St. Thomas's to train and teach in other hospitals. So scandalous had been the nursing care of the sick in these institutions that the entrance of refined, educated, and specially trained women worked nothing less than a revolution. So useful to the hospital proved their practical service that before long other hospitals began to adopt the new idea of training schools and to establish them, not as separate educational enterprises but as working departments under their own management with students as a sort of apprentices.

How far this movement has gone, how schools of nursing have developed, and have been moulded by their development, as parts of the hospital organization, it is one of the main objects of this report to make plain.

The history of nursing education, so far as it has progressed, is indeed the history of most vocational education. For professional, commercial, industrial training in almost all lines had its roots in apprenticeship of one kind or another, and until comparatively recent years apprenticeship was the traditional and accepted method of instruction. But while standard professional education such as law and medicine, architecture and engineering, has long outgrown the apprentice stage, and even such callings as journalism, business and social work are rapidly moving towards an ordered educational scheme, the training of nurses remains one of the few survivals of this earlier and largely outworn type of education. The nurse in the vast majority of cases still receives her professional training not in an educational institution independently endowed and organized as Florence Nightingale conceived it, but in a training school which is a part of a hospital and responsible for furnishing its nursing service. Such a school shares inevitably the essential weakness of the apprentice system; its first liability is service, production, not education. Only within a comparatively short time has the teaching of nursing been in any degree differentiated from apprenticeship, and been placed in part on a sounder educational basis, providing that balance of practical experience and didactic teaching which is the .desideratum in all vocational preparation.

In urging, as this report does, the establishment and endowment of genuine education for nurses, it should not be understood as for one instant underestimating the primal, basic value of the practical training in a field which offers a peculiarly rich, an almost ideal pedagogical opportunity. For here the "motor consequences," as William James termed them, of instruction are reinforced by a motive on the part of the students very different from that animating most vocational training,—the motive to relieve suffering and to save life.

In medicine, law, agriculture, and other professional disciplines the period of apprenticeship training was followed by a too great divorce of theoretical instruction and its practical application, a too great reliance upon formal classroom instruction alone. It has therefore proved necessary in these professions to re-establish practice fields, again requiring, but now as a more carefully integrated share of the training, practical experience on the part of the student.

The fear is sometimes expressed that the obviously approaching breakdown of apprenticeship in nurse training will lead to a similar error, with the loss of practical efficiency in nursing. But in the course of this report it will become abundantly clear that no such danger is evident, that on the contrary it is the forced compliance with hospital needs which has been and continues to be the genuine obstacle to educational advance.

THE DUAL FUNCTION OF THE TRAINING SCHOOL

On entering upon a study of nurse training today we are confronted by this dual character of the training school. It is indeed, as we shall see, the crux of our problem, the heart of our difficulty. For the school of nursing has sought to perform two functions: to educate nurses and to supply the nursing service for the hospital. But in these two functions there lies an ever present possibility of conflict. The needs of training and of hospital services may not coincide, and when the two are in conflict, the needs of the sick must predominate; the needs of education must yield. Whether or not, for instance, a student nurse has completed the services required for her training, whether or not she has had any experience with children or has had sufficient instruction in medical disease, if surgical patients are in need of care, to the surgical ward she is sent, though she may already have exceeded the time set for this service.

Or, again, whether or not she may have learned in a week to mend rubber gloves or learned in a day to wash lettuce for private patients, if gloves are to be mended or lettuce is to be washed, to these services she is assigned for additional weeks.

In a later chapter we shall show how, by providing supplementary services, these needs of the hospital may be met without depriving students of a balanced training; how, by a different organization of the school, the present training of students may be both shortened and enriched. We shall also show in detail the failures in the first principles of teaching found even in the best schools. But at this point in our discussion we must first illustrate concretely how the training of nurses is sacrificed and prolonged in deference to the needs of the hospital. Today this cardinal point is unheeded, unrecognized. Were it once clearly established and its wide implications made plain, the fundamental error in the present relationship of hospitals and training schools would be abundantly evident. In such a showing lies the only hope of improvement. For the bar to progress at present lies precisely in ignorance of the facts. No action will follow until these facts sharply challenge the interest of those in authority; that is, first, the responsible hospital trustees and, behind them, the general public on whose financial support either directly through gifts or indirectly through taxation, the hospitals are dependent.

Hospital trustees form a group which has won an honorable position in American communities in building up a great philanthropic institution. They have given volunteer service and time, without stint, to its up-building. Many of them every year have made up, from their own pockets, the deficits in hospital finances. Yet they are uninformed of the true conditions of the department which, in addition to its educational rôle, has furnished the total labor supply for the great majority of patients. To make known the facts, to show the conflict between education and care of the sick is therefore our first concern.

THE CONFLICT BETWEEN EDUCATION AND CARE OF THE SICK

RECORDS OF ACTUAL EXPERIENCE

What, indeed, is this conflict, and how is it manifested? To many persons, including doctors as well as trustees, it is a new thought that the interests of hospital and training school are not one. That any legitimate conflict exists between the two is almost unthinkable. To them the school of nursing represents merely the department of the hospital, whose function it is to furnish the nursing service. They have tacitly assumed that the student nurses, in the course of three years, learn to care for the sick in the various divisions of the hospital and emerge at the end of that period as trained nurses. Thus the welfare of hospital and training school coincides. The work of the hospital is done and the students are simultaneously and automatically taught. And since a nurse should be equipped primarily for service, the difficulties and hardships of the work, such as they are, form an inherent and perhaps the most valuable part of the training, disciplining the nurse for any emergency as effectively as a more formal method would do.

This assumption has been so generally accepted that it is the more important to show its essential errors.

On what grounds, it may be asked, in the first place, is the existence of such a conflict asserted? How can it be proved? The answer lies in the training schools' own records.

In order to learn the complete disposition of the students' time during three years of training, the daily assignments of students in different hospitals were drawn from the records, analysed and computed, and are shown in Graph 1.

Here we see the range of days spent in different services by students of the same class compared with the time planned by the school as necessary for training in these services. The white columns show the school plan; the black columns its actual performance, by the minimum, median, and maximum amounts of time spent in each service by students of the class most recently graduated.[7]

[7] Two points of statistical importance should be explained here:
1. Here and elsewhere in this report, instead of the usual average (arithmetic mean), the median has been used, that is, the middle value, when all values are ranged in order of magnitude. The special advantage of using the median is that it represents not an abstract figure but the actual record of a specific student, and can thus be effectively contrasted with the records of other students representing minimum and maximum

The striking fact which leaps to the eye in this graph is the extraordinary, the bewildering diversity in the assignments of students of the same class, shown in the range of days spent in the different services, and the equally marked deviations from the time planned by the school for these services.

Thus, for example, in Hospital No. 1, a large municipal institution, each student was supposed, according to the school plan, to need and to receive 7½ months in the various medical services. How was this standard lived up to? As a matter of fact, analysis of the records of one class of 61 students who had completed their training showed that half the class had over 9 months, ranging up to 12½. The student who had least time in the medical services fell short of the time planned by almost 2 months, having only 5¾ months; the student who had the longest medical services exceeded the time planned by exactly 5 months. The difference in medical training between the two classmates was therefore almost 7 months.

In the surgical services the showing is worse. The time planned is itself excessive, being over 4 months longer than the standard set for medical training, 11¾ months as against 7½. Long as was the period planned, all but one of the 61 students exceeded it. This one girl had a week less than the time planned; but half the class had over 14½ months, or approximately 3 months at least in excess of the school plan, while the girl having the longest surgical service (18¼ months) was kept at these duties 6½ months or more than 50 per cent longer than her training was supposed to require.

On the other hand, the assignments to the children's service very generally fell below the desired 2 months. One student had no experience at all with children; half the class had less than 1½ months. In the obstetrical service in this hospital the median amount of time spent coincides with the plan of the school. Yet one student had only 3 weeks of obstetrical

experience. For statistical accuracy the representative character of the median has been proved by its practical coincidence with the arithmetic mean, which has also been calculated for every service.

2. With regard to the inclusion in the various services of time spent in practical work during the preliminary term, the following points should be noted. This inclusion, though in contrast to the prevailing practice of the training schools in reckoning time planned, is necessary to a true picture of the student's actual experience. While indeed it may slightly increase the excess of services already exceeding the school plan, it conversely may partly correct the defect of certain other services falling below the school plan.

GRAPH 1

COMPARISON OF TIME PLANNED IN 7 SERVICES BY 2 SCHOOLS OF NURSING, WITH MAXIMUM, MEDIAN, AND MINIMUM ACTUAL TIME SPENT IN THESE SERVICES IN EACH SCHOOL BY STUDENTS OF ONE CLASS.*

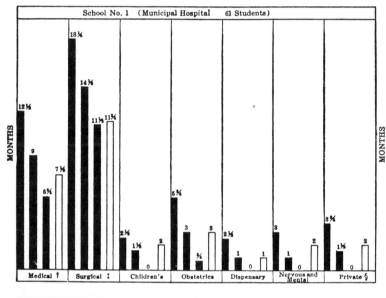

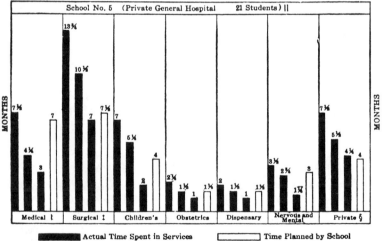

* Excluded from this graph is all time spent in elective services and services which are available for less than half the students of a class.

Time spent in practical work during the preliminary term is included in the designated services.

† Medical service includes all training in general medical, skin and venereal, communicable diseases, tuberculosis, and diet kitchen, and the proportion of mixed service stated by the school to be medical.

‡ Surgical service includes all training in general surgical, gynecological, orthopedic, operating room, recovery, urological clinic, eye, ear, nose, and throat, and surgical supplies, and the proportion of mixed service stated by the school to be surgical.

§ Private service includes special and nurses' infirmary service.

‖ Representative section of class.

training, while at the other end of the scale another student had 5 months more than the minimum.

Similar examples of this extraordinary range of duty among the members of a single class were found in each one of seven schools, in which assignments of students were studied. Variations in night work assignments are shown on page 434.

At Hospital No. 5, a privately endowed hospital with large surgical services, the subordination of the medical training to the surgical is even more extreme than in Hospital No. 1. Here even the girl having the maximum medical experience exceeded the time planned by only 2 weeks; half the class had less than two-thirds of the 7 months planned; the girl with the minimum experience had only 3 months. Significant in this connection is the range of duty in the private service, which is again very largely surgical. Four months are specified for private duty. Yet half the class ranged between 5½ and 7½ months. In the children's service, the unusual length of which partly compensates for the short medical assignments, the difference of time spent by the two students having the minimum and the maximum experience was 5 months.

That in these primary services there should be so wide a range of days for students of one class is in itself an anomaly. In reply, it might, perhaps, be claimed that since girls vary in manual dexterity, and some may take longer than others to master the technical procedures, the length of assignments may vary with the development of the student's capacity. But no such claim can seriously be put forward. Little or no connection exists between the student's educational needs and the duration of these different services. A superior student who had interrupted her training for war service overseas, where she had over a year's surgical experience, found herself on her return to her school, assigned to another long period of surgical duty. Often, indeed, it is precisely because of the student's proficiency in a given branch that she is deliberately kept to it. She is, in effect, doing what should be paid graduate service, often in deference to the wishes and even the demands of attending surgeons and physicians. The head of the school, in many cases known to the writer, has yielded to such demands against her own judgment and against her will. In some cases she has resigned rather than yield.

Mere justice would require that, within reasonable limits, and with reasonable regard to individual requirements, students in the training school, as in other educational institutions, should stand on the same footing as regards their opportunities of training.

It is frequently urged in defense of the excessive duration of certain services that the excess is unavoidable owing to the clinical make-up of the hospital. When, for instance, the surgical beds of a given hospital outnumber the medical beds by a ratio, let us say, of 2 to 1, such a hospital, if staffed entirely by student nurses, must inevitably overweight the surgical training in the same proportion.

Thus, for instance, in a large private hospital the number of beds in the medical and surgical departments represent respectively 21 per cent and 29 per cent of the total bed capacity. Analysis of the allotment of the students' time shows a rough correspondence: 18 per cent and 32.6 per cent of their total training were spent respectively in those two services. The number of beds assigned to private patients comprise 36 per cent of the total bed capacity; and in this service, which in our opinion is of little or no value as a training field, one-fourth of the total time of all students was spent.

But the defense of invoking necessity only admits the domination of student education by hospital needs. The remedy must be found in strengthening the weaker services by means of special case study, as later indicated, and transferring the excessive services in part to a permanent paid body of graduate nurses.

On the other hand, it is sometimes asserted that excess of time devoted to one service is compensated by defect in another, and that the common content of training in the major services, such as surgery and medicine, makes any disproportion of time between the two a matter of comparative indifference. That is to say, since so large a proportion of elementary nursing duties, such as bed-making, bathing, etc., are the same for both medical and surgical patients, it is of little importance in which service the student obtains this training. But this claim ignores the essential point that after a comparatively short period of intensive training in such elementary nursing duties, the educational advance of the student depends precisely on the differentiation of her training in the special services. Suppose the "common content" of medical and surgical training to occupy two months of the student's time, a three months' assignment to medical service will leave but one month for the needed characteristic training in medical disease, and will certainly not be balanced by the existence of an eight or nine months' surplus for special training in surgical disease.

Causes of Irregular Assignments

At first sight it would appear as though the chaotic assignments of students reflected directly upon the responsible head of the training school, the superintendent of nurses. In the school she is apparently in complete authority, exercising powers of control over her students greater than exist in any other educational institution of similar grade, and backed by a tradition of obedience unknown outside of military or religious orders.

Without reference to her control of the students' living conditions, elsewhere treated in this report, the superintendent or her deputy disposes absolutely of their schedules and services, excepting only for a limited number of elective courses open to third-year students in some hospitals. How then, it may be asked, does an educator so situated countenance assignments such as those illustrated above, so unjust as well as detrimental to training, graduating students who have in effect served the hospital in some services far beyond the needs of training at the expense of their experience in other services equally important?

On reflection, however, it becomes readily apparent that responsibility for the present status of teaching rests on no single individual but in a complex and baffling situation. It is again the dual function of the training school which must be held accountable for its deficiencies.

The Dilemma of the Training School Superintendent

Indeed the superintendent of nurses, the so-called autocrat of the school, in her own person typifies concretely the conflict between education and care of the sick. She is at once head of the hospital nursing staff and principal of the school. Her responsibilities are dual: to patients and students, to provide nursing care and to provide the education promised by the school in its printed program.

In proportion as the superintendent is able and conscientious, imbued with the rights of both patients and students, her difficulties and the conflict in her duties increase. An equitable solution is often obviously impossible, and to the imperative demands of suffering all other considerations must yield.

It is, in one sense, to the lasting honor of the nursing profession that this solution of their problem has so far been accepted; that the tradition of "humanity first" has been the guiding principle of their training. The devotion which no other element of training can ever replace is thus inculcated in the very choice of alternatives.

But, on the other hand, the ultimate wisdom of pursuing this course is more than open to question. This devotion to duty may be too dearly bought. It is after all possible that, were the facts known outside the school of nursing, a different solution might be found; the sick might be cared for without sacrificing the very object for which the training school exists, the education of new generations of nurses. When, in addition, it appears that the sacrifice of education is actively defeating the aims of the school—alienating instead of arousing the devotion of students, contributing to decreases in the number of applicants, turning out nurses of ill-balanced, widely diverse training, unfitted to meet modern needs—then the sacrifice of education wears a very different aspect.

The Relation of Superintendent and Students

If the superintendents of nurses are to be criticised in this connection, it is not so much for what they have perforce done, as for what they have left undone. They are subject to criticism for their failure to make articulate and bring home to others the impossible nature of their task, the irreconcilable conflict in the schools. Undoubtedly, as we shall see, the difficulties of bringing home the facts to their superiors in the hospital have been almost insuperable. But to their subordinates, who are also the persons most immediately concerned,—that is, the student nurses,—the superintendents might before this have made plain the system under which they have been obliged to operate. How much smothered discontent and friction might be avoided if students were taken into the confidence of their instructors and made to feel that their irregularities of assignment are in large part due not to indifference or injustice but to economic compulsion, and the need, hitherto undisputed, of staffing the wards and meeting the primary needs of the hospital as distinguished from the training school.

That such explanations, instead of undermining loyalty, would go far to arouse it was shown at a recent unique meeting of superintendents and students from a large number of schools. The meeting was held to celebrate the completion of training begun as a war-time service by the Vassar Training Camp for Nurses.[8] For the first time in the history of nursing the principals, instructors, undergraduates, and recently graduated nurses from a variety of schools met on an equal footing to discuss professional problems. The young nurses, perhaps for the first time as a group, were articulate and voiced their grievances, an almost unheard-of innovation. Many of the superintendents answered inquiries and criticism, not *ex cathedra*, but as human beings, themselves subject to rigid restrictions in the conduct of the schools. "With the realization of this fact," says the official students' account of the meeting, with youth's generous response to a new appeal, "much of the misunderstanding and criticism of training school days was wiped out and the young nurses realized the problems they too would soon be called upon to face in their new work." [9]

For one such epoch-making meeting and many individual instances of openness towards students on the part of superintendents, there exists the traditional, the accepted rôle of the head of the school as unapproachable autocrat and judge. Only a determined effort to change this rôle will enable superintendents to establish with their students the more democratic human relations which other educators find successful and a matter of course. In the gradual establishment of self-government for student nurses, more fully treated in another section, lies the best hope of changing from the inherited cloistral traditions to a more democratic basis. But to an interested outsider at the Vassar meeting, the failure of various superintendents adequately

[8] Established at Vassar College, June, 1918, where three months' intensive teaching was given, preliminary to two years' training in co-operating hospitals. 418 students were accepted. 169 have graduated.
[9] The Thermometer. Published occasionally by the Graduates of the First Vassar Training Camp for Nurses. March, 1921.

to seize upon the need for a fundamental change in their approach to students was abundantly evident. One prominent leader voiced a general feeling. Her weekly office hour for students, newly open to all, had been unappreciated and had met no response. No students came to utter the complaints they were invited to make. That this innovation had been established only a short time, and the students were in no way prepared to come at short notice into new and confidential relations with an official hitherto hedged and inaccessible, appeared to be wholly unrecognized.

For their subordinates, then, the responsible heads of the school could do much at once to explain and render more tolerable, if not to change, the often non-educational routine demanded by the present organization of the school.

In nursing circles the facts are well known, and frankly discussed. With their colleagues and associates the heads of the school are open regarding the submergence of education. The literature of nursing is full of it. Year by year, at their annual conferences, the leaders debate the issue with chagrin, with impatience, even with passion.

"It is entirely certain," said one of them at a recent meeting, "that we cannot long continue to conduct our schools of nursing on the old basis of almost pure apprenticeship. The disheartened women who have been struggling valiantly with this system for the past 25 or 30 years know well that it cannot survive. Its day is past, and we must build on such parts of our structure as are sound a new and equitable system that will guarantee the maintenance of modern educational methods." [10]

For one state, New York, it was reported at the same meeting by an official of the State Department of Education, that of the 144 registered schools in the state, 60 had changed superintendents at least once during the year 1919. While various reasons contribute to this deplorable turnover, such as unfitness for the position and the attraction of capable women by large hospitals away from the smaller ones, yet one highly important factor is what was termed "the impossible demands of the hospital," that is, precisely, the conflict of duties upon which we have dwelt.

[10] National League of Nursing Education, Proceedings of the 26th Annual Convention, 1920. Pages 157-158.

THE SUPERINTENDENT OF THE TRAINING SCHOOL AND HOSPITAL ORGANIZATION

Yet for the superintendents to make known these difficulties of their position to their superiors in the hospital is, as has been intimated, a profoundly difficult undertaking. In the hierarchy of hospital organization, the immediate superior of the superintendent of the training school is the superintendent of the hospital. This superintendent is himself an executive burdened with many problems, responsible to the hospital trustees for the financial as well as the technical direction of the institution. As a rule his primary interest, so far as concerns nursing, is naturally the nursing service of the hospital, that is, the care of patients and the satisfaction of the medical staff.

The hospital superintendent is an expert along many lines, but in most instances he is not an educator. Yet he is practically in control of the pedagogical methods of what purports to be an educational institution. Generally the superintendent of the hospital appoints, or, what amounts to the same thing, recommends for appointment, the superintendent of nurses. In most cases his power of veto or of approval over the policies of the training school is absolute, for it is only through him that the head of the training school has any access to the final authorities, the hospital trustees. Finally, he is usually a physician; she a nurse. The etiquette of the profession, discipline, and the hard-worked plea of "loyalty" to the institution effectually prevent any direct appeal to the hospital board.

It goes without saying that in many instances the relations of hospital superintendent and the head of the training school are thoroughly harmonious. He relies upon the judgment of the head of the school in educational matters, supports her policies, and presents the financial needs of the school to the hospital board. Yet the system which gives over the control of education to an official unacquainted with educational problems, and carrying heavy executive responsibilities is obviously unfair to the students. Their needs are not adequately represented to those who ultimately determine them.

The hospital trustees in their turn are charged with many diverse duties towards patients, medical staff, nurses, the community. They are over-burdened with the business of running the hospital.

Of conscious exploitation of students by hospital boards, ex-

cept in commercial hospitals run for profit, there is clearly none
or little. But we must bear in mind that nursing, like teaching,
is a function of public service. More and more, for its own
comfort and safety, the community has a stake in the education
of new generations of nurses. Scarcely less disastrous than
exploitation, from this point of view, has been the total ignorance
on the part of hospital trustees of the facts of student training
under their own roofs. To make the facts known, to voice the
needs, the legitimate claims of the school, the obligations of
hospital boards, this is the first need! But whose duty? It
is clearly unreasonable to expect that hospital boards themselves
or hospital superintendents amid their varied responsibilities
should give first consideration to the function and needs of the
training school. On the superintendent of nurses these needs do
press, but as we have shown, she is debarred or has so considered
herself, under present circumstances, from giving them precedence or even from effectively voicing her dilemma. Here, then,
is the need and the rôle in the hospital organization for what
is known as the training school committee.

The Training School Committee

In a later chapter we shall show that the best organization of
a school of nursing is totally separate from the hospital. Hospitals are philanthropic or charitable institutions, raising with
difficulty their own budgets; the school of nursing is educational.
Its management and its endowment should be independent of
the hospital in whose wards the students receive their clinical
training. Since classroom training can best be given in a purely
educational institution, the endowment of university schools of
nursing is an indispensable part of progress in nursing education.
In such schools there would be trained primarily the leaders
of the profession, teachers, supervisors, superintendents of
schools, and public health nurses.[11] There is also the possibility
of the endowment of separate schools of nursing not necessarily
under university auspices but as independent technical schools
of high type, such as Drexel, Pratt, Armour, etc. Such schools
would of course also send their students to the hospitals for
their professional training, and work in close co-operation with
them. Other possible types of organization should, furthermore,
be fully explored, as for example the possibility of a county

[11] See Chapter VII.

school of nursing supported by county funds, making available for the students whatever clinical resources the special geographical area may afford. These resources might of course need to be supplemented by outside affiliations.

But for the present, undoubtedly, the great majority of training schools will retain a close relationship with hospitals, of which they are now departments. It is therefore of paramount importance that the relationship should be at least readjusted in the interest of the minimum claims of education.

In such hospitals, then, as continue to keep the training school as part of the hospital organization, there should be appointed by the board of trustees a training school committee composed of both men and women. This committee is to lay down educational policies, to advise with the head of the school, and above all to represent the school on the board of trustees. Its primary function is to direct education: subcommittees should deal with the budget, the nurses' home, recreation, etc. It should ideally be composed of representatives of the board of trustees and of the medical staff; of persons known to have had experience in education; and of members of the alumnæ of the school. The superintendents of the hospital and of the training school should be *ex officio* members.

The establishment of training school committees, while still comparatively recent, is increasing throughout the country. But for the most part, the composition of these committees at present is totally unsatisfactory. Often the committee is composed wholly of members of the medical staff of the hospital. This is obviously a mistake, since such physicians are commonly not in touch with modern educational movements, and represent, moreover, only one aspect of the school, the nursing service already over-emphasized. Or the committee is often composed wholly of women who have neither educational training, nor sufficient influence with the board of trustees to be of value in representing the school.

Too often the committee is concerned not with the complex educational problems which confront the schools, needing for their solution all the wisdom which can be brought to the principal's aid, but with petty details of management, such as, for instance, the discipline of the students. The discussion of the principles of discipline and student government are clearly within the province of such a committee. "But if I cannot judge how to deal with the mistakes and discipline of the girls better than the busy medical men of whom my committee is composed, I had better resign my position," said to the writer a vigorous and able young superintendent, who had indeed quietly taken into her own effective hands such details formerly solemnly discussed in council.

Too few training school committees meet regularly, and at the frequent intervals which the seriousness of their function demands, to be of real constructive service. Their potential service to the cause of nursing education can scarcely be overestimated, and it is a service urgently needed.

It cannot be too strongly emphasized that the progress that has undeniably been made in nurses' training has been made by the nurses themselves, practically without help and without thanks. If there is today any coherent, any integrated system of training to meet the insistent public demand for nurses, it is owing mainly to the patient, constructive efforts of the heads of training schools, who have stood out against the needs of the moment in the interest of genuine instruction. It has been a progress made in the face of obstacles that would have daunted less resolute enthusiasts, in the face of indifference, of negligence, and of active opposition from those who should have been the first to encourage it. It has been a progress moving squarely against the vested interests of hospitals long in control of the destinies of nursing education. "Ordinarily, the nurse has been a source of profit to the hospital and too often has the training school been exploited for its benefit," says a candid critic of the hospital training school, himself one of the few medical men who have treated the problem of nursing education with vision and sympathy.[12]

Of these vested interests of the hospital and its traditional appropriation of the school as a nursing service purely, we are next to speak.

The Cost of the Training School

FINANCIAL RELATION WITH THE HOSPITAL

We have pointed out the fact that one of the prime duties of the training school committee is to represent the school on the

[12] The University Education of the Nurse. Richard O. Beard, M.D., Professor of Physiology, University of Minnesota. Bulletin V. Published by the Committee on Education of the National League of Nursing Education. November, 1919.

hospital board of trustees, effectually to voice to the board of trustees the financial needs of the school. It is evident that the dilemma of the training school is at bottom a financial one. Its failure—the worst failure of which an educational institution can be guilty—is the failure to teach. Now the cause of this failure is primarily the lack of money, without which the school cannot provide teachers, nor teaching equipment, nor even a place to teach; without which it is impossible to supply the supplementary nursing service to staff the wards while the students are given the classroom instruction that is to accompany, interpret, and illuminate their practical ward training. In a word, without sufficient funds, the wisest educational program must be frustrated.

Under the present system the school as a department of the hospital is given an allowance limited to the barest necessities, as viewed not from the standpoint of education, but of the hospital needs. A single striking instance illustrates this point. In its recent efforts to raise an endowment fund, a leading school of nursing points out that during its 31 years of existence it has grown from 17 to 250 students, and has graduated almost 1,000 nurses. During that period, says the appeal, the school of nursing "has provided through her student body the entire nursing care of the larger number of the 132,589 patients who have been admitted to the hospital." In addition to this it "has provided nursing supervision for the 2,000,000 patients who have come to the dispensary . . . and has extended this supervision beneficially into the homes of many of these patients."

Additional dormitories, the appeal continues, have been provided to meet the steady increase in the number of students. And "almost every year since the hospital was opened has seen either the expansion of existing services or the creation of entirely new ones," such as the psychiatric and the children's departments. "But no additions to any building have been made, no single new class or lecture room or laboratory has been provided, to supply the increased teaching facilities needed. The school outgrew its teaching equipment long ago." It has never been able to afford a librarian or clerical staff, and has urgent need of more teachers and supervisors.[18]

The appeal is careful to state that the hospital of which it is a part has not had resources available to meet these neces-

[18] The School of Nursing of the Johns Hopkins Hospital and a World Need. 1921.

sities of the school; that hospitals in general have great difficulties in meeting their current expenses. It is indeed undeniable that the financing of hospitals is often supremely difficult. Yet funds are found, money public and private is procured for new buildings, new services, new equipment, as a public service indispensable to the community. In the acquisition of funds, the needs—even the irreducible minima—of the training school, as we have shown, have never been adequately voiced even to the hospital board, much less to the general public.

Yet far from weakening the appeal of the hospital for support, the inclusion of the training school's needs would go far to strengthen it. The hospital might wisely capitalize the school as an asset, instead of submerging it. That the appeal for education has not lost its force the successful school and college "drives" of the last few years have demonstrated, the growth of high schools throughout the country testifies. But the hospital board, uninformed of the struggle for education carried on under its own roof and burdened with the direct hospital work in its charge, is undoubtedly losing a legitimate opportunity for greater public support.

The publicity sense which is so admirably exploited in behalf of other needs of the hospital might be as effectively enlisted in behalf of the training school, if the board were in command of the facts, and if the public were aware of its stake in nursing education. For we face here a problem not only of education but of nursing service, and consequently of the public safety or danger. The hospital which uses students for its sole nursing staff, without adequate teaching, supervision, and suitable conditions of living, in effect jeopardizes the lives committed to its charge.

THE BALANCE BETWEEN COST AND SERVICES RENDERED

Now in estimating the cost of the training school to the hospital, it is evident that two sets of figures are needed. First, the total cost of instruction, including maintenance of students as well as tuition; second, the money value of the services rendered by students and staff of the school. Plainly, it is only by striking a balance between these figures that the true cost of the schools can be stated.

The first figures, showing cost of the school, are usually available in the hospital budget; the second, showing income or contribution from the school, by an extraordinary anomaly, are never currently and consecutively kept, even by the leading and most efficiently run hospitals. It would appear a mere matter of course that, in the recent reorganization of hospital cost accounting, the true cost of the training school should be a matter of regular and public record, supplying as the school has, so preponderant an item of hospital expense as the main labor force and nursing personnel for the great majority of patients. But in fact, to the amazement of the lay inquirer, it is only by special study and analysis of its budget that any hospital can today estimate the cost of the training school. The items constituting income or outgo are not even agreed upon. What is the money value to the hospital of the probationer, of the first-, second-, or third-year student? Is she an asset or a liability? What is the money value to the hospital of the ward head nurse and supervisor? In how far would the administrative officers need to be retained with a corps of graduate nurses? Clearly the answer will vary with the organization of the school and with the varying duties assigned to students and supervisors. In hospitals, for instance, in which, as we shall see, the probationer has no regular ward duty, and only a limited amount of simple ward work such as bedmaking, she must be counted almost wholly a liability. In other hospitals where students from the start perform duties otherwise needing paid service, their services should clearly be credited to the school. Yet at what rate? Is the service performed of graduate nurse grade, or of the grade of maid's service, or of that of the trained attendant?

In any true estimate of the school cost, these points and many similar must first be satisfactorily settled. In general the hospital's point of departure must be the cost which *would be* entailed for the nursing service without a school of nursing to draw on.

It has been proposed that student nurses instead of being maintained by the hospital in return for their services, should pay for their board and lodging during training and themselves be paid for services rendered in excess of those which are strictly educational. Such a reorganization, difficult as it may be to work out, may ultimately be accomplished and would undoubtedly react to the advantage of student training. It is obviously, however, a proposal unrealizable at present and probably for many years to come.

THE OBJECTIVES OF TRAINING

Whatever its weakness in organization and errors in educational policy, we yet must return to the clinical facilities of the hospital as the unique field for the training of student nurses. It remains, what Florence Nightingale found it, the incomparable opportunity in its congregation of clinical cases.

Before analyzing in detail the content of the present training and the fundamental reorganization to be recommended, it will be clarifying to set down the objectives of student training and some of its main tendencies. At the outset we should state clearly the type of student under discussion.

Our study of the function of the nurse in public health and private duty has made clear that two types of education are needed: one for the fully trained graduate nurse, the other for a less skilled subsidiary nursing worker. In our subsequent discussion of the nursing aide or attendant, we shall outline the minimum requirements for the education of this worker, who is as much needed in her own field as the fully trained nurse in hers. But the education here at issue is that of the graduate nurse, trained to care for acute disease, capable of carrying out the doctor's orders, giving all manner of nursing treatments to patients in his absence; responsible for the basis of the doctor's judgments, that is, the exact and intelligent reporting of symptoms, often obscure enough; responsible also for meeting emergencies in the doctor's absence; for protecting herself and others from infection; above all, in her rôle of public health nurse, responsible for the teaching of health to the families in her charge, a teaching which rests on the nurse's alertness for all that is divergent from health, in these families and homes.

To meet these objectives, to furnish this equipment, the nurse's training should primarily be aimed to develop certain powers, such as technical skill, observation, mental alertness, judgment, personality. We have already pointed out how the low educational requirements for admission defeat or render impossible the success of professional training. In many states the only educational requirement is completion of one year of high school. This means that the student is too ignorant to grasp the essentials of nursing education. Schooling which has ceased at 14 or 15 years is no preparation for a professional training and fatally handicaps nurses in their later careers. Completion of four years of high school is therefore the minimum on which the course can properly be based.

2. Clinical Facilities in Hospitals of Different Type and Size

It will become evident throughout this report that no single norm can be dictated as obligatory to the various types of hospitals considered. Plainly, large hospitals with rich clinical facilities offer possibilities of training which cannot be duplicated in smaller institutions. Many, indeed, of these latter, comprising as we have seen almost 40 per cent of the total number of schools of nursing (1,800), are maintained by hospitals too small to offer nursing training. In a subsequent chapter we shall raise the question whether, provided the patients are safeguarded by an adequate graduate service, these restricted hospital opportunities might not be utilized for training the less highly skilled nursing aide or attendant increasingly necessary to supplement the expert nursing service.

The adequacy of clinical facilities is of fundamental importance to the equipment of the nurse; they are the laboratory in which the student receives her practical training. Is a given school able to offer students experience in all essential services? Is the experience adequate? Its rank as a teaching field must abide by the answers to these questions, whatever the excellence of its classroom instruction. If training in all major services is provided for, its value must still depend on the guarantee of variety and adequacy afforded by the number of beds they contain or the acuteness of the service.

In attempting briefly to summarize the clinical facilities offered by the hospitals studied we shall take into account not only the four accepted services, medical, surgical, pediatric, and obstetrical, but two services, communicable, and mental and nervous diseases, in which the modern demands on nursing make training increasingly necessary. The fact that 10 in every 100 persons are victims of tuberculosis, that an only slightly smaller percentage suffer from syphilis, to mention only one of the venereal diseases, and that in the state of New York, for instance, one adult out of every 10 enters a state hospital for mental diseases before he dies has made these diseases special points of attack in the public health campaign. The urgency, therefore, of including communicable diseases and mental and nervous diseases in the nurse's training is scarcely open to question. Unfortunately, suitable facilities for training in these services have been and still are very difficult to secure.

CLINICAL FACILITIES OFFERED IN 23 HOSPITALS STUDIED

Eleven schools of our special group provide adequate clinical facilities for student training in the four major services, either in the home hospitals or by affiliation. Five of them offer a more nearly complete teaching field by making in addition provision more or less adequate for training in communicable and in mental and nervous diseases.

Of the major services, pediatrics seems to be most frequently neglected in student training among the hospitals studied. Five schools make either no provision or no adequate provision for a pediatric training service.

All but one of the 23 hospitals provide more or less adequate facilities for training in obstetrics, either at the parent hospital or by affiliation. It is a growing practice in this department to estimate the student's experience not by number of beds or length of service, but by the number of deliveries at which she has assisted. Such a measure is a long step towards standardizing the nurse's obstetrical training, and should be adopted by every school.

Five hospitals of our group offer clinical opportunities for training in mental and nervous diseases. One of these maintains too small a department to be adequate as a teaching field; the others have services ranging from 27 to 312 beds.

About two-thirds of the 23 hospitals of our group offer student training in communicable diseases. This is provided for in several ways. Eight hospitals maintain communicable disease services of their own of suitable size for training, or supplement their own facilities by arranging affiliations for at least part of their students; 8 more give training in communicable diseases by means of the contagious cases cared for in pediatric services of varying size, or further, in one or two instances, by skin or tuberculosis services. Nearly a third of the group (7) offer no practical experience in this essential branch of student training.

But the value of clinical facilities for student training does not depend wholly on the range of services offered or on their adequate size. Another index of their value in training at any hospital may be found, as we have already indicated, in the acuteness of the several services. Thus a service of large bed capacity occupied chiefly by chronic patients may be of less value educationally than a service of fewer beds which affords opportunity for the study of the acute stages of disease. The character of the services, whether active and acute or preponderantly chronic, will be found to depend somewhat upon the type and size of hospital in question.

TYPE AND SIZE OF HOSPITALS STUDIED

On a previous page of this report (page 190), we have already shown the hospitals of our study to be divided into certain typical groups: municipal hospitals, large private general hospitals, small private general hospitals, special hospitals, and university hospitals. The type of clinical facilities presented by each group is roughly characteristic of schools similarly organized throughout the country.

MUNICIPAL HOSPITALS

The 4 municipal hospitals included in this study have a total bed capacity utilized for training ranging from about 500 to 2,000 beds. Clinical facilities are offered in the four major services, medical, surgical, obstetric, and pediatric, abundant enough to insure a well-rounded student training. Two of the 4 offer in addition training in nervous and mental service; 3, excellent facilities in communicable disease; and 2, a fairly good experience in dispensary work. The high value of these hospitals as a training field, with their relative completeness of service and the richness and range of clinical material naturally presented by their large numbers, is limited by two things: the tendency to large chronic services, of little benefit to student training, and the common understaffing and lack of supervision which results in overwork, careless technique, and lack of case study. On the other hand, the waste of time in the large private services maintained by private hospitals is eliminated in municipal institutions.

LARGE PRIVATE GENERAL HOSPITALS

The 10 large private hospitals of our study, with a bed capacity utilized for training ranging from 150 to 621 beds, offer for the most part excellent facilities for training in major services. The preponderance of surgical over medical beds in this type of hospital leads naturally, however, to the over-emphasis of surgical experience already noted in this report. Student training in these schools has not the drawback [14] of large chronic services as at the municipal hospitals, and the smaller bed capacity is compensated for by the greater activity and acuteness of the services. Thus, in this group, the average stay per patient ranges in the several hospitals, in proportion to the activity of their services, from 12 to 19 days. In half these hospitals the stay was less than 2 weeks (13½ days). At the municipal hospitals of our study, the average stay ranges from 12 to 32 days, the midpoint for these hospitals being 22½ days or more than a week longer than the average stay shown by the private group. A disadvantage to training, on the other hand, is the high proportion of private service with its limited educational value.

Seven of these schools are maintained by hospitals of notably high medical and surgical standards, of which 2 are affiliated with medical schools and 3 used as teaching fields for medical students. One of the 7 offers an adequate teaching field for mental and nervous diseases; 1 has a communicable disease service of sufficient size for training, the 6 others supplying this training in large part through the pediatric service and but 1 of them offering an elective affiliation for communicable disease training in the senior year. In 3, obstetrical service is given by affiliation.

Three schools of this group, with access to respective hospital capacities of 150, 250, and 300 beds, are markedly inferior to the others of the group in the training offered. They are indeed not representative, like most of the others, of the best schools of the country, but representative rather of schools least fitted in clinical or educational facilities to train students. At these hospitals the surgical services preponderate over the medical in the proportion of 3 to 1. They maintain no communicable disease service, no separate pediatric service which might take its place, or a negligible one, no nervous and mental service, and in one case, even, no obstetrical service and no affiliation to take its place. Obviously, an extensive system of affiliation is needed before such schools as these can offer adequate training.

SMALL PRIVATE GENERAL HOSPITALS

The 5 small private general hospitals included in our group, with a capacity of 50 to 150 beds, are also representative of the inferior schools of the country. In these an adequate basic training even in the major services is by no means assured to

[14] With one exception.

the students. Three small schools make no separation of medical and surgical wards and no permanent assignments of beds within the two services to men or women. As the great majority of hospital cases are surgical, there can scarcely in these hospitals be any but the most meager facilities for training in the medical service. In the surgical service, moreover, the shifting numbers of men and women patients make a student's experience in gynecological or genito-urinary nursing highly uncertain. Adequate facilities for training are wanting also in this group in pediatrics and obstetrics. None of the 5 provides training in mental and nervous diseases; 1, by affiliation, provides an excellent experience in communicable disease service.

These small schools labor under the disadvantage for student training of an even larger relative assignment of beds to private service than do the larger private schools. In the previous group, the hospital with the median number of private beds gave over 25 per cent of its total bed capacity to private service. This is the highest percentage generally held to be compatible with good training, but 5 hospitals exceeded this mid-point and the maximum assignment was 36 per cent. In the present group of smaller hospitals, the median number of beds in private service is 30 per cent of the total bed capacity, with a maximum rising to 53 per cent.

It is worthy of note that 2 of these schools offering so inadequate a training in the fundamental services nevertheless require a 2-months' course in public health nursing, while a third offers the service as an elective to a small group of students. It is scarcely necessary to point out the fallacy of attempting to give training in a nursing specialty to students wholly unable to profit by the experience in view of their lack of grounding in the basic clinical services.

SPECIAL HOSPITALS

Two special hospitals included in this study attempt at present to give a 3-years' course in general nursing. At one of these, a maternity hospital caring for obstetrical and gynecological patients only, students spend 2 years and 3 months of their course, while 9 months (the maximum allowance) spent in affiliations at two other hospitals constitutes their only opportunity for training in all other essential services. The other, a children's hospital, trains students in its own specialty for all of its course but 11 months, into which it crowds preliminary teaching at an allied college and affiliated training in general adult services. Practically no training is offered by either school in communicable diseases and none in nervous and mental service.

Such schools thus require a student to spend more than 2 years in a specialty which in a well-balanced, course would take from 4 to 6 months' training. This more than dubious procedure from the educational view-point is in sharp contrast to the practice of two other special hospitals which make no attempt to maintain courses in general nursing but offer a highly specialized training to affiliates. To provide training of high grade in their specialty for students from general nursing schools, —such should be *par excellence* the function of the special hospital in nursing education.

Of the 2 university schools studied, one, with a capacity of 850 beds, offers clinical facilities as complete and abundant as those afforded by any of the municipal hospitals. The other hospital, with a much smaller bed capacity (190 beds), offers a teaching field in the four major services but makes no provision for nervous and mental training except through such cases as may occur in the medical service, and gives training in communicable diseases only through the pediatric department, the skin cases in the medical service, and an affiliation for tuberculosis offered as an elective to all seniors.

In schools of this type it should be noted that defects of clinical facilities are largely compensated for by an improved use of material for training. Case study is made the general basis of student assignments, and even the limited material afforded by the smaller hospital is made more valuable for training by means of careful selection than the larger facilities of many schools less advanced in educational methods.

CONCLUSIONS

It is evident from this brief summary that many of the schools, even in our picked group, are unfitted, as at present conducted, to offer a 3-years' nursing course. It is evident also that only by an extension of the system of affiliations already successfully in operation in certain services can hospitals with limited clinical facilities make good their missing types of experience.   Elsewhere in this report we shall discuss at greater length the possible solutions of the problem of the smaller schools.

The elimination of the schools least fitted to survive, a country-wide extension of affiliations with special hospitals such as maternity and children's hospitals, institutions for mental and nervous cases, for tuberculosis, etc., and the restriction of these special hospitals to training in their specialty would go far to standardize nursing training.   It would preclude on the one hand the present widely differing equipment of nurses, many of whom are now, unknown to the public, without experience in essential services; it would obviate the over-emphasis of specialties now incident to training at special hospitals.   Lastly, in place of their own student service, now provided at the expense of a one-sided training, it would supply the special hospitals with service by consecutive groups of affiliates from different schools.   We postpone to a subsequent chapter discussion of the permanent graduate staff without which no student service can be maintained at a proper educational level.

In the light of these primary considerations, let us now consider in detail the actual nursing training given, or approximated to, in the 1,800 schools of the country.

3.   Entrance Requirements

EDUCATION

In regard to the educational requirements of the training schools, the Bureau of Education report on these schools for the year 1917-1918 shows a striking decrease between 1911 and 1918 in the number of schools requiring the full high school course for entrance, but as marked a rise in the number requiring one or two years of high school.   Thus, of 1,592 training schools affording data, the percentage requiring the completion of high school fell from 40.6 in 1911 to 28.1 in 1918.   On the other hand the percentage of schools requiring one year of high school work for entrance rose in the same period from 24 to 42.7, and the percentage requiring two years from 3.3 to 16.5.[15]

In the limited group of our study, 23 training schools reporting gave the following data on minimum entrance requirements:

[15] U. S. Department of the Interior, Bureau of Education.   Bulletin No. 73, 1919.   Nurse Training Schools, 1917-18.   Page 36.   (Advance Sheets from the Biennial Survey of Education in the United States, 1916-1918.)

13 training schools required 4 years of high school
3 "   "   "   2 "   "   "   "
6 "   "   "   1 "   "   "   "
1 training school reports that it attempts to meet
the state requirement of one year of high school.

Of the 13 schools requiring four years of high school, 2 university training schools required, one, college matriculation, and one, an added preliminary course.

We have called attention to the fact that the inclusion of a number of training schools of the first rank, raises our group decidedly above the average. We should therefore expect to find the educational equipment of entering students above the entrance requirements of the rank and file of the country's schools. To tally with the entrance requirements of the 23 schools here considered, the percentage of their students qualified for college entrance should be about 56. How many of these students exceed the entrance requirements is indicated, however, by the fact that of 2,082 reporting from a total of 23 schools the high percentage of 78.2 had had four years of high school or its equivalent, and were qualified therefore for college entrance. This figure is raised by the fact that all students were qualified in the schools requiring completion of high school, and that in 3 others the number qualified rose above 90 per cent.

At the lower end of the scale, the percentage of high school graduates in some of the smaller schools fell as low as 15 and 22, and at three schools conducted under sectarian auspices ranged between the figures of 25 and 36.6.

Even in our selected group of schools, then, it must be emphasized that some 22 per cent of the students were not high school graduates, and fell below, therefore, what should be the minimum requirement for the nurse's professional training. For the completion of but one or two years of high school leaves the student too ignorant to grasp many of the essentials of this training, and handicaps her heavily in her whole future career.

That the schools themselves realize the need of adequate schooling as a basis for the training course, is shown by the fact that in various states in which too low a standard is specified by law (viz. one or two years of high school), this standard is voluntarily exceeded by various schools. Of the 23 schools of our study, only 7 merely met the varying state requirements; 15 exceeded the state requirements by from one year to four years;

11 exceeded by three years the requirement of one year of high school.

Thirteen of our training schools numbered college graduates among their students. The percentage of these for all schools was 9.1, the figures in certain schools rising as high as 16.3, 17.8, and 22.5. These high figures were undoubtedly greatly influenced by the presence of members of the Vassar Training Camp in the hospitals studied.

AGE

According to the survey of training schools made by the Federal Bureau of Education for 1916-1918, over 40 per cent (42.9 per cent) of the 1,700 schools reporting, maintained by general hospitals, required 18 years of age for admission. Over 70 per cent (70.5 per cent) required either 18 or 19 years.[16] An earlier report on training schools, that of 1911, showed that about the same proportion of schools (71.7 per cent) at that time required 20 or 21 years as the age of admission. Thus, in the space of seven years, the age requirement for entrance has been lowered two years.

In the selected group of our present study, of 23 training schools affording information, an even higher proportion, 86 per cent, required 18 or 19 years for admission. The age requirements were distributed as follows. Of the 23 hospitals,

> 12 required 18 years for admission,
> 8 "   19   "   "   "
> 2 "   20   "   "   "
> 1 "   21   "   "   "

Of the students actually in training at these 23 schools (to the number of 1,993 for whom data were secured), 46 per cent were under 21 years of age, 35 per cent were between 21 and 25, and 19 per cent were over 25 years of age at entrance. Thus, over half of the superior group of schools studied required 18 years for admission. Nevertheless 3 schools of high standing still retained the older age requirement.

It is important to remember in this connection that 18 years is the normal age of graduation from high school. To recruit students, it is therefore important that, with completion of high school required for entrance, the age of admission to training should coincide with the age of graduation.

[16] Op. cit. Page 21.

TUITION FEES AND ALLOWANCES

It has been the tradition of the school of nursing not only to make no charge for tuition, uniform, board and lodging, etc., but to give the student in addition to her training, equipment, and living, a monthly money allowance. This practice is a surviving mark of the apprenticeship system out of which nursing as a professional training is slowly evolving. Schools of more advanced educational standards tend increasingly on the other hand to omit these allowances and to charge tuition fees. Thus in the picked group of our study, of 21 schools affording information, one-third charge tuition or require some fee at least for the preliminary period.

One school affiliated for its classroom instruction with a neighboring technical college charges $100 for the preliminary term and $100 for each subsequent year. Other schools ask fees for the preliminary term only; 2 of high standing charge $50,[17] 2 others $25, and 2 others still a so-called "breakage fee" of $10. Two further schools charging no tuition fees but making no money allowance bring the number discarding such allowances up to 9.

Of the 12 remaining schools all pay money allowances to their students, ranging in amount from $4 to $15 a month, frequently in an ascending scale from year to year. The largest sums are paid by the municipal hospitals; these allowances mounting as high as $150 or in one case $190 in addition to room, board, and laundry.

How little the giving of allowances counts in the group of schools studied as an inducement to candidates and how little the charging of tuition acts as a deterrent is shown by the relatively large enrolment of students in the schools charging tuition and making no allowances. The better educational and living advantages appear to outweigh the comparatively small money inducement in attracting candidates of good calibre.

PREVIOUS PAID OCCUPATIONS OF STUDENTS

From 15 schools with records of the paid occupations of their students previous to entrance, it appears that about half of the total number enrolled (1,200) had worked before entering training. About two-fifths of those previously employed (41.8 per

---

[17] One of these charges also a breakage fee of $10; this is repaid the student if there are no charges against her on her leaving the school.

cent) had been teachers, a profession with no high age requirement for candidates, though requiring educational qualifications, a profession, too, whose need for recruits is systematically made known to high school students. Somewhat over two-fifths (46.7 per cent) of the students reporting had been in wage-earning occupations, largely clerical, industrial, etc. The remainder (11.5 per cent) had been employed in occupations more closely allied to nursing which may have given them an interest in the subject, that is, as doctors' or dentists' assistants, as governesses or children's nurses, in social welfare, etc.

Number of Groups Entering Yearly

One of the obstacles to efficient teaching in the training schools is the surviving tradition of admitting candidates at almost any time in the year. It is common to admit groups of probationers three times, four times, five times, six times a year, and not infrequently even oftener. The number of groups actually permitted to enter each year at 20 schools of our group affording data is shown in the following table. It is significant that the school allowing candidates to enter 10 times during the year, or almost every month, is also the school that clings closest to the apprenticeship system.

Number of Groups Entering Each Year at 20 Training Schools

Number of Training Schools	Number of Groups Entering Yearly
6	2
4	3
4	4
1	5
3	6
1	7
1	10
20	

Under the apprenticeship system it may be possible to teach students satisfactorily who are all or nearly all at different stages of training. A very different situation exists where a professional education has been evolved, depending on class instruction as well as on experience in the wards. It has long been an accepted academic practice to admit students to schools or colleges twice in the year, and it is customary either to begin new courses at the half year, or so to plan longer ones that new students may enter them without serious handicap to themselves or appreciable detriment to the older students in the class. But it is not within educational possibilities so to arrange a course that it can be interrupted repeatedly by the entrance of new students and still serve their best interests and those of the older students as well. The foregoing table shows that two-thirds (14) of the 20 schools reporting allow students to enter more frequently than the two times yearly sanctioned by success-ful academic practice.

An extreme example taken from one of our municipal hospitals may suggest the wide-spread damage to teaching that results from this system. Here, after completing a short preliminary course as probationers, students enter the advanced class in anatomy and physiology at whatever point the class may have reached. This course continues for nine months, and, as pro-bation classes may enter the school at seven different times dur-ing the year, it is evident that the course may be interrupted by the entrance of new groups of students no less than seven times. As no pedagogical ingenuity could adapt a well-taught course to such conditions, it is perhaps as well that the instructor at this school is conscious of no difficulty, and remarks somewhat naïvely that it "makes no difference in anatomy, as one part is not dependent on another."

Credits for Advanced Standing in Nursing Schools

From our brief statement of the entrance requirements of the schools and the actual preparation of candidates it is clear that students entering nursing training represent very different de-grees of education, ranging all the way from the unformed girl with a year or two of high school to the normal school, college or university graduate who in certain schools constitutes already so large a percentage of the student body. It is a mere matter of justice that some adjustment shall be made whereby a girl with a thorough college training, for example in science, shall not be obliged to spend unprofitable hours in a comparatively elementary course in the nursing school. It is scarcely less obviously fair that there should be some allowance for previous training in the case of a student, who after a year or two of work at some training school of good standing desires for ade-quate reasons to continue her course and seek her diploma at another.

Such adjustments will naturally tend to be made rather on

the merits of individual cases than by hard and fast rule, in view of the wide variation in the quality of college courses, and the diversity of methods and standards in training schools.

CREDITS FOR COLLEGE COURSES OR COLLEGE DEGREES

As a matter of fact, the tendency is general in the nursing schools to give credit for college work in required subjects. Of 13 schools giving detailed information in the matter, almost all (11) give credit for subjects covered in college courses. Of the 2 remaining schools, one is a school of the highest standing, with an unusually large proportion of college graduates among its students. It allows as a rule no advanced standing for college courses. Exceptions have been made, but in the experience of the school, the students, it is stated, prefer to repeat the work in required subjects.

It is much less general to give specific credit for college degrees, though the view is not infrequently held that the training involved in a college course, irrespective of the subjects studied, deserves some recognition and some abatement of the length of time required in the nursing school. Only 7 of the 13 schools affording data definitely state that they give such credit. Eight schools for which data on this point are unavailable are situated in a state where the law provides "that college graduates may be granted an advance credit of eight months in nursing practice in the training schools."

Though in general, as we have noted, the assignment of credits is governed according to the merits of the individual case rather than by any fixed rule, it is nevertheless of interest to see by one or two concrete examples what credit for advanced standing may amount to at individual schools and according to what standards it may be granted. Thus at a prominent municipal hospital school, credit, which is granted "at the discretion of the superintendent," may amount to a curtailment of six months of the required training course. "The requirements for graduation," according to the school statement, "are based on a system of credits for academic work" which "would permit a student to complete the course in a minimum period of 30 months." At a representative school in the East a college degree in science may cut down a student's nursing course by a full year; a degree in Arts by nine months; a shorter time in college by lessening credits.

CREDITS FOR PREVIOUS EXPERIENCE

Credit is less commonly granted for previous training than for ground covered in college classroom or laboratory. This is due to the unstandardized condition of technique in the training schools and the natural feeling that a school can guarantee only its own teaching methods. Out of 18 schools reporting, only 11 grant credit for experience. In certain cases the responsibility for such decisions is taken out of the hands of the schools; 6 of the 11 just quoted, for example, are located in a state where the Board of Examiners passes on the question of whether experience in one school is worthy of credit in another.

4. The Period of Preliminary Instruction and Probation

The subject to which we must next give attention, a subject which is still one of the vexed problems of nursing education, is the disposition of the student's time during the first three to six months of training often known as the preliminary term. How shall the prospective nurse be introduced to her actual subject matter? How shall she learn to nurse?

Here we have on the one hand a student, inexpert and ignorant of the new world she is to enter, at best an eager learner; on the other hand, what is known in the slang of the medical profession as the "clinical material" of the hospital, in its wards, clinics, and dispensary. What instruction is needed before an inexperienced girl can be entrusted with even the simplest care of human beings singularly dependent by helplessness or suffering on her skill, sympathy, and judgment? Shall she be introduced at once to the wards, and learn as an apprentice by working under her elders? Such has been the system in large part in the past, and such it remains in many hospital training schools. For, as we have seen, it is only within a comparatively short time that the teaching of nursing has been to any degree differentiated from apprenticeship, and been placed in part on a sounder educational basis.

DISADVANTAGES OF THE APPRENTICESHIP SYSTEM

Gradually it has become apparent that the old system is a slow and cumbrous method of education; that it often has not even the virtues of a true apprenticeship wherein pupils work directly under the eye of a master. For in the hospital ward the immediate superior of the new student is the head nurse, responsible for the management of the ward unit, large or small according to circumstances. Her duties are principally executive; as a teacher she is rarely equipped. With the best teaching equipment, she must in any case, after satisfying the imperative claims of ward management, have but the scantiest margin of time or attention available for the students. Often, indeed, she is herself a student learning administration, the practical running of a ward with its countless details as to supplies, assignment of nurses, household management, etc. How under such circumstances shall the new-comer be really taught; learn not only the practice but the principles of nursing to guide her in the emergencies which are a part of all serious illness, principles equally essential in her future work of prevention and health teaching?

It is true that even under the old system of training now slowly being superseded, the superintendent of nurses or her assistant spends some time on the wards in teaching new nurses and also devotes some hours each week off the wards to instruction in elementary subjects. But if the head nurses are too much absorbed by administrative duties to have any adequate time for teaching, this is no less true of their superiors who are responsible for the whole nursing service of the hospital.

Moreover, when no regular provision is made in the students' schedule for such class instruction, when lessons or lectures are merely added to a full day's hard work, it is clear that little profit can accrue. The physical demands of their duties, the early hour of rising, the unaccustomed hours of standing, and the consequent excessive fatigue of girls entering upon a new and arduous career make study a farce. They might better be asleep in bed than half asleep in the classroom.

Health suffers as well as study. Few reliable statistics are available on the morbidity of student nurses, as shown by their days of absence from duty. But it is well established that absence from duty is most common during the first year; that the common ailments of the new-comers, such as flat-foot and other trouble with the feet due to long standing, throat trouble such as tonsilitis or laryngitis, are most common to the early months of training.

THE PRELIMINARY TERM

Accordingly, in the best schools (and increasingly even in those less good), a preliminary period is being introduced with a larger amount of time allowed for systematic classroom instruction in elementary nursing and allied subjects before any care of patients is required or permitted.   Of 23 training schools 22 had a preliminary period of some kind, varying from two to six months, with at least 110 hours of classroom instruction, and with hours on the wards varying from two to eight.   The movement for the preliminary term, though still rudimentary in the country at large, is well established.   In an unpublished survey of schools in a western state it was found that of 48 training schools, 13 or more than a quarter had such a term.

The Period of Probation

It must be remembered that besides being a period of preliminary instruction, this term is also designed to serve as a period of probation.   It is generally known that candidates do not enter the training school at once as undergraduates, but are accepted as probationers during a specified period of some months.

During this time they are to prove their fitness, in health and calibre, for their future work.   This is and should be a period of genuine probation, testing the metal of the prospective student through hard and often distasteful manual work, initiating her into the ways of an institution where discipline is demanded by the ever-present issues of life and death.

A Program for the Preliminary Term

A successful educational program for the preliminary term has still to be achieved, and leading schools are only at the beginning of experiments testing how best to use the time.   Unquestionably, the essential step forward is taken when probationers are not given regular ward duties, and are not obliged to waste their time in merely "picking up" nursing technique without preliminary study.   The problem is to afford these young students sufficient contact with patients to give point to their classroom studies, and not so much ward work that it must necessarily, owing to their inexperience, be merely routine repetition of disagreeable duties to relieve the older nurses.

According to the newer system with the preliminary term, the general plan followed, at least in theory, is somewhat as follows: Either at their very entrance upon training or after one or more weeks of classroom instruction, the probationers are sent on the wards for routine manual work and some practice of easy procedures, usually at first for a period of several hours a day which is later increased to full-time duty. This arrangement, though an appreciable advance on the apprenticeship system, is still far from an ideal or even an intelligently graded training. Too much time and energy is still spent in routine service, "to get the work done." As we shall presently see, in merely practising on the wards under supervision the lessons learned and first practised in the classroom, from cleaning and polishing service rooms to bed-making and simple nursing procedures, there is ample opportunity for all the hard manual work and repetition of tasks which the probationer needs to test her spirit and to render her automatically perfect in her duties. Indeed the repeated performance of manual tasks, which later in her career is wasteful and serves only to delay her education, may be for the probationer an essential part of her training. But for the probationer, as well as for the older student, the test of the reasonableness of her duties should clearly be their educational value.

At other hospitals the practical training outside the classroom is confined to work which amounts to no more than pure maid's service, in such departments as the diet kitchen or surgical supply room. The principle underlying this division of duties is to postpone introducing probationers to the wards until a later point in classroom instruction, and to vary their practical experience. But such an arrangement is evidently open to abuse, and the probationers' time is as plainly misused as in excessive ward work when they spend weeks in making surgical dressings for the hospital which they could learn to make in a week, or waste months in the diet kitchen preparing salads for private patients, cooking in quantity for the wards, or cleaning vegetables.

Such time is worse than wasted, for the unreasonableness and monotony of such assignments naturally tends to chill the beginner's enthusiasm and responsiveness in the first flush of interest in her new career. She loses even the stimulus of actual contact with patients, the incomparable personal appeal of her profession, which at least was offered under the old apprenticeship system.

An effort to preserve this stimulus, and yet to release the students from the fatigue of ward duty in the interest of better study has been made at a well-known school connected with a university. Here two- to four-month periods of classroom instruction are made to alternate with equal periods of ward duty, not only in the preliminary term but later in the course, though even during the classroom periods students are sent back to the hospital for one or two half-days a week. A defect of this particular experiment lies in the fact that four months of work on the wards precede any instruction in the basic sciences.

In many schools the turnover of probationers is high, rising to 50 per cent of the entering class. It it doubtless inevitable that even under a reorganized system there should always be a certain proportion of withdrawals, some girls failing to meet the test of probation owing to temperamental or physical unfitness. But this normal percentage is undoubtedly heightened by the ill-considered training and the unnecessary hardships of the preliminary term.

On the other hand the withdrawal of probationers is unquestionably due in large part to the present low standards of entrance requirements which admit to many hospitals candidates obviously incapable of training.

We may now take up in detail the subject common to all schools in the first year, that is, the teaching of nursing procedures.

5. The Teaching of Nursing Procedures

Their Central Importance

Nursing procedures include all the simple duties of daily nursing care as well as the nursing treatments for the cure or prevention of disease which the doctor prescribes and for the performance of which the nurse is, usually in the doctor's absence, responsible. The procedures thus range upward in difficulty and responsibility, from such simple matters as bed-making according to hospital standards, through the daily activities of bathing and feeding patients and keeping them comfortable in bed, taking temperature, pulse, and respiration, to the more advanced procedures such as hot and cold packs, stupes, douches, various forms of irrigations each with its own technique, catheterization, taking cultures or blood for tests, operating room technique, and the care of obstetrical patients, charting, etc.

Obviously, the degree of responsibility involved in these treatments varies with the severity of the disease: in dangerous cases even a simple procedure such as taking the pulse may require a high order of skill and judgment. Upon the nurse's accuracy in observing symptoms and keeping records, the doctor's diagnosis, basis of all treatments, may be dependent; on the adequate performance of the nursing duties life or death may hang.

The teaching of practical procedures is thus in a sense the center of the nurse's training, the basis of her future professional usefulness. Indeed the "theory and practice of nursing," as this subject is usually called, is more far-reaching and inclusive than appears at first sight. For in it are implicit practically all the other important subjects of the nurse's curriculum.

In the practical procedures the nurse *applies* concretely all her other teaching: broadly speaking, it is only for such concrete application that the rest of the curriculum exists at all, that the nurse must have instruction, first, in the preliminary sciences, and later, in a wide range of professional subjects, such as the nature and treatment of disease, the symptoms to be watched for, the drugs to be administered, and the effects to be observed and recorded.

To provide the necessary conditions for teaching the theory and practice of nursing is therefore a prime requisite of the training school. Many different methods of instruction are used, varying from the most haphazard, unworthy the name of instruction, to carefully graded courses, correlating after the preliminary period instruction in the nature and treatment of disease with the study of nursing technique begun in the preliminary term. From a study of the various methods encountered in different types of hospitals, the main points in the teaching of nursing procedures emerge clearly enough, and owing to the central interest of the subject they will be treated in some detail.

System of Teaching

When well taught, instruction in this subject consists of four stages:

1. Class work, in which the teacher describes and demonstrates the procedure in question, beginning usually with bed-making.
2. Demonstration of the same procedure by the students, generally known as "demonstration back."
3. Practice by the students between lessons, preferably under careful supervision.
4. Practice on the wards, under supervision of the teacher or her assistants, of what the student has learned in the classroom.

Not until she has successfully passed through these four stages is she regularly assigned to give even the simplest care to patients independently. The teacher certifies to the head nurse in writing exactly what treatments the new student is capable of performing, and until so certified she is not allowed to perform any.

From this brief outline of the four stages of training, it is evident that for the adequate teaching of the theory and practice of nursing there are minimum requirements which may in turn be summarized. There are needed:

An instructor who shall have proper assistance in the use of material;

A demonstration room with adequate equipment and supplies;

Approved methods of class teaching with demonstration by instructor and students;

Opportunity for practice between lessons;

Prompt application of class teaching on the wards under careful supervision;

A certificate of fitness for each procedure learned.

In contrast to these minimum requirements, we shall find that, while excellences along one line or another are variously found in the hospitals studied, few or none provide all the necessary conditions for successfully teaching this subject.

INSTRUCTORS

It would seem self-evident that in this central subject of the nurse's training, a subject demanding for its proper treatment such prolonged hours of instruction, demonstration, and supervision, and fraught as it is with heavy responsibilities, the instructor should be free from other claims to devote herself to her teaching. Yet in more than half of the training schools giving information on this point, nursing theory and practice is taught by an administrative officer of the hospital whose executive duties must in case of conflict take precedence over the demands of instruction. Of 17 training schools, nursing classes in 10 were taught either by the superintendent (1), the acting superintendent (2), an assistant superintendent (5), or by a head nurse [18]

[18] It should be noted that the combination of practical instructor and head nurse while a difficult one, proving for the most part unadvisable in practice, has its advocates because of the opportunity it offers for careful and effective supervision, good correlation, and standardized technique. This is deliberately planned at the 2 training schools spoken of. On the other hand, with management as her primary responsibility, it seems impossible that the instructor's classroom work should not be

(2). It is impossible under such conditions that the claims of student training shall not be sacrificed to the immediate urgencies of the hospital service. The training in nursing procedures, which should be the focus of the whole education of the student nurse, can be safe from interruption, irregularity, and forced slighting, only by the appointment of a special full-time instructor.

At smaller hospitals, such as we have in the main so far referred to, the appointment of special instructors may seem in view of financial difficulties a counsel of perfection, yet it marks clearly, as has been pointed out, a step in the evolution of a professional training from the earlier and more casual type of nurse's education.

The 7 remaining schools—3 large, 3 small, and 1 of medium size—have teachers of practical nursing whose primary business it is to teach. They may not be always teachers of high grade. At one municipal hospital the nursing instructor had, at the time of inspection, held her position a few weeks only, was not a high school graduate, and had never taught before; she was moreover expected to teach an elementary science class as well as her classes in nursing practice. But the gain in principle of an arrangement which allows a teacher to concentrate upon her teaching work remains a great one. Two of the 7 hospitals, and one of them a small one, have recently appointed full-time teachers of practical nursing. At several others there is one instructor in elementary nursing procedures or general nursing practice and another or others for advanced courses, special branches, or for review.

One of these schools has the honorable distinction of employing the services of two exceptionally well-equipped teachers in its practical nursing course. One of them, who is also assistant director of nurses, is a normal college graduate and holds also a degree in teaching. The other, who carries the larger share of the practical instruction, holds the same pedagogical degree.

ASSISTANCE IN THE USE OF PRACTICE MATERIAL

In teaching which involves the use of so much demonstration and practice material as the classes in nursing procedures, the

hampered by her administrative duties. At one of these training schools, it is planned that the head nurse of the adjoining ward shall relieve the head nurse-instructor for her classroom duties.

expense of time and effort demanded in its care, in taking out, clearing up, and putting it away, is inevitably very great. Even if we discount the instances where material must be collected from the wards or brought over from the hospital when the demonstration room is situated in another building, the tax on time and energy is very considerable. It would seem only reasonable for the training school to provide some paid assistance for such largely mechanical service in the interest of the instructor's time and strength, which should surely be conserved for the essential purposes of her work.

Yet in but one of the 20 training schools offering data is good paid assistance furnished,—a private hospital where an intelligent "maid on classrooms" helps in preparing material for the classes and in afterwards putting it away with the assistance of the students.

In another large training school the nursing instructor is relieved of the care of demonstration material by her two student assistant teachers and by the students in her classes. These assistants place a list of needed articles on the board; the students get them out, prepare them for demonstration, and put them away.

But in the majority of cases, the main burden is carried by the instructor, a state of things unfortunately too common to arouse comment. At 17 out of 20 schools the instructor prepares the material alone; at 5 she does the whole work of clearing up and putting away material as well. At 2 she has occasional assistance, and at 4 others regular assistance from her students in putting things away. At the remaining 7 schools the students are made responsible for putting away material after class, and at one of them they even assist the instructor in preparation.

The extent to which a teacher's time may be exploited in such unconsidered mechanical service may be seen by way of extreme example at a training school constituting a department of a large university. Here a thoroughly able instructor is said to spend often 2 to 3 hours in preparing material for class because of the necessity of assembling equipment and supplies left scattered by the students. The waste of an expert's time on work which could equally well be performed by an intelligent maid must revenge itself by lowered efficiency in the duties where an expert is irreplaceable.

We have spoken of the waste of the instructor's services. But the fact that the only relief afforded her in 19 cases out of 20 comes from the students is also in need of comment. It should be remembered that time spent by the students in the routine care of material beyond the minimum advisable for training is time lost from an educational point of view and further emphasizes the need of paid assistance.

PROVISION OF A DEMONSTRATION ROOM

The successful teaching of the theory and practice of nursing depends largely on the character of the facilities provided for instruction. A special demonstration room is one of the primary needs.

Where there is no special room, recourse must be had to the best substitute. The resourcefulness of the teacher may enable her to make good use of makeshifts, to teach the students good technique in a general classroom, in a room off the ward, or in any other place which is available. But it is readily evident that such teaching is precarious and may be interrupted by any contingency, that the lack of a special demonstration room impedes teaching in one way or another, interferes with the storing of adequate supplies, and above all makes undue demands on the teacher's time and strength in improvising what under good management should be regularly available. While therefore good teaching may be done without the special demonstration room, no training school should hold itself justified for being without one.

Undoubtedly in teaching nursing, as in any other applied science, a mechanical efficiency alone is worthless. Demonstration room, equipment, and supplies may all be of standard perfection and the teaching may yet be routine and devoid of the spirit without which it can never produce fine nursing. A mechanical efficiency may even be damaging if it leads to a lessened emphasis on the student's personal care and consideration for patients. Fortunately it is not an alternative which confronts us: the emphasis is safe in the hands of the good teacher, and it is clearly the combination of good teacher plus good equipment which is the desideratum.

At half of the training schools studied, large and well-lighted special rooms are provided for demonstration. Ideal conditions for teaching are offered at a school connected with an eminent private hospital where an entire ward unit, occupying a floor of the newest hospital building, is in use as a demonstration room.[19] The ward setting is reproduced at 2 other schools. Demonstration rooms elsewhere, not so complete, imitate at least some features of the model ward; thus, a training school connected with another municipal hospital has a "well-equipped service room, reproducing a ward service room, adjoining its demonstration room."

Other hospitals provide demonstration rooms of varying merits and defects. At only 2 schools offering data on this point are the special rooms provided too small and crowded to be adequate.

Six of the training schools under consideration provide no separate demonstration room. One special hospital makes no attempt to replace it and does all practical teaching on the wards. At another training school a large assembly room, formerly the chapel, now serves a variety of purposes and among them that of nursing classes. At 4 other hospitals the instructor must teach nursing procedures as best she may in the general classroom used for all, or nearly all, of the other classes. In one case, at least, the room is "crowded with material" used in connection with other courses.[20]

EQUIPMENT OF THE DEMONSTRATION ROOM

For teaching nursing procedures adequate equipment and supplies are also essential, such as running water to teach proper cleaning of utensils, etc.; a gas or electric stove, bed, crib, blackboard for graphic descriptions, desks for the students, and a sufficient supply of linen, rubber gloves and sheets, glassware, and drugs.

Even good demonstration rooms are not always well-equipped. Of the 10 schools furnished with good special rooms for demonstration, only 4 can be picked out as having in addition adequate equipment and supplies.

Of the 22 schools reported on, only 10 provide both running water and a gas or electric stove in the room used for demonstration. Seven lack both of these essentials and 5 either one

[19] Even here, however, these model conditions are the result of chance rather than of intention. At the opening of the new building there was not enough money to open the ward in question, and it was therefore temporarily assigned to the training school for the teaching of the theory and practice of nursing. The school has accordingly only a precarious hold on this ward unit.

[20] Even special demonstration rooms, it should be noted, are not always in the undisputed possession of the training schools. Thus the large demonstration room at a certain university hospital is said to be sometimes in emergencies demanded by the doctors for the use of patients.

or the other. These major defects often coexist surprisingly with an otherwise high standard of equipment. Two large municipal hospitals, generally well-equipped, lack respectively running water and stoves, and in each case must depend on facilities "across the hall." More serious difficulties are found at a large private hospital; here the lack of running water and stoves in the demonstration room forces the class to use when necessary the diet kitchen, where they often interfere with other classes. A still worse system obtains at one of the university training schools studied. Stoves and running water, not provided in the demonstration room, are said to be "near by," but the heavy ward work "may cause inconvenience or delay in their use." These facilities are in fact in the ward service room, and the demands of student training are expected to run their chance with the more imperative necessities of the ward patients. This is a thoroughly bad example, in a school of high standing, of the conflict elsewhere discussed between the claims of hospital service and of student training. A large university training school of deservedly high rank, in sharp contrast to excellent facilities for science teaching, undertakes to teach nursing procedures in a classroom lacking running water and stoves, and without adequate supplies.

At other schools demonstration room, equipment, and supplies are all inadequate. The teaching of nursing practice is handicapped not only by the inadequacy of the room, but by the absence of teaching equipment. In one school, for instance, a bed must be brought into the room when needed. At others, material even for demonstration must be brought from the hospital.

ADEQUACY OF SUPPLIES FOR DEMONSTRATION AND PRACTICE

Besides demonstration by the teacher and "demonstration back" by the students, the acquisition of good technique requires opportunity for practice by the student. For such practice, obviously, additional supplies are needed.

Only about one-third (7) of the 20 training schools affording data supply adequate material for individual student practice as well as for demonstration by teacher and students. Even at these the material required is not in all cases ready to hand but may involve in its assembling considerable expenditure of time and effort. At one of them, a university training school where lack of storage space in the demonstration room makes it impos-

sible to keep on hand sufficient supplies, for example, of drugs
and glassware, material enough for individual practice is always
secured, but often with much labor on the part of the instructor.
At another, the training school holding nursing classes in its
assembly room, certain expensive equipment is always brought
as needed and at much loss of time from the wards near by.
A considerably larger hospital makes a practice of sending for
treatment trays and some other demonstration material to the
wards, in the interest, it is said, of uniformity. In several cases
drugs are wanting, and must be borrowed from the wards.

Half the schools provide sufficient material for demonstration
by teacher and students but not enough for individual practice
by all the students. At 5 of these the supply is sufficient for a
limited individual practice, made possible by the assignment of
small groups or by allowing certain students to practise while
others observe. By a peculiarly grudging policy in one large
training school, all linen must be brought to the demonstration
room from the hospital and is brought in quantities only sufficient for demonstration.

At two smaller hospitals which make use of the general classroom for demonstration, not enough material can be kept on
hand even for demonstration by the teacher. At one of these,
material for the use of both teacher and students must be carried by the teacher from the hospital to the nurses' residence,
which contains the general classroom; at the other, a small special hospital, where demonstration is done by the teacher only,
supplies are said to be brought from the wards when needed.

Teaching Methods in the Classroom

Classroom instruction in the theory and practice of nursing is
given in all but one of the 23 training schools studied. At this
one, class work had been temporarily suspended at the time of
inspection, but was to be resumed for the next entering class.

At the various schools various methods, ranging from modern
to obsolete, are selected or combined for didactic work in the
classroom: lectures or dictation, recitation from textbook assignments or reference reading, outlines, the keeping and correcting
of notebooks, etc. Of 18 schools furnishing specific information
more than two-thirds (13) use textbooks either alone or in combination with other methods.

But any one of a number of methods of class presentation of

the theory of nursing may undoubtedly be adequate and effective in the hands of an able and skilful teacher. It may be said in general that in such a subject as this, class time may be economized by the use of textbooks or reference books, and that mimeographed outlines are a gain in precision as well as time over dictated notes. At one special hospital, to take a vicious example of waste and probable inaccuracy, the class presentation consists of questions and answers dictated by the superintendent from a notebook compiled many years ago, supplemented only occasionally by reference reading. At another special hospital of much higher educational rank, more than one-third of the time in the class observed was devoted to dictation of technique in a new subject, the only check on the student's accuracy in note-taking being an "occasional inspection of notebooks and a requirement of weekly synopses." It seems obvious here that more exact instruction could be obtained by the use of outlines of technique as well as more time released for other class activities. At the same hospital the proportion of time devoted to demonstration in the class observed was found to be only one-sixth.

On the other hand, the abuse of the textbook method may be seen at a private hospital where the student's first acquaintance with a treatment is gained from reading and she is asked in recitation to describe methods read of but never seen. The too frequent result is the bad pedagogical fault of a wrong first impression which must be corrected by the instructor. Another source of confusion at this training school is that the theory studied in the text and taught in the class does not always correspond with the methods taught in the demonstration room and used in the hospital.

DEMONSTRATION

The indispensable part of the teaching, the pivotal part of the course, must inevitably be the use of demonstration. The procedure or treatment under discussion must be not only described but seen and practised until automatically perfect.

At the great majority of schools studied (18), demonstration is performed, as it properly should be, by students as well as teachers. In over half of these schools the students demonstrate in return.

Three training schools, however, 2 of them ranking high, are thoroughly unsatisfactory in this regard. The teacher demonstrates alone, there is no demonstration by the student, and no

arrangement for supervised practice in the classroom.   In one of
them, a university training school, the admirable facilities for
work in the basic sciences contrast oddly with this inadequate
and ill-planned course.   Another training school connected with
a leading municipal hospital is little better, in that it offers,
besides demonstration by the teacher, opportunity to only one
student in a section daily to "demonstrate back" the procedure
taught by the teacher the day before.   Here, again, the very
limited chance for the student to learn the technique of her profession is not reinforced by any period for supervised practice.

All but one [21] of the schools affording data (21) are provided
with a doll or dolls for demonstration.   More than half of them
(13), moreover, make use of students as subjects, and one with its
course in process of organization plans to do so.   Patients, too,
are used for demonstration at 12 of the hospitals studied; at 5,
on the wards and at 7, in the demonstration room.   At 1 hospital
an entire ward unit is to be given over to the instruction of
students.   Patients are brought to the demonstration room and
used in one school "quite freely," in another for "any treatment," in a third for certain procedures such as bathing and
hair-washing, in 3 others "occasionally," and in another sometimes for practical examination of students at the end of the
junior course, in the application of treatments.   At 8 schools
no use is made of patients for demonstration.

SUPERVISED PRACTICE IN THE CLASSROOM

Of the 18 training schools which provide for demonstration by
both teacher and students, 11 still further emphasize the need
for an expert and finished technique by providing also for periods
of supervised classroom practice.   In some of these, however,
this practice is held in part of the class period and is not perhaps
to be distinguished from "demonstration in return."   The value
of having practice thus closely linked with demonstration is
obvious; on the other hand it seems improbable that under this
arrangement the time allowed the individual student can be
adequate.   At one of these schools the fraction of the practice
period given each student is said to average only 15 to 20 minutes daily under supervision.   At 6 of the other hospitals providing for definite periods of classroom practice, time is assigned
varying from 3 hours a week to 4 hours daily.   One of the smallest hospitals visited allows an hour's practice daily except on

[21] The special hospital giving all practical teaching on the wards.

Saturdays. Another small hospital is said to require 3 hours' weekly practice of probationers and 3 hours of juniors and seniors by way of review; but even this scant allowance the observer notes as doubtful, owing to the cramped space of the demonstration room.

A different arrangement obtaining at a leading private hospital entirely separates student demonstration as well as student practice from demonstration by the instructor. Here the instructor demonstrates to the entire class for 3 periods weekly; the class is then divided into 3 sections, each of which meets separately for demonstration in return and practice. Each student is said under this system to be allowed 9 hours a week for supervised practice. At another training school where the course in nursing is unusually well taught, no definite practice periods are assigned but supervised practice is held between nursing classes and the study hour is frequently used for the purpose.

At 12 schools, however,—more than half of those affording data,—no arrangement whatever is made for supervised classroom practice. In 3 of these cases the defect is the more glaring because students are given no opportunity for demonstration; the whole acquisition of technique is, in other words, relegated to the wards and takes place at the expense of the patients.

At another school connected with an eminent municipal hospital, where a minimum of student demonstration is allowed, the same failure to impress by practice goes far to neutralize the benefit of the fine teaching equipment provided. Here the potential value of the demonstration room, admirably equipped as a model ward, is peculiarly high precisely because the equipment on the wards is old and incomplete. But the opportunity offered by these facilities to fix the ideal method in the students' minds before their practice with the inadequate equipment of the wards is twice lost: first, through failure to allow any sufficient amount of student demonstration (since but one student in each group daily has the chance to "demonstrate back" the procedure taught the day before); and second, by defect of provision for any supervised classroom practice. Optional student practice is indeed allowed here, as at one or two other schools, but, as "any such practice is done voluntarily by the students in their free time and without supervision," we can hardly suppose it to amount to much in time or value.

It is significant of the widespread disregard of what should be an essential policy of student training in this subject that at another well-known hospital students are said to be "permitted to practice in the evening, *if they wish to*" and, again, unsupervised. An exact parallel would be a science course in which students were permitted "if they wished" to work in the laboratory! A small third school, where nursing classes are obliged to use the general classroom, apparently allows voluntary practice, but assigns no definite times, and the room is naturally often in use for other purposes.

APPLICATION OF CLASSROOM INSTRUCTION ON THE WARDS

Not less important than the close correlation of practice with theory in classroom instruction is the prompt application on the wards of the theory learned and technique practiced. The successful transference from the classroom to the wards of a smooth, finished, and intelligently accurate technique is at once the crowning achievement and the final test of a well-correlated course in the theory and practice of nursing.

It is self-evident that the young student should be assigned to only such treatments on the wards as she has been already taught and has thoroughly mastered in the classroom. It is as obviously of prime importance in the interest of standardized technique that the ward experience should be given as promptly as possible after the classroom instruction and practice. It is no less clearly essential that this ward practice be given under supervision as rigorous and competent as that of the classroom until the student's technique is assured.

Need of Prompt Application on the Wards

The need of immediate application on the wards of procedures learned in the classroom seems in the majority of cases affording information to be very indifferently regarded if not entirely ignored.

Conspicuous examples of carefully planned correlation of ward practice with class instruction are offered by only 3 training schools. These 3, it is worth noting, belong also to the group making careful provision for student demonstration and classroom practice. At all of these the level of classroom instruction in nursing practice is notably high.

At one of them, a large private hospital of high standing, a system obtains by which the two student assistants to the instructor find out daily from the head nurses what treatments are to be given, and arrange to have certain cases assigned to the probationers. At another, ward practice in any treatment is given only on notification to the head nurse by the practical instructor that the student is ready, and careful assignments are then made to the same procedures on the wards as have just been learned in the classroom. The third, a university training school, conspicuous not only for able teaching of theory but for liberal provision for classroom demonstration and practice, makes sure that each student has mastered all procedures and that classroom training in each procedure shall be reinforced by ward practice by a rigorous system of checking. Instruction must always precede the giving of treatments on the wards, and, especially in the more difficult treatments, supervised ward practice is made to follow as directly as possible upon practice in the classroom.

At 8, at least, of the training schools studied, practically no correlation is attempted. These schools do not neglect a problem; they fail to recognize its existence. Thus at one school the student may have no opportunity to practice a procedure on the wards till long after her classroom work. At another the probationers for their half-time ward duty (4 hours) are "assigned to all wards in rotation, *regardless of coincident theory,*" and may be able to make practical application of their class teaching only after an interval of weeks.

Certain schools, moreover, fail all along the line in the vitally important task of binding practice closely to theory. The extreme of unsatisfactory method is illustrated in institutions which by neglecting to provide either for student demonstration or supervised student practice in the classroom, leave, as it seems, to chance the transition from class instruction to ward practice.

But it is left for the special hospital cited before as giving all practical nursing instruction on the wards to offer an example of non-correlation so glaring as to be almost grotesque. Here no attempt is made to correlate classroom theory with ward practice, either in method or time. Theory and practice are taught by different women, differently trained, and wholly without conferences. No plan or schedule is followed. Procedures are taught on the wards as opportunity arises, without reference to class instruction, and either before or after it as the case may be. No record of this practical teaching is kept and no relation is established with classroom topics.

But the most carefully planned transition from classroom instruction to ward practice must be as carefully checked to insure a standardized technique. Chief among the means of insuring such standardizing is supervision, as detailed and exacting as that in the classroom. This should be given primarily by the practical instructor who must follow her pupils to the wards to inspect their work, and further by the supervisors and head nurses. It is clearly only by a good understanding and close co-operation between these various agents that the desired result of a standard hospital technique can be achieved.

The urgent character of this need of supervision has only to be stated to be fully recognized. Yet we see school after school letting slip the gains of painstaking instruction, imperilling the whole carefully acquired and not yet fully established technique of the student by failing to enforce it during the difficult period of her adjustment to practical service on the wards. For it is evidently at this point that the careful habits are fixed or the careless ones substituted which will characterize, in all probability, the student's professional life.

For however carefully trained and however much on her mettle to succeed, the young student on the wards is subject to innumerable temptations to bad or slipshod work. Inferior equipment will in many cases make the standard practice of the demonstration room difficult if not impossible; the frequent understaffing of the wards with the general atmosphere of urgency to cover the utmost work in the shortest time is the worst possible influence for technique, and the forced tolerance on the part of her superiors of carelessness and slighted work has a disastrous repercussion on the student's *morale*.

Of 24 schools affording data on this subject, there are but 7 or 8 at most where the supervision of student practice on the wards can be called satisfactory or adequate.

Examples of Successful Supervision

Three of these are, as we should expect, the 3 already mentioned as making ward practice follow promptly upon demonstration and practice in the classroom. At one of them the practical instructor herself devotes 6 hours daily to very careful supervision of her students' work on the wards, observing especially all new procedures whether given by probationers or advanced students. This personal attention goes far to make possible the uniform excellence of technique observed at this hospital. At another, the university training school quoted, the work of ward supervision and instruction is shared by instructor and head nurses, between whom there is close and constant co-operation. The ward staff at this hospital, as is too rarely the case, is large enough to allow the head nurses time for these essential duties. The instructor is further assisted by the assistant superintendent, one of the two seeing every patient and observing every nurse each day. Even at night students are under careful observation by the night supervisor who makes a detailed report to the office.

At the third of these schools, the duty of supervision is delegated by the instructor to her two student assistant teachers, to the head nurses, and to the senior nurses on the wards. While this method of procedure may not appear as satisfactory as supervision by the head of the department herself, the lack of her personal observation is largely offset by the careful system of checking followed, and the fact that her insistence on exact methods during a long period of teaching has built up a standard of practice accepted throughout the hospital. This method of supervision seems justified, furthermore, in a school where the preliminary group is so large that adequate personal supervision by the instructor of the practice work of all members of the class is physically impossible.

Excellent methods of supervision are found at the largest of the municipal hospitals studied, together with a degree of individual attention from the practical instructor remarkable in an institution of such size, and accurate record is kept of each student's work. During 1919 the amount of personal supervision given students averaged more than 2 hours daily. The instructor's work is supplemented by the graduates in charge who give much of their time to the supervision of the student nurses. This is made possible by the notably generous allowance of clerical help at this hospital. The assignment of a clerk to each ward releases the head nurse from the petty duties of ward administration, and enables her to devote a much larger share of her time, as an expert in nursing, to supervision of the detail of duties of both junior and more advanced nurses.

At other schools the instructor generally observes all first treatments, depending variously for further supervision on floor supervisors, head nurses, and office staff. At the small hospital where the practical instructor is also head nurse of one floor, the problem of sufficient supervision is easily solved for the small numbers involved.

Examples of Inadequate Supervision

In the cases of more than half of the schools observed, on the other hand, the supervision of ward practice must be ranked as definitely inadequate or poor.

At 5 of the smaller hospitals insufficient or ineffective supervision is the almost inevitable result of combining an administrative office with the position of practical instructor.

At a better-known hospital, the practical instructor, while she holds no other position, has been given a schedule so heavy that she has not time enough for adequate supervision even of the probationers. No effective co-operation with the head nurses has been established, and for 2 hours at least daily (half the ward duty of the probationers) students are on the wards practically without supervision.

At none of these schools has any satisfactory substitute been worked out for the personal supervision of the instructor. At one of them it is stated quite simply that the students are relied on to supervise each other!

Lack of Good Management

Other reasons militate against successful supervision at other hospitals. In some cases it is a matter of unintelligent planning and lack of system. At a large university school offering, as we have seen, neither first-rate facilities nor a high grade of teaching in this essential subject, the practical instructor who gave the supervision had apparently no systematic way of checking up the procedures observed. At another well-known institution the instructor gives 2 hours daily to supervise the work of the probationers, but her lack of intelligent method makes much of her supervision valueless. Her morning rounds seem to be largely a matter of routine, unvaried to permit observation of procedures of varying difficulty. Thus, on the day of our visit, the probationers under supervision were doing merely elementary procedures such as bed-making and bathing; the advanced and difficult treatments, to be observed had she timed her rounds differently, must have gone unsupervised.

Lack of Co-operation

Lack of co-operation may elsewhere defeat the ends of supervision. Thus, at the large municipal hospital where the ward practice is regarded "merely as part of the ward work," the cleavage between the teaching staff of the school and the supervisory staff of the hospital is almost absolute. This unfortunate state of things dates back to a political appointment and a difficulty between superintendent and instructor which closed the wards to the latter. The present instructor is trying to combat this deplorable tradition by herself beginning again the interrupted supervision of ward practice, but she is young and inexperienced and a proper co-operation of head nurses, supervisors, and office staff will probably be a thing of slow growth.

Here at present, as all too frequently at other hospitals, instead of a unified policy directed to the common end of an efficient training, we find a divided interest and purpose among the several persons supposed to supervise the students' work. The head nurse is concerned primarily not with technique but to see that the work on her ward is done; the office assistant to see that ward and service rooms are clean and orderly, to collect time slips, special reports, etc.; the instructor, whose available time is trifling compared with the need in so large a hospital, is left unsupported in her effort to enforce a standard of nursing practice. If these various persons responsible for the students' work could stand unitedly behind the educational policy of the training school, the burdens of the instructor would at once be greatly lightened and a long step taken towards the standardization of nursing practice at the hospital.

Inadequate Staffing

Finally, no system of supervision, however carefully planned, and no effort on the part of the instructor can hold its own against the understaffing of the wards and the consequent overwork of the head nurses. This pressure of immediate need leaves them no margin of time to enforce their standards, forces them to emphasize quantity rather than quality of work, and demoralizes the students by seeming to belittle at the outset of their practical experience all the technical perfection so laboriously inculcated in the classroom. This is the situation both at the hospital just quoted, and in even greater degree at another large municipal hospital where the instructor, in spite of the excellent provision for classroom teaching, feels that her work is rendered nugatory by hospital conditions, and has resigned in discouragement.

We have spoken of the signal importance of co-operation between the instructor and the head nurses. One of the most interesting means observed for securing this co-operation is the plan of instructing head nurses in supervision, just adopted at one of the smaller institutions. Here each new procedure, or any change of method to be introduced, is demonstrated in the classroom to the head nurses responsible for the nursing technique of the students on their wards. Thus a close link is forged between classroom instruction and ward practice.

The same close linking less elaborately brought about is to be noted at a larger hospital in another city where the instructor notifies the ward supervisor of any changes to be made in procedure, and no such change is permitted unless authorized by the school office.

Of methods or devices other than supervision for securing standardized technique, 13 of the hospitals under consideration make use of none whatever; at almost all of these supervision, too, is faulty, inadequate, or lacking.

Use of Nursing Practice Card, Etc.

Most common of the devices elsewhere in use is the nursing practice card. This card, carried by each student, is checked by the instructor as each procedure is satisfactorily performed, and constitutes therefore a complete record of the student's progress.[22] Nine of the hospitals observed use these cards; they are a valuable means of making certain at the same time that each student has had practice in all procedures and that her technique is up to the school standard. Two other hospitals while not using the nursing practice card make use of methods as accurate for checking the students' progress; one of these uses record cards, kept presumably in the possession of the instructor; at the other the student assistants who take the instructor's place in supervision carry notebooks in which each

[22] A curious and unsatisfactory divergence from this method is found at a school where the student herself is allowed to record on the practice card the procedures she has done on the wards.

student is credited with successive procedures as they are properly performed under their supervision.

Among other means of value adopted to standardize nursing practice is the provision by certain hospitals of an outline placed on each ward or floor of the technique of all procedures. Such an outline is available for reference at 2 hospitals and is being compiled at a third.

It need scarcely be said that the provision of standard equipment alike in the demonstration room and on the wards is of essential importance for uniformity of technique. So important is this matter that at 3 large municipal hospitals uniform application of classroom technique is said to be difficult if not impossible, because of inadequate or unstandardized equipment on the wards.

TIME ALLOWED TO THE TEACHING OF THE THEORY AND PRACTICE OF NURSING IN 22 SCHOOLS [23]

In the 22 schools studied, the time allowed to the teaching of nursing procedures ranges from 55 to 222 hours. The average allowance is 135. The schools are grouped in the following table according to their assignment of hours.

THEORY AND PRACTICE OF NURSING

Number of Hours	Number of Schools
50- 99	4
100-149	9
150-199	7
200-249	2
	22

6. The Case for the Basic Sciences

In the foregoing study of the teaching of nursing procedures, we have not yet touched on a cardinal and controversial issue. If the teaching of nursing procedures is the center of the nurses' training, it would appear indispensable that the student be given the background of knowledge necessary for intelligent understanding and application of the subject. This necessary knowledge is a grounding in the basic sciences: anatomy, physiology, chemistry, and bacteriology,—subjects usually taught, to some

[23] For purposes of classification (see page 393) includes also bandaging, massage, and hospital housekeeping.

extent at least, during the preliminary term or, in schools having no such term, during the first months of training.

Our next point for discussion is the legitimacy, sometimes challenged, of including these sciences in the nurses' training. "Why basic?" it is sometimes asked: "How related to the nurses' training, and why necessary at all in their curriculum? What need of the laboratory branches to teach nurses to be clean and deft?"

In entering upon this question we may profitably raise a more fundamental query and ask why sciences, such as chemistry, biology, physiology, are recommended and taught in the best high schools throughout the country. Obviously, aside from the vocational use of these subjects, as necessary prerequisites for agriculture, medicine, engineering, dietetics, and other callings, instruction in the basic sciences is meant to give boys and girls some elementary conception of the world they live in, some elementary grasp of the nature and processes of life and growth. As a basis for the further teaching of hygiene and the principles of health and of sex, which the high schools are beginning to undertake, these elementary sciences are obviously indispensable.[24]

If these sciences were well taught in all high schools, and if all nurses in training entered with four years' high school preparation including these sciences, the nurses' training schools might be in large part relieved from the necessity of teaching them. There would still be needed special applications of these sciences to the work of the nurse, but much would be gained if students entered trained in even one science, such as chemistry. Now, however, a large percentage of nurses in even the better schools begin their training with no knowledge of any science, either subject matter or method. Only a few who come from the best high schools and have chosen their subjects therein to include sciences, have had any adequate grounding in either chemistry or biology, while the student who has had good courses in both these subjects is a rare exception. Furthermore, the high school courses are usually taken while the student is still very young, often not more than fourteen or sixteen, before she has any serious aim, and for these reasons the value and significance of the work is not realized.

[24] For a statement of the objectives of science instruction, see U. S. Department of the Interior, Bureau of Education, Bulletin No. 26. 1920. Reorganization of Science in Secondary Schools.

It may be that in the future, by giving credit for previous instruction in at least chemistry and biology, or by making some instruction in science prerequisite to entrance, the training schools may be freed from the necessity of devoting as much time and attention to science as is now indispensable. The development of central schools for teaching the sciences and other subjects, to which students from various training schools are sent, offers perhaps the most hopeful solution of the difficulties encountered by the training schools in providing adequate science teaching. Progress in establishing such central or joint courses in various communities is discussed at the end of this section. But first the actual need for science teaching in the nurses' curriculum demands our attention.

GENERAL BENEFITS FROM SCIENCE TRAINING

From adequate science teaching, aside from acquiring specific information, the student nurse, like other students, acquires certain general benefits which may be briefly summarized: training in accuracy of observation and of statement; training in manual dexterity through the exact use of material and apparatus; training in patience of observation and judgment in drawing conclusions. Of all these benefits, it must be clear, the nurse stands in special need. Accuracy of observation, manual skill, patience, and judgment are qualities primarily demanded by the issues of life and death and by the complexity of human relations among which the nurse is soon to play her part. True, her years of training within the hospital in actual contact with disease are designed to develop precisely these qualities. But in the science courses, given while she is as yet too inexperienced to be trusted with the care of actual disease and where the consequences of lost time, of error, or of failure are less serious than on the wards, she may obtain invaluable preliminary training.

NEED OF SPECIFIC SCIENCES IN NURSING EDUCATION

Besides these general benefits, a knowledge, sound though comparatively elementary, of certain specific sciences and laws of science is indispensable for the nurses' training. In making this contention let us state bluntly at the outset that it is not to make nurses into doctors, but for the intelligent discharge of strictly nursing duties that this grounding in science is held indispensable. At best, only a relatively short time can be available for these courses. At best, they will be only elementary as compared with the intensive training of the physician or research worker. But we are concerned now not with the extent of courses but with the establishment of a principle, the need of adequate science teaching for nurses, often denied, often grudgingly provided for, rarely given its due weight in hospital training.

WHY THE NURSE NEEDS ANATOMY AND PHYSIOLOGY

It is clear that without a knowledge of anatomy and physiology the nurse cannot even be taught the manifold curative and preventive nursing treatments, on the teaching of which we have dwelt at length in the preceding section. On·this point no further words need be spent.

A second point is the gaining of accurate knowledge, vivid and dependable, of the reactions of the healthy human organism. On her recognition of the deviations from the normal rests, in large part, the nurse's intelligent co-operation with the physician; on her report of things unseen by him must often rest his important decisions. From the study of anatomy and physiology, she is to obtain the background of the normal against which the picture of disease is projected. Without such a grounding she cannot be taught to recognize with quick intelligence significant pathological symptoms, to discriminate between the trivial and the vitally important; yet for the appreciation of just such variations and for the reporting of them she will be responsible. "The doctor does not want the nurse to call him every time the patient coughs," remarked an intelligent nurse in a discussion of the value of the elementary science courses which she was taking as a postgraduate, to supplement her deficiencies of training. "He expects her to give intelligent attention to her cases, an impossibility without some scientific background. The doctors who do not want nurses trained to use their intelligence, and regard the nurse as a machine, are the first to complain if she shows lack of comprehension." On the other hand, a science teacher interested in the adequate training of nurses writes:

"It is the human body upon which the nurse focusses most of her attention, and it should certainly be made possible for her to understand this main point of interest. This knowledge of the patient can come only through a comprehension of the chemical and physical processes involved in the performance of the bodily function." [25]

"The student who has dissected a sheep kidney, identified the parts and worked out a diagram of the microscopic structure, will undoubtedly take a more intelligent interest in the next kidney or bladder case she has on the ward," writes another teacher.[26]

The nurses themselves realize their need of a sound knowledge of anatomy and physiology. They are eager for such knowledge. Another nurse now at Teachers College for further training said of her postgraduate work in science: "I'll be a better nurse if I am more intelligent. I may not rub a patient's back with any more affection, but of course I'll do it better if I know more about vertebræ and what may be wrong with them." This nurse had been in charge of a hospital nursing staff in France and had made financial sacrifices to go to Teachers College, yet she felt so strongly the need of basic instruction that she, like hundreds of other nurses, has returned to take elementary science courses.

More and more, with the advance of medical science, its terms become a language which the nurse as well as the physician must understand. The nurse's comprehension of the fundamentals of anatomy and physiology makes a few sentences of explanation from the physician full of meaning; the case stands before her, a problem rich in scientific and human significance, even though her part is concerned only with the care and cure planned by the physician.

The same argument obviously holds true of bacteriology.

WHY THE NURSE NEEDS BACTERIOLOGY

"Why," asks the critic, "is it not enough to teach nurses to be clean? Why teach bacteriology?"

"Being clean," however, in the surgical sense, and for the aseptic technique demanded in the care of disease cannot be really taught by mere rule-of-thumb directions. To apply in private homes, often under difficult conditions and with im-

---

[25] A Course in Chemistry for Student Nurses. C. A. Mills, Ph.D., Instructor in Bio-Chemistry, College of Medicine, University of Cincinnati. American Journal of Nursing, April, 1921. Page 461.

[26] National League of Nursing Education, Proceedings of the 26th Annual Convention, 1920. Interest in Class Work. Katherine Ink, Visiting Instructor, New York City. Page 127.

provised means, the technique learned in the hospital, to protect herself and others, the nurse needs a sounder basis of fact.

The case for the basic sciences in her curriculum does not involve an exhaustive or even an advanced study of bacteriology. It means, for example, sufficient instruction in the fundamentals of bacteriology to make her acquainted with the nature of bacteria, to make her ever aware of the living things which her unaided eyes cannot see but whose presence on an unsterilized instrument may mean the death of a patient. The student who has seen her cultures become contaminated in the laboratory because of a moment's carelessness on her part, who has seen bacteria multiply overnight in countless hosts, who has come to realize by daily experience in the laboratory what sterilization and asepsis mean, has been awakened to a new, stimulating appreciation of the sources of infection, of those ever present enemies of health and recovery from which it is her province to protect her patient, herself, and the community.

She has not learned mere rule-of-thumb directions about cleanliness, scrubbing and the like, to be forgotten or wrongly applied in emergencies or under conditions differing from those under which she was taught. She has, if well taught, been grounded in principles of asepsis which can guide her safely to improvise means and recognize and meet new conditions.

WHY THE NURSE NEEDS CHEMISTRY

Behind physiology and bacteriology, and behind dietetics as well, and indispensable for making them intelligible, is chemistry.

Physiology, for instance, teaches that life involves a continuous change of structure, this in its turn being inseparable from a long and complicated series of chemical syntheses and decompositions which we call metabolism. Clearly, the student who is to have a working knowledge of what the simplification of food in digestion means, must have some acquaintance with the phenomena of chemical change. If she has performed laboratory experiments in which before her eyes substances were oxidized, heat evolved, carbon dioxide formed; if she has seen that some substances will pass through membranes while others will not, she has gone a long way toward a comprehension of certain groups of bodily changes which are of vital importance. The nurse to whom "oxygen" means nothing can scarcely make much headway in understanding the plight of the body with

leaking heart-valves, particularly if in addition she has never
seen a normal heart valve and has no comprehension of how it
works. Her intelligent co-operation in the care of such a case
rests on her chemical, her anatomical, her physiological
foundations.

The nurses' course in chemistry must be one of reasonable
thoroughness. It cannot consist, as it often does now, of a few
lectures and perhaps two or three demonstrations, if it is to give
her a truly basic knowledge. Equipment is expensive and
teachers are hard to find, but no training school should consider
these reasons adequate for the retention of ridiculously brief,
stereotyped courses in so important a field. As years pass it
may indeed be true that more and more dependence can be
placed on the preparatory courses in high schools, but such
courses will need for a long time specific adaptations to the
problems which confront the nurse.

Without a grasp of elementary but basic scientific conceptions
in these various lines, the student can only learn in parrot
fashion, repeating words which cannot penetrate or lead to intelligent action. But action, as we know, is precisely the aim
and end-all of these courses. It is because of their direct application to her future work that the nurse needs them in her
training.

A single example illustrates the point at issue. Take, for
instance, so simple a task as the giving of a nasal douche. Here
is a common enough procedure, ordered by a doctor as a routine
treatment. Yet in one of our leading hospitals, eleven different
student nurses were observed on different days, using for a nasal
douche a supersaturated salt solution, ignorant of the anatomy
and physiology of the affected parts, and hence careless of the
proper technique for the douche and the danger of forcing the
solution into the eustachian tubes. Instruction in the proper
administration of the douche, if given, had been readily forgotten, where a knowledge of the structure and function of
the passages would have enlisted the student's practical intelligence. Instead of relieving an excessively painful inflammation,
the student succeeded in introducing undissolved salt into tender
membranes.

To these students, variations in the strength of salt solutions
as related to living tissues had no significance. This was in a
hospital where chemistry was taught very briefly, and where

there was no laboratory work in physiology. Some of these 11 students may not have had the course in drugs and solutions. They were trusted with the patient and the treatment, yet they had not been scientifically fortified. Nurses' errors would fill a large volume, yet no analysis has been made to determine how many of them would probably become all but impossible were nurses given the scientific basis underlying the procedures which they use.

Why Scientific Teaching Should Precede Instruction in Disease

Equally important is the point that often, for lack of grounding in the preliminary subjects, the nurse's later teaching, her training in strictly professional subjects, is hopelessly hampered. For after the preliminary term, comes her instruction on the wards, which we are presently to examine in detail. After her four-months' grounding in the simpler nursing procedures and the sciences, she is now to receive her professional training in the actual care of the sick, and be taught the care of all kinds of patients—medical, surgical, obstetrical, pediatric, and whatever other varieties of cases the hospital affords. In lectures, quizzes, and clinics she is to be taught something of the nature and significance of the symptoms, diseases, or conditions which she is encountering every day and every hour on the wards.

We shall presently see how inadequate, in most hospitals, is the allowance of time for this professional instruction; but even more serious an obstacle to its success is the lack of proper preliminary instruction of the students. Without the grounding in the fundamental sciences for which this chapter argues, the clinical instruction of the nurse on the ward and in the classroom, which is the essence of her training, is practically unintelligible to her. The doctors and nurses who give her this instruction have an impossible task to perform, making bricks without straw. The lack of an elementary but sound grounding in scientific conceptions hampers them in their classes at every turn.

7. Teaching of the Basic Sciences

The basic sciences generally included in the early months of training are anatomy, physiology, bacteriology, and chemistry. Of the 23 training schools whose curricula have been studied,

20 gave courses in all four of these sciences. Three are lacking in one or more of the subjects.[27]

GENERAL CHARACTERISTICS OF THE SCIENCE COURSES

The common defects of scientific instruction in the training schools studied are the lack of good teachers, the neglect of laboratory work, and the insufficient allowance of time.

LACK OF WELL-EQUIPPED TEACHERS

Any criticism of the nurse instructors of science must be prefaced by noting the great educational advance made in the comparatively recent appointment of any special teachers for these branches, hitherto taught mainly by the superintendent of the school in addition to all her other duties. Only a few years ago, at the 1917 meeting of the League of Nursing Education, the status of these teachers in the training school hierarchy was seriously discussed as a new problem.

That the number of properly prepared nurse instructors of science is totally inadequate can hardly be a matter of surprise. Unless they have studied science before entering training, the science courses in the training school have not offered any adequate preparation for teaching, even in the subject matter of the courses, much less in any methods of teaching. Until very recently, moreover, there has existed practically but one school in the United States to prepare teachers for the training schools— Teachers College at Columbia University. The influence of Teachers College in training and sending out nurse instructors has been countrywide,[28] but to supply trained teachers of science to all or nearly all the training schools of the country has obviously been beyond its possibilities.

LACK OF LABORATORY TRAINING

Even with good science teachers, instruction in these branches is hampered by the lack of laboratory equipment. In teaching nursing procedures the ingenuity of the teacher may improvise many appliances. In teaching science courses ingenuity can be used to improvise, to a certain extent at least, methods of demonstration in class. But no ingenuity can replace the lack of

[27] In one hospital where the subject is lacking, a course was planned but had not yet been begun at the time of our visit.
[28] For discussion of the influence of Teachers College on nursing training, see Chapter VII.

scientific laboratory equipment for individual work, such as microscopes, fresh material, chemical reagents, etc. Yet individual laboratory work is admittedly the center of science teaching.

INADEQUATE TIME

Moreover, neither a high grade of teaching nor the best facilities for laboratory work can make up for insufficient time. In most of the courses offered the wholly inadequate allotment of hours makes superficial work practically inevitable.

ANATOMY AND PHYSIOLOGY

A course in anatomy and physiology is included in the curricula of 22 of the 23 hospitals.

HOURS AND YEAR WHEN GIVEN

The hours given to the teaching of this science vary in the 22 schools from 30 to 150 with a median of 60 hours, as against 90 hours suggested in our proposed course. The importance of placing the work in anatomy and physiology in the early weeks of the training course is manifestly very great. An intelligent knowledge of the human body is an indispensable preliminary to the theory and practice of nursing, if our standard of the nurse's training is to include an intelligent understanding of what she is doing as well as a merely mechanical efficiency.

The great majority of these schools place the subject near the beginning of the curriculum. Thus, 20 schools give courses in anatomy and physiology during the first year, and 16 of them give part or all of the course in the preliminary period. One eminent training school connected with a famous private hospital gives all of its 110 hours during this period; a university school of high standards does the same with a course of almost maximum length (144 hours). Seven schools follow the plan of beginning the course in the preliminary months and extending it into the latter half of the first year, but most of these place the major portion of the work in the preliminary period.

Seven other schools, in addition to earlier elementary work, give advanced courses in the second or third year. Only one, however, a school where little attention is paid to preliminary theory in any branch and the probationers are put at once on full ward duty, postpones its entire course to so late a period.

A strange exception to the general practice of giving anatomy and physiology, or at least a part of the course, in the preliminary period is found at an important municipal hospital of high standing. Here this science is not given until the second year. Even then, as the course is given but twice in the year and as classes are admitted four times, a given student may not receive this elementary instruction until she has been actually nineteen months in training—more than half her course.

A special cause of postponement is found at small training schools which are sometimes led, "owing to the small number in classes," to combine two or more classes for one lecture course. Thus, a small private hospital gives anatomy and physiology for preliminary, first year, and second year students combined. Students at this school may accordingly pass their whole first year without the basic training involved in this important preliminary study.

STAFF

Of 34 teachers mentioned in connection with these courses:
   5 are superintendents or assistant superintendents of the training schools,
  12 are resident instructors (women),
   5 are internes or physicians of the hospital staff,
   2 are visiting physicians,
   1 is a visiting instructor (physician) from a near-by university,
   1 is an instructor in the affiliated college where the course is taken,
   8 are professors or instructors in the medical schools or universities of which the training schools are part.

Thus, 10 of these instructors are specialists in the subject and professional teachers as well; 7 are specialists with or without any ability for teaching. A third of the whole number of instructors are resident in the training schools as teachers of theory, but, as we shall see in a later chapter, they may or may not be equipped for teaching, since they range from women with a university or normal school degree to women without even a high school diploma; they may or may not, again, be overburdened beyond the possibility of good teaching. The 5 remaining teachers are administrative officers of the training school and almost inevitably must subordinate education to executive duties.

METHODS OF TEACHING

The usual method of class teaching shows various combinations of the following: lectures, more or less informal; recitations on text or reference reading; daily or frequent quizzes, written or oral; demonstration by the teacher in classroom or laboratory.

The adequacy of class teaching without one or other of these means obviously depends upon the skill with which the other methods of presentation are employed. Lectures, indeed, may be successfully dispensed with when lessons are assigned in a good text and students participate in recitation and discussion, with reviews of difficult points under the guidance of a broadly trained instructor; and textbooks are in fact in use in the majority of schools considered. For explanation in class, demonstration, however, is indispensable.

We postpone until a later section the discussion of the fundamental importance of laboratory training and equipment.

USE OF DEMONSTRATION IN CLASS

It is gratifying to find that in 21 out of the 27 classes studied such demonstration plays a part, variously combined with lectures, recitations, or quizzes, and in some cases with topical reports from the students.

Obstacles to Good Teaching

But this general approximation to good method may be rendered nugatory in a number of different ways. Thus, one of the hospitals studied is provided with full classroom and laboratory equipment, and employs lecture, recitation on text, quiz, and demonstration in classroom teaching, together with individual laboratory experiment. But these advantages of adequate equipment and satisfactory method are all but nullified by the short-sighted management which crowds the classes beyond the point of efficient teaching and so overburdens an able instructor that she has no vitality to put into her work. Small wonder that the class observed, with too many students to follow the discussion and with a teacher harassed and exhausted nervously, "showed a tendency to drag and lack interest."

Again, a competent instructor may be hampered by an unintelligent policy on the part of her superiors. Such a situation exists at a large and prosperous private hospital with high-grade students, which shows a carefully arranged plan of instruction, including textbook assignments with class recitation, and discussion, topical reports, quizzes, and demonstration. But the narrow educational policy of this institution limits demonstration by excluding all mammalian dissection, and thus curtails its value for the understanding of human anatomy. An expert and ambitious instructor is on the point of leaving because of lack of freedom to develop her science course.

Examples of Unsatisfactory Teaching

On the other hand, lack of training or of educational experience on the part of teachers may prevent them from making the most of opportunities that exist or from initiating improvements. The weakness of apparently well-planned courses in the two following instances is plainly due to the limitations of the instructor.

In a certain school in which the class appears on paper to be well conducted, the lecture was found to be extremely automatic and entirely lacking in interest, and the blackboard sketches, which took the place of models for demonstration, to be so inaccurate as to give no correct idea of the organ under discussion. In addition to the teacher's disability, moreover, equipment for demonstration was meager and fresh material was confined to a few bones and organs from the butcher.

In another school, where the advanced class at least must be included among those nominally taught upon approved lines, observation showed the instructor to be entirely unfamiliar with modern scientific teaching methods. The quizzing here is of the most perfunctory question and answer type, with the same set of questions and answers used year after year, and the demonstration merely the exhibition of a few bones, charts, and microscopic slides. Preserved specimens from the pathological laboratory of the hospital are available, but it has never occurred to the instructor to make use of them. Little use, moreover, is made of a small laboratory which, in the opinion of our investigator, might be used to good advantage. The instructor expressed great repugnance to the use of frogs, cats, or rabbits for dissection. She occasionally demonstrates an eye or a heart but dislikes it greatly. Apparently there is almost no use of fresh material in the class. It is doubtful if even fresh bones are obtained, as the instructor does not consider the use of fresh material necessary.

This school is attached to a large municipal hospital peculiarly rich in human material for study. But the opportunity it offers must be in large part lost to students coming to their work with the second-hand and meager knowledge of fundamental physical facts afforded by the course described, as a background for their observation.

Still worse than this failure to teach anatomy by demonstration with fresh material is the attempt to teach it by dissection at another training school, on the part of a teacher herself ignorant of anatomy and untrained in dissection. In the class observed, some of the students were making a dissection of two guinea pigs supplied by the pathological laboratory while the rest of the class stood around and asked questions. The instructor could give the students almost no guidance in technique and a guidance at best uncertain in matters of fact. She mistook the sex of the animals and failed to point out important organs. The whole "demonstration" was a hit or miss performance.

But even with the best of teaching, good work in the class visited must have been impossible because of the lack of needed instruments. For at this school the course is handicapped not only by the teacher's inexperience but by totally insufficient equipment. The room used for demonstration is without water, gas, or sinks, and is located one floor above elevator service. Most of the equipment used must be borrowed and assembled from other departments and carried up the stairs to the classroom. Under such handicaps of inconvenience and difficulty, the class seen by our field agent should not perhaps be too severely criticized. To be sure, the material and equipment needed was such as it is easy to obtain at a hospital, and might no doubt have been procured in spite of difficulties by a teacher of sufficient enterprise and with a less heavy schedule. A full set of Harvard physiological apparatus, moreover, was later found by the investigator in the pathological laboratory, evidently quite unused.

Examples of Resourceful Teaching

It is not difficult, on the other hand, to quote examples of schools with limited opportunity which obtain apparently successful results through the resourcefulness of teachers with training and vision.

For instance, among the most interesting classes observed was one in a school entirely lacking in laboratory facilities. The instructor's skill showed itself in her explanatory amplification of the textbook assignment, the use of the blackboard for illustrative drawings in class by pupils as well as by herself, the encouragement of creative effort among the students in the preparation of special illustrative reports; e.g., diagrammatic studies of a kidney tubule and its blood supply, of the processes of digestion, etc., made from descriptions in assigned medical reference texts. The room used for demonstration has insufficient daylight and is not supplied with water, gas, or sinks. In spite of these drawbacks, valuable demonstrations are given, not only with a manikin and various models, but with fresh material from a near-by medical school and from the butcher. Special trips are arranged to a medical museum for the study of preserved specimens.

But much time is wasted by this instructor in preparing and putting away demonstration material, and the success of her teaching without proper equipment for demonstration and laboratory work is at the cost of enormous and wearing personal effort, which should be conserved for legitimate use.

A further example of an instructor's efforts to compensate for the total lack of laboratory facilities is found at another school, highly reputed indeed, but meagerly equipped even for demonstration.

In the class observed on bones the teaching was in every respect as good as could be done without individual laboratory equipment. The illustrative material for demonstration was distributed and placed on four tables in different parts of the room so that it could be available without too great crowding for the thirty students in groups. Through the exertion of the instructor in assembling scattered materials, this included many fresh bones sawed to the best advantage, sawed dry bones, Nystrom charts, a skeleton, several skulls variously cut, a good temporal bone to show the ear, and other bones in abundance. Four borrowed microscopic slides were placed under microscopes with explanatory cards by each. All possible pains were taken to make the exhibit clear, but as the subject is intrinsically difficult, the method was at best but an unsatisfactory substitute for individual laboratory work, and the whole admirable makeshift was achieved at undue expense of time and effort on the part of an expert teacher already burdened by heavy responsibilities.

In an institution where every means is at hand to develop the teaching service to the highest perfection, it is surely bad policy as well as unreasonable to ignore the urgent plea of the instructor for adequate laboratory facilities, and to continue to exploit her ingenuity and strength in the maintenance of make-shift methods, however good as such.

The remaining 6 classes are conducted almost entirely without the very important benefit of demonstration.

In one of these the lack of demonstration is not serious, as the teaching is well planned and conducted, and the course provides for thorough individual laboratory work. The 5 others are more meager, consisting in several cases exclusively of formal lecture or other stereotyped form of presentation. Of these, 2 are especially barren, depending actually on the mere dictation of typewritten questions and answers, unsupplemented by either demonstration or laboratory work. One is a probationers' class of 24 hours.[29] No textbook is used. Questions and answers are dictated to the class from a notebook used for many years; these notes are committed to memory by the students at a supervised study hour held just before the class; and the teacher's presentation consists wholly in reading these questions from the book before her and hearing the answers, also typed. It cannot be a matter of wonder that the recitation is parrot-like, with little or no interest evinced by the students. In another hospital a similar course is offered, partly in the second and partly in the third year, to students who have had no previous instruction in either anatomy or physiology, except incidentally in the teaching of practical nursing. There is no textbook, no demonstration or laboratory work. The students take almost verbatim notes of a stereotyped lecture which are inspected and corrected in lieu of a textbook.

Two other courses given in a small hospital of good standing are of higher grade, but consist almost wholly of formal lectures, the first offering a very little demonstration only (e.g., circulation), for which the class is taken to the completely furnished laboratory of a co-operating university; the advanced course giving no demonstration of any kind.

Six classes in anatomy and physiology in which, as we shall see, there are also good facilities for laboratory work, are all

---

* This preliminary class is followed by a course in the latter part of the first year, where somewhat less crude, though still entirely inadequate methods are followed. See page 261.

well provided with material for class demonstration, that is, fresh material and preserved specimens, bones, charts, models, slides, and microscopes, etc. Eighteen classes which have no laboratory work at all are variously supplied with demonstration material. In 12 of them fresh material is used for demonstration. One of these uses no fresh material in anatomy but gives its students the perhaps greater advantage of observing human dissections in the dissecting room of a medical college.

Of permanent equipment—bones, charts, models, apparatus— only 3 or possibly 4 collections described can be called ample; 8 or 9 are meager. Five schools have no microscopes. In additional cases they are available only by borrowing from other departments. Three have practically no technical equipment, and must rely solely on fresh material brought in for whatever demonstration they do.

THE ESSENTIAL NEED OF LABORATORY TRAINING AND EQUIPMENT

Whatever the method by which the subject-matter of anatomy and physiology is presented in the classroom, it would seem superfluous to urge the indispensable importance of individual laboratory observation in familiarizing the student with the actual structure and activities of the various tissues and organs studied. For the future nurse the value of laboratory work lies precisely in the practice given in the orderly, definite, exact use of material and apparatus, in the observation of structures, of chemical changes, of living complexities. Dr. Flexner's incisive criticism of methods of science teaching, emphasizing the central importance of laboratory work, is as applicable to the limited instruction of the nurse as to the strenuous laboratory discipline of the medical student:

"In methods of instruction there is, once more, nothing to distinguish medical from other sciences. Out-and-out didactic treatment is hopelessly antiquated; it belongs to an age of accepted dogma or supposedly complete information, when the professor 'knew' and the students 'learned.' The lecture indeed continues of limited use. It may be employed in beginning a subject to orient the student, to indicate relations, to forecast a line of study in its practical bearings; from time to time, too, a lecture may profitably sum up, interpret, and relate results experimentally ascertained. Textbooks, atlases, charts, occupy similar positions. They are not, in the first place, a substitute for sense experience, but they may well guide and fill out the student's laboratory findings." [30]

For laboratory work in anatomy there should be an abundance of material: bones for the student to handle, with definite assignments so that her time may be given to observing in particular, not to looking at things in general; dissection of fresh mammalian material, since the conception of the normal living body does not come readily from rigid pickled material or from models, though demonstration of human dissections, of preserved specimens, and of models are helpful for comparative purposes; and the study of a certain amount of microscopic material.

In physiology the student should perform a sufficient number of experiments to make vivid to her some of the most significant facts in digestion, respiration, circulation, the action of nerves and muscles. Frequently by the performance of one experiment, a whole series of bodily phenomena becomes understandable and significant. Such, for instance, would be the careful working out of a simple series of experiments on salivary digestion, which might serve to illuminate the whole subject. Oftentimes important physiological experimentation can be done by the students on each other, for example in respiration and circulation, thus supplying valuable observations on the normal organism which may serve as a background for later accurate observation of pathological states. The equipment essential for this physiological study is not elaborate, but the mode of approach, through carefully planned and well-supervised laboratory work, is of great importance in the nurse's training. Demonstrations by the instructor may supplement but they cannot replace the personal performance of experiments by the student herself.

LABORATORY FACILITIES IN THE SCHOOLS STUDIED

That the necessity for individual laboratory work for student nurses has been almost wholly unrecognized by the hospital authorities is shown by the small number of schools at which such opportunity is provided.

Two-thirds of the hospitals whose teaching facilities were studied (15 out of 22) make no provision whatever for individual

[30] The Carnegie Foundation for the Advancement of Teaching. Bulletin No. 4, 1910. Medical Education in the United States and Canada. Pages 60-61.

laboratory experiment, though in several cases such provision seems to be entirely feasible. Only 6 make definite provision for individual laboratory work in both sciences. One other provides excellent laboratory experience in its course in physiology, but none in anatomy, though the latter course, which includes frequent demonstration, is apparently of high educational value in spite of this incomprehensible omission (see page 268).

Of these 7 classes supplied with laboratory facilities, 4 have laboratories belonging to the training school, available for individual experiment in anatomy and physiology, 2 make use of the laboratories of allied medical schools, while another sends its students for the entire preliminary science course to a well-equipped technical college where individual laboratory work plays a large part in the students' training.

Some of the most glaring defects in the provision for laboratory facilities are found not in schools of scanty resources but in well-endowed hospitals in the main of deservedly high reputation, where equipment in other departments is for the most part generous and intelligently planned. Thus, one of the leading schools of the country makes indeed some provision for individual laboratory experiment but under the handicap of very limited equipment. Among other things, material for microscopic work is very meager, and even a complete set of slides owned by the instructor cannot be used to advantage because of the lack of sufficient microscopes.

In certain other prominent schools the situation is very much worse. One large training school with the prestige of affiliation with a medical school of great reputation teaches its students their anatomy and physiology entirely without laboratory experiment.[31] The burden thus thrown on an able and conscientious teacher in trying to make demonstration take its place has already been pointed out (see page 262).

In an eminent private hospital with lavish equipment in certain departments, the absence of all laboratory facilities is due to the fact that the school is comparatively new. The plea is made that laboratory provision is included in future plans. Nevertheless, the subordination of science teaching in the minds of those in control of the school's policy is shown by the fact that so far, for a period of several years, the science classes not

[31] A very few experiments in digestion done in the clinical laboratory are negligible.

only have been conducted without individual laboratory facilities, but have been allowed to remain of distinctly low grade in other respects.

In one school constituting a department of a large university with a well-equipped medical school, the course in anatomy is illustrated in the classroom entirely by demonstration of bones and anatomical models instead of actual dissection.   These models are very numerous and excellent, and if it is anywhere possible to substitute models for dissection, it is undoubtedly so here.   The lack of dissection is, moreover, to some extent compensated for by the opportunity given the students from time to time to observe human dissections made by medical students. But with laboratory facilities at hand, it is difficult to understand why the present plan is followed.   The student suffers the disadvantage of nowhere gaining any conception of normal fresh material.   When she comes to surgery in the hospital the conditions are almost entirely abnormal.   She may thus always lack a normal basic conception for comparative purposes.

The course in physiology in the same training school, on the other hand, is greatly in advance of the work observed at most other hospitals.   It provides comprehensive classroom instruction by a university professor as well as extensive laboratory experiments involving the use of elaborate physiological apparatus.

USE OF OUTSIDE FACILITIES

Autopsies

To supplement the first-hand experience of demonstration and individual laboratory work, it is arranged in some hospitals that students should attend autopsies.   In 12 out of 22 hospitals studied the custom is followed, but attendance is variously reported as "seldom," "sometimes," "frequent," and in most cases the use made of the visit is not altogether definite.   One hospital arranges only one visit to an autopsy, but requires a full report of this as part of the regular class work.

Perhaps more valuable than casual attendance at autopsies are the visits made in 2 hospitals to the medical school dissecting rooms while medical students are making human dissections. In one case 10 or 15 minutes are given to such visits after nearly every class, and students have an opportunity to handle and become familiar with the organs and tissues they have been studying.   This is only feasible, of course, where the hospital is closely allied with a medical school and where a friendly feeling of co-operation exists on the part of the medical school authorities.

Medical Museum

Medical museums may also be available as rich fields for study. In 6 hospitals visits to such museums are arranged for, but the chief use of the medical museum is to furnish preserved specimens for class demonstration. In many cases, of course, no museum exists near enough to make such co-operation feasible, and study of preserved specimens must be limited to those that can be furnished by the collection of the hospital's pathological laboratory.

X-Ray Room

Only one school of our group is known to plan class visits to its x-ray room. Probably this means of illustration could be used to advantage in many other hospitals.

BACTERIOLOGY

Like anatomy, bacteriology is included in the curricula of nearly all the hospitals studied. Of the 23 hospitals reporting, 21 show bacteriology among the introductory sciences.[32]

HOURS AND YEAR WHEN GIVEN

The hours vary from 11 to 80, the median school, however, showing only 24 hours. In our proposed plan, the allotment of hours is 45. The outstanding fact here is the entirely inadequate amount of time allowed in the majority of schools. When half of the courses are less than 24 hours and even three-quarters of them are less than 36, it is clear that not even the elementary facts of bacteriology, or more than the most superficial handling of laboratory material, can be taught.

In 10 hospitals the work is given entirely as a preliminary subject. One hospital gives an advanced short course in the first year in addition to the preliminary course at an affiliated college. In the others the course is variously distributed over the preliminary period and the latter part of the first year, but in no case is any of the work postponed to the second or third year. This is as it should be, since the purpose of the course is primarily to insure as early as possible in the student's practical

[32] In one hospital where the subject is lacking a course is planned but had not yet been begun at the time of our visit.

experience a comprehension of the theory of asepsis and the part played by bacterial life in determining physical welfare or disease.

Of the 21 instructors in charge of these courses:

9 are resident women instructors,
4 are the pathologists of the hospital,
4 are internes or attending physicians,
4 are professors or instructors of allied or affiliated medical schools or colleges.

Only 4 of the number of outside instructors are professional teachers whose positions in educational institutions offer as well the presumption of competence in their subjects. The 8 hospital officers and physicians are presumably expert in the subject-matter taught, but their teaching qualifications are uncertain. In the case of the 9 resident instructors, as we have seen in connection with anatomy and physiology, equipment and teaching ability, in default of specific knowledge of their preparation, are likewise uncertain.

METHODS OF TEACHING

For 20 hospitals [33] data are at hand regarding methods of teaching. There are two instances of the combined use of text, lecture, recitation, quiz, demonstration, and individual laboratory work, and one more school using all these methods except a text.

In bacteriology as in anatomy and physiology, the outstanding weakness of the courses observed was the lack of individual laboratory work. Yet bacteriology is a science that lends itself least profitably to classroom methods, except as they are supplemented by individual laboratory experiment. The value of the courses given in the various hospitals may therefore be gauged chiefly by the laboratory facilities offered and used. As a substitute for individual laboratory work, demonstration is less valuable in bacteriology than in either anatomy, physiology, or chemistry. It is disappointing, therefore, to find that, although 17 of the 20 courses include more or less valuable demonstration by the instructor in connection with classroom work, only 7 make any provision for individual laboratory practice.

---

[33] One other provides all its preliminary science through affiliation with a neighboring college, which affords excellent laboratory facilities.

FACILITIES FOR LABORATORY WORK

Of the 7 training schools in which laboratories are used for individual work, 2 make use of the excellent facilities provided by the universities of which they are an integral part; 3 other schools have their own laboratories, and the remaining 2 use the pathology laboratories of the hospitals. Two of the 3 laboratories belonging to the training schools are entirely modern in plan, adequate in size, and excellently equipped for all the sciences. The classroom work in bacteriology in these 2 schools is generously supplemented by thorough individual laboratory experiment. Entirely satisfactory laboratory practice is not possible in the third of these training schools, owing to bad light, inconvenient arrangement of fixed furnishings, and inadequate equipment.

Of the 2 pathological laboratories in which individual work is done, 1 is admittedly a makeshift used pending the completion of a school laboratory included in the plans for a new nurses' home. The present quarters are cramped, storage room insufficient, and equipment only fairly adequate. The second of these pathological laboratories belongs to a hospital used as a teaching field for medical students, who occupy the laboratory in the afternoon, leaving it free for the nurses' use in the morning. Opportunity here should be excellent. Space and equipment is satisfactory, but the entire storage room for individual supplies is monopolized by the medical students. Student nurses' supplies have to be kept in boxes which have been provided through the ingenuity of an enterprising instructor, and the work is carried on under these circumstances with very great inconvenience both for the students and for the instructor.

It is worthy of note that this is one of the few pathological laboratories that offer adequate accommodations for a class of any size. In most cases, where the room has been planned solely for the hospital analyses, it is too limited in space and in duplication of implements to be entirely adequate for class use.

EQUIPMENT

For good laboratory work equipment is assumed to include sterilizer, autoclave, incubator, icebox, individual work desks well placed for light, and sufficient storage space for individual supplies. Supplies should include individual implements (forceps, needles, etc.), glassware, chemical reagents, culture media, microscopes, and microscopic slides, and various fresh materials for bacterial examination and study.

Gauged by this standard, of the 7 schools offering individual laboratory work, 5 are well equipped (except for the lack of storage room in one pathological laboratory noted) and 2 are unsatisfactory.

EXAMPLES OF GOOD LABORATORY TEACHING

A good class in bacteriology was observed in a well-equipped school connected with a private hospital. The hour began with a brief written quiz and lecture developed by questions on diseases and conditions which predispose to infection. This was followed by laboratory tests made on a guinea pig inoculated with tuberculosis. Sputum specimens from tuberculosis patients and from suspect cases, made by the students themselves, were studied. A tuberculin test of 5 students was made by one of the class. The investigator comments as follows:

"A splendid example of good teaching, from the standpoint of scope of subject covered, content, variety, thoroughness, interest, and power of arousing independent thought of students. This instructor gave encouragement to the student without in any case suggesting the answer when she could think it out by herself. The ill-effects of bad nursing on conditions described were pointed out, and correlation with other aspects of the subject were noted continually."

Throughout the class the students followed closely every step in the development of the lesson, showing themselves alert and ready with prompt replies, even when considerable thought was necessary for the answers. Such interest and understanding on the part of the students would hardly be possible, without the intimate personal knowledge that comes from direct observation of laboratory experiment.

Another good class was visited in a university course for nurses. A short period in the classroom was spent in a review quiz on different types of cell structures previously studied. Assignments for laboratory work were then given, with explanations of what the students were to look for and details as to how to prepare their slides from the fresh material. Although this was only the third laboratory period in the course, the students took hold as if they knew how to proceed and within half an hour seven of the ten had actual specimens under their microscopes, illustrating the points previously discussed. Each examined the slides of the others as well as her own and made drawings of what she saw. "Not one," the observer reports, "but was absorbed with interest in the work of the hour; and not one seemed at a loss to understand the meaning of what she saw."

The practical value of the laboratory method in exemplifying a lesson clearly and forcefully was well illustrated in a series of homely experiments observed in one of the leading training schools, where, as one of their laboratory exercises, the students inoculated agar plates from their hands, (1) with no washing, (2) after a ten-minute scrub, (3) after an iodine treatment. The plates were laid away for examination after the proper period of incubation. The efficacy of various methods of sterilizing the thermometers was also made a matter of ocular demonstration.

It is safe to say that even an elementary course, accompanied by such practical laboratory experiment, would result in more substantial scientific understanding than a more elaborate course based on exposition and discussion alone, or even illustrated merely by demonstration by the instructor. Such experiment brings home to the student, as no mere lecture can, what has been well said by a teacher of bacteriology: "The culture is the detective that reveals the criminal nurse." The laboratory illustrates for the student the essential duties of disinfection and sterilization.

DEMONSTRATION BY THE INSTRUCTOR ONLY

Ten schools have no individual laboratory work by the students, and use laboratories for demonstration by the instructor only. Weak as this method is in comparison with student experimentation, the instructors have at least a minimum of scientific apparatus and material with which to demonstrate.

In 3 other schools the instructors give demonstrations in an ordinary classroom with only such material as can be brought in. This amounts to little more than the showing of microscopic slides which the students have had no share in making. One of the schools is connected with a large, wealthy hospital able to provide whatever facilities the authorities may approve, but the school is dominated by a board apparently without appreciation of the necessity of laboratory practice in any of the sciences.

In another of these 3 schools the bacteriology course given to first-year students is thoroughly unsatisfactory and barren. Like the class in anatomy in the same school (see page 264), bacteriology is taught by perfunctory questions and answers. In the class visited the teacher read aloud a chapter on malaria from a popular book called "Insects and Disease." There was no correlation with any other subject nor with any of the students' practical work, and naturally enough no interest was shown on the part of the class.

Yet in the same hospital a small laboratory in the basement of the nurses' home is utilized by second-year students in a course on laboratory technique. Although the room is so small that it can accommodate only six students, individual experimentation is carried on by students working in pairs. The work includes urinalysis, examination of stomach contents, feces, blood, and sputum, and making slides for examination of blood, sputum, and bacteria. On the day of our visit slides of tubercle bacilli were being made by the class. The students were questioned both on methods of making slides and on the importance placed in diagnosis on finding the bacillus; there was keen interest and active participation. This work, while not of high quality, showed clearly enough that the existing laboratory facilities, meager though they were, might have been used to good purpose in the bacteriology course of the first year.

One instance where the opportunity for individual laboratory work is incredibly neglected is in a training school using the laboratory of an associated medical school. Although the room is fully equipped for individual work and is so used by medical students for part of the day, the nurses' training school is not allowed to use the equipment and owns none of its own. The equipment used for demonstration to the nurses (microscopes, etc.) is actually borrowed by the physician-instructor from another laboratory!

In another case, the hospital pathological laboratory, is described as ample and the equipment complete,[34] but in spite of the facilities ready to hand no individual laboratory work whatever is arranged for. The scarcely final excuse given is that the microscopes are all in use by medical students.

Again, individual laboratory work in one school was at the time of our visit abandoned temporarily owing to the burning of the pathological building of the hospital. Apparatus and ma-

[34] Apparatus of the pathological laboratory can be supplemented from that of the co-operating medical school.

terial from the hospital pathological equipment was used for one demonstration only during the course. Yet arrangements to continue individual work in temporary quarters might undoubtedly have been made, as the hospital is allied with a large medical school amply equipped for the instruction of its medical students.

While demonstration of any sort is better than none, and while skilful demonstration may be illuminating to a high degree, it must be again insisted that an intelligent understanding of the processes of bacterial life and the relation of microscopic life to the condition of grosser organisms is peculiarly dependent on an opportunity for the minute observation and careful study of individual experiment. By no other method can the ordinary mind connect intelligently an invisible cause with an apparently unrelated result. In view of the value of such experience in a nurse's training, it is surely not too much to expect of the schools that their course in bacteriology shall provide at least a fair amount of individual laboratory practice, such as we have described at certain schools.

CHEMISTRY

Courses in chemistry are given in 19 of the 23 training schools investigated. In one school where it is neither included in the curriculum nor required for entrance, it is reported that as a matter of fact the majority of entering students have had a course either in high school or college.

HOURS AND YEAR WHEN GIVEN

The hours of the courses given cover the astonishing range of 10 to 135. That this maximum is isolated is shown, however, by the median, 24, which is fairly representative of the grudging time allowed this science by the majority of schools. Only two courses are over 40 hours in length. Our proposed plan, on the other hand, allows for 60 hours. In all but one school chemistry is given as a preliminary. In that one, a course of 18 hours is given in the second year. The subject cannot be logically postponed beyond the earliest period of training, as the principles of chemistry are essential to an intelligent study of the other basic sciences, anatomy and physiology and bacteriology, as well as to an understanding of the action of drugs.

INSTRUCTORS

Of the 20 instructors mentioned in connection with these 19 schools:

4 are resident nurse instructors. (One of these is the acting superintendent, another the dietitian.)

3 are hospital internes or attending physicians.

1 is the hospital pathologist.

2 are hospital pharmacists. (The resident pharmacist of one hospital teaches also in the second hospital as visiting instructor.)

3 are instructors at an allied or co-operating medical college.

2 are instructors in universities of which the training schools are part.

4 are instructors in affiliated high schools.

1 is an instructor in an affiliated college.

Half of these instructors, then, are professional high school, college, or university teachers. The teaching ability of the 6 hospital officials is uncertain, and the adequacy of the 4 nurse instructors making up the rest of the list depends on whether or not they have had specialized instruction.

METHODS OF INSTRUCTION

Class work with recitations and quizzes based on lectures or assigned text forms part of the course, as in other sciences. Individual laboratory experimentation is much more general in chemistry than in any other of the sciences, though in chemistry better than elsewhere it may be supplemented or in part replaced by classroom demonstration. Thirteen out of 17 schools reporting make use of laboratories for individual work combined with demonstration. In 2 others, small laboratories are used only for demonstration by the instructor; only 2 schools depend for illustration on such demonstration as can be done in the classroom.

LABORATORY FACILITIES AND EQUIPMENT

In 4 schools the classes use the finely equipped laboratories of allied universities, medical schools, or the pathological laboratory of the hospital is made to serve in one case; 4 training schools have their own laboratories; and 4 more use the standard equipment of neighboring high schools.

The facilities thus variously provided range from very elaborate equipment including individual desks with sinks and hot and cold running water, exhaust hoods, and complete individual supplies of implements and materials, to simpler and less complete furnishings. Yet in only two cases, one a training school laboratory, the other the pathological laboratory mentioned, was there reason to consider the facilities inadequate.

Lack of equipment cannot then be blamed for any general shortcomings in the teaching of chemistry. The undeniable weakness of this subject in the training schools is primarily due to two reasons: lack of adequate time, and the unstandardized and generally overcrowded character of the courses. In some cases incompetence and lack of vision on the part of the teacher is a contributory cause.

CONTENT OF COURSES: THE ELEMENT OF TIME

The niggardly allowance of time given chemistry in most of the training schools has already been pointed out. In one school which actually allots only 12 hours to the subject, the major part of the course is given to domestic chemistry, 4 lessons only being devoted to the rudiments of general chemistry. It is small wonder that the observer of a class in bacteriology in this hospital found the students lacking in a background of chemistry, and inclined to confuse microbes with molecules!

From this meager scrap of preparation the content of the courses in other schools is found to cover increasing amounts and in some to include the whole field of general chemistry. By far the best course observed was that of a training school belonging to a well-known university, in which, contrary to the rule, generous time is alloted. Of the 135 hours given to the course, 90 hours are spent in laboratory demonstration and experiment. The remaining 45 hours of the course are spent in classroom instruction as follows:

Inorganic Chemistry .... 18 hours
General Organic Chemistry .... 16 hours
Physiological Chemistry .... 8 hours
Chemistry of Urinalysis .... 3 hours

The lesson observed was on carbonates as the basis of many organic compounds. The instructor developed the subject broadly, showing the relations of specific compounds to their groups, and of the groups to each other, thus giving to the students at the start an underlying knowledge upon which to build later details. A strikingly successful feature of the laboratory experiments was the illustration of ordinary reactions by the use of physiological (organic) compounds and drugs, instead of the usual chemicals used in the regular college laboratory classes, which the student seldom meets outside of a chemical laboratory. This correlation of the subject with the practical needs of the nurses was undoubtedly the cause of the absorbed interest shown by the students.

CRAM COURSES

In two other large schools the instructors are faced with the problem of covering the entire subject of chemistry in 32 instead of 135 hours. In attempting to condense the course, it is difficult for any one who realizes the indispensable value of the subject wholly to omit any important topic. The temptation is therefore to crowd the whole subject matter into the utterly inadequate time allowed. In the hands of an experienced teacher such condensation may be skilfully and ably done,. and yet remain far above the heads of elementary students. A case in point is seen in a training school where a highly condensed course is conducted by the instructor of an allied medical school. The classes are held in the medical laboratory, where full equipment is available for demonstration and individual experiment. The course consists of 15 lectures of 40 minutes each, accompanied by 6 three-hour laboratory periods. Like the university course covering 135 hours, these lectures cover the entire field of chemistry including inorganic, organic, physiological chemistry, and the chemistry of excretion and urinalysis. But such a course, however brilliant as a *tour de force* on the part of the lecturer, must be largely wasted through the inability of untrained minds to assimilate so much in so short a time.

Evidence of a similarly mistaken policy is afforded by another chemistry class for student nurses in a large university of which the training school is part. The outline of the course, with the time to be allotted to it, is designated by the superintendent of nurses, reluctantly accepted by the dean of the department, and administered with equal reluctance by the university instructor. These officers protest that with the best teaching it can be nothing but a cram course, absolutely superficial and entirely unfair to the student. They maintain that the outline asks altogether more than can even be touched upon; there can be no adequate treatment of any part of the course. The examination which the students were taking on the day of the visit perfectly illustrated the instructor's point. The questions involved a knowledge of facts which required a much longer course for their proper discussion. From the course as given, the students could have no real knowledge of the topics called for. Yet the instructor felt that the students were worthy of a course of genuinely university grade and was ready to co-operate in giving it whenever the training school curriculum should allow sufficient time for it. Students as well as instructor expressed dissatisfaction with the superficial character of this overcrowded course, some of them saying that girls with a preparation of high school chemistry had had better work than was offered here.

The fault of this training school must be squarely laid to lack of educational standards on the part of the superintendent of nurses. According to our investigator,

"She showed little comprehension of the time requirements of thorough science teaching, probably because her own training was superficial, and because she has been familiar with the toleration of very superficial courses by most nurses' training schools."

This toleration of inadequate courses is doubtless due not only to educational inexperience on the part of training school directors but to the crowding demands of the hospital for student service, and to the temptation to emphasize the practical side of the nurse's training. The need for thorough training in chemistry is perhaps less obvious than in other subjects. Yet it must be reiterated that with the modern development of the study of bacteriology, physiology, dietetics, and the action of drugs, a scientific knowledge of chemistry is the foundation of an intelligent understanding of these subjects also. That its importance is belittled, or but vaguely appreciated, could not be more conclusively proved than by the almost universal allotment of time absurdly inadequate for the proper teaching of the subject.

COURSES OF LIMITED SCOPE: LOSS OF IMPORTANT SUBJECTS

Another way of meeting the difficulty of time than by merely giving a cram course was observed in one of the affiliated high schools. The instructor is one well-known in the city and highly respected as an experienced and able teacher. The laboratory facilities of the school are ample and excellent. The course has been specially adapted for the student nurses, as the time allowed (30 hours) is very much less than that given to the regular high school course, and a definite effort is made to render it of real value to them instead of trying to cover an outline, as is done with such disastrous results in the university school just cited. In order to cut down the standard course and bring it within the time allowed, organic and physiological chemistry are entirely omitted. We have seen that, in the extensive course of 135 hours given so successfully at one of the university schools, this was the very portion of the course which was emphasized as being particularly applicable to the nurses' work; yet with only 30 hours in which to cover the entire subject, something of vital importance must necessarily be sacrificed. Considering the handicap of time, this was held to be one of the best courses seen.

Yet at present it is evident that the problem of chemistry is not being successfully handled in most of the training schools. The dilemma seems to be absolute. If the teaching of the subject is not to continue a failure, either more time must be found for it on the curriculum or chemistry must be made an entrance requirement.

CHEMISTRY AS AN ENTRANCE SUBJECT

It has been pointed out that 3 of the 23 schools studied tacitly assume a training in chemistry as an entrance subject and do not include it in their curriculum. Two of these are large schools of deserved reputation which attract the highest quality of student nurse. The attitude of these schools toward chemistry is that it is a high school subject on which time should not need to be spent within the training school. The verdict on the success of this omission is, however, not unanimous. It is true that in one of these training schools, while the subject is neither required for entrance nor included in the curriculum, it is asserted that most of the class have had chemistry in either high school or college, and that one period of chemistry as a "review" in physiology is sufficient as a basis for intelligent work in the other sciences. This satisfaction does not exist in the other 2 schools. In one of these the head instructor, the dietitian, and several senior students who were interviewed, expressed themselves as feeling that the subject was a fundamental one greatly missed in the nurse's training.

That it cannot generally be assumed that students entering the nursing schools have had previous training in chemistry is very sure. One school may be cited, of less prestige than those mentioned above, where in two classes totaling 59 students only 3 had ever studied chemistry in high school. Even in one of the large schools allied to a university, where the students are recognized as of high grade, many in the chemistry class had had no previous high school chemistry. Plainly, then, we cannot count with assurance on any previous training in chemistry among candidates for the nursing schools.

In view of the already overcrowded state of the training school curricula, it is easy to understand that a longer time allowance for chemistry seems to the authorities a well-nigh impossible demand. The requirement of chemistry for entrance is, on the other hand, beset with difficulties. One prominent hospital which tried the experiment was forced to give it up because of the resulting loss of candidates. Moreover, even if the technical requirements are met by the schools, there is no assurance in the present unstandardized state of the high school curricula that the standards of teaching will be uniform, or that the student "entering with chemistry" will have any adequate practical knowledge of the subject as an equipment for her training school work.

If these difficulties can be met, it would seem best to require of candidates a high school preparation in chemistry. As we shall presently see, chemistry is not the only science which might ultimately be made an entrance requirement and thus relieve the training school of the teaching of first principles in science.

DIETETICS [35]

Scarcely less essential than the four basic sciences already discussed is the inclusion of dietetics in the preliminary term. A thorough course in dietetics should aim to give students through class teaching and laboratory practice a sound fundamental understanding of the principles and methods of cookery. It should make them familiar with the nutritive values of food and with the essentials of well-balanced daily meals for normal health and for convalescence. It should, moreover, train them to high standards of cleanliness and sanitation in relation to food, and of appetizing and dainty service. Fancy cookery as such has no place in such a course, though dainty garnishes and attractive variations of typical dishes should be included. Every effort should be made to direct the students' work to the concrete and practical rather than to the theoretical and abstract aspect of the subject. They should be taught to apply their

[35] Acknowledgments are due for conference and discussion on the subjects treated in this chapter to the Sub-Committee on Teaching Dietetics to Student Nurses of the American Dietetic Association.

knowledge of food values to the planning of the day's diets, and to think in terms of the daily meal service. Their lessons should be based as far as possible on the preparation of actual meals and the setting up of trays, rather than on isolated masses of facts on food values and preparation. The objective in teaching should be not a memorizing of recipes, but a knowledge of general principles and proportions in cooking.

It is important also that the instructor in dietetics should keep in touch with the preliminary sciences directly related to her subject, such as chemistry and physiology, and should correlate her course with them as closely as possible. The course should include a review of the physiology of the digestive processes, and some classification of foods according to their composition and value. It should further give practice in measuring and computing these values, and offer an introduction to the simpler forms of hospital diets.

Furthermore, since the best instruction must be enforced by opportunity for practice, and since even a thorough laboratory course can allow only for limited applications of the principles taught, the course in dietetics must be fortified by a brief period of service in the diet kitchen in which the student by repeated practice of the invalid cookery she has been taught in classroom and laboratory shall acquire a reasonably sure technique in the preparation of simple dishes.

This should be sharply distinguished from the diet kitchen assignment proper, and should be strictly regarded as an extension of laboratory training. As in nursing procedures, a system of definite checking should be adopted so that each student's proficiency should be progressively certified. This will furnish an assurance on the one hand that the necessary ground is covered, and safeguard the student on the other against being made use of at the convenience of the hospital merely to "get the work done."

An adequate basic training in classroom and laboratory in the principles of nutrition and the practice of cookery, thus reinforced by a certain amount of further practice in a short diet kitchen assignment, is an indispensable preparation for effective later training in special diets with accompanying lectures on diet in disease. Weakness in the preliminary course involves waste of time and duplication later, inasmuch as part of the time set aside for intensive professional training must be reassigned to elementary work supposedly already mastered. Thorough preparatory training, on the other hand, in normal nutrition and simple cookery sets the time of the diet kitchen service free for the specialized work properly belonging to it.

HOURS AND YEAR WHEN GIVEN

Instruction in dietetics is given in all of the 23 training schools studied. Not less than 60 hours of lectures and laboratory work with laboratory periods of at least 2 hours in length should be considered adequate for this basic instruction in nutrition and cookery. This should be followed directly, preferably in the preliminary term, by a short period of practice in the diet kitchen.

But in fact the hours allowed for the teaching of dietetics vary almost as widely as do those for the basic sciences. Omitting an isolated maximum of 135 hours allowed at a university hospital, where the general subject of nutrition is treated together with special diets in the second year, and the next highest number, 66, allowed at a large municipal hospital adopting a similar plan, the range is from 17 to 64 hours, and the median 34. Curiously enough the minimum allowance is found not only at a special hospital where instruction is notably weak but at a training school of wide educational distinction. The maximum, 64, again at a university hospital of advanced educational standards, barely passes the minimum allowance which we believe to be essential for classroom instruction, leaving out of account the added hours of practice in the diet kitchen.

In more than four-fifths of the training schools studied (19 out of 22), the course or courses in dietetics are rightly given in the preliminary period or in the first year. Of 22 schools affording information, 9 place this work in the preliminary period, and the remaining 8 either divide it between the preliminary period and the later part of the first year, or place it wholly in the later part of this year. Beyond question this subject, if it is to have its highest interpretative value in the student's experience, should be given as a preliminary; and certainly before the end of the first year. Yet 2 schools, one of them where the instruction in dietetics is notably good, divide this work between the probation period and the second year, and 3 others place it wholly in the second.

NURSING AND NURSING EDUCATION

As the development of modern medicine makes the subject of dietetics more and more important in the training school curriculum, the choice of instructors is a matter of increasing moment. It should be taught by trained dietitians, graduates in household science from accredited schools, preferably, moreover, with hospital experience.

At 16 of the 22 schools giving data in the matter, the courses in dietetics were found to be in charge of one or more regular dietitians. At 4 of these the dietitians in charge are assisted by one or more student dietitians; at another the chief is given two assistant dietitians. A large university school supplements the teaching of two hospital dietitians in the elementary course by instruction in the advanced course by a household arts instructor and a home economics professor from the university. Of the remaining schools, one well-known special hospital sends its students for dietetics training, as for the preliminary sciences, to a neighboring vocational college; 2 others send their students to Young Women's Christian Association classes under Young Women's Christian Association instructors. Nineteen schools, then, give their students the benefit of instruction by specialists in dietetics; at 4 schools at least they are trained teachers as well. At 2 others the courses are in charge of "assistant dietitians," and at the remaining one, of a non-resident dietitian no further described, and of a physician.

There is, of course, no assurance that a trained dietitian will be an efficient teacher. One of the dietetics courses poorest in quality and least educational, though given at a school of generally high standing, is taught by the first assistant dietitian. At another school the appointment of a "special resident dietitian, young and inexperienced" as instructor holds out dubious promise for the work she is to teach.

We must bear in mind, moreover, that in the schools of the country as a whole the qualifications for teachers of dietetics are likely to be much less standardized than in those of our picked group. For example, in the schools affording information in a certain western state, 21 teachers of dietetics were trained dietitians while 18 had no special training. Yet the fact that special training for a specialist's position is accepted as indispensable in the teaching of dietetics in the great majority of a group representing the better practice of nursing education in the country, marks in this subject, in contrast with too many others, a long step towards the establishment of a minimum standard, and opens the way for further selection.

METHODS OF INSTRUCTION

Dietetics is taught with few exceptions in the training schools by the usual lecture and laboratory method with varying use of quizzes, recitation, and demonstration. Two-thirds of the schools where the point was noted (10 out of 15) use textbooks; about the same number are adequately equipped with charts and other illustrative material.

Lack of a textbook involves here, as we have elsewhere noted, very often a waste of time in taking notes on what might better be learned from a standard text. At its worst, the lecture system degenerates into mere dictation, as was observed at several of the hospitals visited. At a leading university training school, indeed, and at one of our most distinguished private schools, where educational standards might be expected to be of the best, the dietetics lesson was compared by our investigator to a dictation exercise. Where no textbook is used, the students' notebooks are generally handed in and corrected.

The Need of Laboratory Training

If laboratory practice is essential to the best teaching of the basic sciences, it is even more obviously indispensable for any successful teaching of dietetics. In dietetics, no less than in nursing procedures, the success of the teaching must depend on its opportunity for direct practical application. No one has maintained that cooking can be acquired by didactic instruction or by demonstration. It is of the essence of the subject, as it is again of nursing practice, that the student not only must understand but must directly apply the theory learned in the classroom, and must acquire technique by practice.

Three training schools, 2 of them strangely enough of high standing educationally, leave out entirely the essential training of laboratory work. One of these gives in other respects a wholly inadequate course, the other 2 make some attempt to supplement their didactic instruction by a certain amount of demonstration. The more distinguished of these 2 schools gives one of the worst courses observed during our study, short, elementary, and dull, with little use of illustrative material and a minimum of demonstration, and throws the whole weight of practical instruction in cookery on a long assignment to the diet kitchen. Small wonder that the probationers so assigned, many of them college women, instead of professional training find their diet kitchen work equivalent to the merest maid's service, spend long hours in washing lettuce or preparing salads, and are obliged in wearisome repetition to make toast, cook eggs, make coffee and cocoa, spread bread, and serve meals from the steam table.

In one middle western city where an enlightened effort has been made to improve academic standards by a system of centralized teaching, the classroom work in dietetics is wholly unsupported by any provision for laboratory work and the students' practical work consists in plain cooking in the hospital kitchen for 152 patients.

Tendency to Over-Emphasize Cookery

It has been a standing temptation of the training school to plan the teaching of dietetics for the practical convenience of the diet kitchen service rather than for the student's ultimate education. Thus we may trace a general tendency among the hospitals studied to emphasize simple cookery at the expense of the basic principles of nutrition, and still more to subordinate to it the more advanced professional instruction in caloric feeding, weighing and calculating of diets, etc. Instances of this general criticism of the work in dietetics at the various hospitals visited may be found in the comments of our investigators at 2 prominent training schools. At one of these the class visited seemed "more a cooking school hour than an intelligent course in nutrition," at the other the work was qualified as "needlessly superficial," and "really a cooking course rather than a course in scientific dietetics."

In certain instances of "fancy cookery" observed in the classes visited, the object of a basic course in dietetics seemed to have been wholly forgotten. At one important training school where a scanty 34 hours was allotted for the entire course, a part of one of these precious hours was found to be devoted to the making of candied cranberries.

At other schools our observer noted a higher standard of work and a more scientific attitude. At a university school visited the lecture on nutrition was noted as of regular college grade, while at a large municipal hospital the dietetics given seemed to be "a thorough-going course of much value to the students" and the class heard "fully equal in value to the average college teaching."

LABORATORY EQUIPMENT

For adequate laboratory training in dietetics, facilities must be provided for individual laboratory work. These should include individual equipment of desks, drawers, stoves, and, where possible, ovens, individual cooking equipment, dishes, and utensils. There should be adequate provision of sinks with hot and cold water, a range with a large oven where individual ovens cannot be provided, an ice-chest, and a good-sized store closet. For individual attention and satisfactory class teaching, not more than 16 students should be included in a section.

Six of the hospitals studied provide well-fitted dietetic laboratories with more or less complete individual equipment. Four others arrange for excellent facilities for their students outside the hospital. Thus one university school shares with the home economics department of the university the use of a "beautiful, newly equipped class and laboratory room" in one of the university buildings. The laboratories of an affiliated college used by the classes of another training school are of standard excellence, and the Young Women's Christian Association courses attended by the students of two schools under sectarian control have at their disposal the usual laboratory equipment with individual appliances.

Three of our group of training schools are entirely without laboratory facilities for the teaching of dietetics. At all 3 the courses given are in any case meager and inadequate. At one of them the very limited instruction consists wholly of classroom work. At another, 5 periods of demonstration, supplementing the didactic work, are given in the regular diet kitchen, quite without equipment for teaching purposes. At the third, the inconvenience of arranging demonstrations either in the dark basement classroom, or in the diet kitchen during the evening hours when it is not in use, results in a minimum of demonstration.

Between these extremes, the facilities offered by the other hospitals vary widely. One well-known university school offers an example of the frequent subordination of the nurses' work to that of other departments of the university. Here the dietetics laboratory, a large room well fitted for individual work, has been recently taken for a graduate laboratory in physiology. The laboratory equipment, without notice to the training school superintendent, was transferred to a small room lacking light and ventilation, entirely inadequate for the requirements of the class, and used, moreover, for other purposes. Overcrowding is a serious problem at this university, but it has been allowed to work a peculiar hardship on the teaching of dietetics.

One of the smaller schools provides for a teaching laboratory a kitchen in the nurses' home, formerly a private residence, equipped with individual sets of portable equipment, but without individual stoves, desks or drawers.

The 5 remaining training schools of our study use the regular hospital kitchens for their laboratory work in dietetics. Some of these are provided with teaching equipment; others are quite without it. Three schools, and schools of considerable distinction, have nothing to offer but the equipment of the ordinary kitchen. At one of these the lack of suitable accommodation and of common utensils, such as sharp knives, is noted by our observer as making good work by a large section really out of the question.

It can scarcely be wondered at if such lack of primary facilities is reflected in discouragement and lack of interest on the part of teachers and students alike. At one of the small, ill-equipped schools, the teacher of dietetics, though keenly interested in her work, is described as "discouraged by the lack of suitable facilities." Another teacher, at a larger school, forced to conduct her classes in the regular kitchen without special teaching equipment, expressed strongly her feeling of the need of a regular dietetics laboratory. The lack of interest observed on the part of class and teacher alike may not be unnatural at the university school where dietetics has just been banished from a good and well-equipped laboratory to a crowded and inconvenient room. Even the barren and valueless course, already described as conducted at a distinguished training school where such teaching should be an anomaly, is undoubtedly deadened and robbed of whatever interest it might have by the lack of laboratory facilities and the "inconvenience" which renders even demonstration for the most part a prohibitive difficulty.

TIME ALLOWED TO THE TEACHING OF THE PRELIMINARY SCIENCES
IN 22 SCHOOLS [36]

To the preliminary science courses the time allowed in the 22 schools studied shows the great range of 52 to 510 hours. The

[36] Including anatomy and physiology, bacteriology, chemistry, dietetics, and hygiene.

latter number, an isolated maximum, is found at a single university school. The average for all schools, 180, indicates very clearly the wholly inadequate time given by the majority to instruction in these basic and indispensable subjects. The following table shows the grouping of the schools according to the hours allowed these courses.

PRELIMINARY SCIENCES

Number of Hours	Number of Schools
50- 99	3
100-149	7
150-199	7
200-249	2
250-299	..
300-349	2
350-399	..
400-449	..
449-500	..
500-550	1
	22

LABORATORY ASSISTANCE IN SCIENCE TEACHING

In all the preliminary sciences the deplorable custom obtains, already noted in connection with the teaching of nursing procedures, of throwing on an often overworked instructor the chief burden of preparing and clearing away the laboratory and demonstration material required for the science classes.

The situation in the teaching of anatomy and physiology may be taken as typical. At 8 out of 12 training schools affording data, the work of preparing for classes and experiments in these subjects is done almost solely by the instructor, and in only 4 of them is she even relieved, and then largely by the students, of the mechanical work of clearing up and putting away material after class. At a ninth school where much use is made of the student assistant teacher, such an assistant, among her other duties, relieves the instructor of much of the care of laboratory material. In one school only, which uses the laboratory of an affiliated medical college, is adequate paid assistance given by the laboratory janitor. In several others provision is made for some assistance, slight and occasional or more nearly adequate, by an orderly, maid, or other helper.

The economic and educational waste of taking the time and strength of either hard-worked instructors or hard-working students for duties which can equally well be performed by paid assistants has been already remarked in our study of the teaching of nursing practice. To add the mechanical tasks of a laboratory boy to the heavy professional responsibilities of resident instructors or the crowded schedules of student nurses is a policy as short-sighted as it is unjust.

UPKEEP AND EXTENSION OF EDUCATIONAL EQUIPMENT

The need of an independent endowment for the training school is notable in the matter of funds for the upkeep and extension of its educational equipment. Such provision, indispensable as it is for any educational institution that seeks to keep in line with modern progress, seems to be rarely made in schools of nursing. Out of 12 schools reporting on this point, only one has a definite appropriation for the upkeep of its various departments in the hospital budget. It is highly significant that this school, and one other with a small private fund and generous backing, are the only ones of our group possessing their own laboratories fully equipped for individual experiment in all the sciences.

The 10 remaining schools must make special requisition, as their needs arise, generally on the hospital treasury and through the superintendent. This plan carries the obvious disadvantage that a business administrator, as the superintendent almost without exception is, and not an educational expert, must pass on the educational needs of the school. Results of this system may be noted at one of the foremost hospitals of the country: here the educational director of the training school reports any new supplies or improvements as exceedingly hard to obtain because neither superintendent nor school principal realizes the pressing need of better educational equipment, especially for some of the science courses.

At another large hospital, the science department of the training school makes requisition for needed supplies on the general house fund, here quite separate from the hospital in management. Unfortunately, however, no special sum is set apart for educational needs, and as the disbursing agent has varied demands to satisfy, a request for laboratory fittings or new books must press its claims against the immediate emergencies of housekeeping.

BOOKS

For the purchase of books as well as of other supplies there is little definite provision in most of the hospitals. In but two training schools of those affording information is there a special library fund.   At another already cited, the regular appropriation from the hospital budget for the supplies of each department includes of course the need of books.   Elsewhere (in 7 schools) books are obtained only by special requisition, and in most cases with considerable difficulty.   At one distinguished school the instructor has been driven to appeal to the Ladies' Board for the few books she needs; at another the faculty have themselves met the difficulty by the purchase of new books at their own expense.

SCIENCE REQUIREMENTS FOR ENTRANCE AND CREDITS FOR SCIENCE

From a survey of the field it is clear that, except in training schools connected with universities which can provide science teachers and laboratories, science teaching in the separate schools is carried on under great difficulties.   Even where the need of this teaching is recognized, the cost of providing and maintaining several different laboratory courses is a comparatively large item of expense for the training school.   The difficulty of obtaining science teachers has already been emphasized.   In some cities an attempt has been made to meet the scarcity of instructors by having two or more schools share a "visiting" teacher.   But this plan does not go far enough to be of constructive value.

We have raised the question whether some of the science teaching might not be required as prerequisite for entrance to the training school, at least within a given number of years.   Chemistry, for instance, which requires separate laboratory equipment and in our proposed curriculum a minimum of 60 hours, is taught in many high schools.   The same is true of dietetics.   It is true as already intimated that these subjects, even if required for entrance, would still need amplification in the training school and special correlation with the ends of nursing.   But the time and effort needed to relate such basic knowledge more closely to nursing would be slight as compared with the present need of teaching students who enter ignorant of a single conception or even definition of science.   The requirement for entrance of high school courses in biology would also greatly aid, and somewhat reduce the time needed for subsequent teaching of bacteriology.

The objections to requiring science for entrance are, as we have seen in the case of chemistry, twofold: the danger of losing good students who have not had these courses, and the difficulty of obtaining scientific instruction of uniform grade in high schools throughout the country.

The first difficulty might be met by allowing a reasonable margin of time to elapse before such a requirement should go into effect. It obviously could not apply at once. But with notice given in advance that such a step is contemplated, students might prepare themselves in time for the requirement.

The second is a more serious difficulty. Especially in small communities, the high school is often as ill-equipped to teach science as the hospital, both in teachers and in laboratories. The shortage of teachers is a topic even more burning than that of nurses. To expect the small high school to provide laboratory courses in chemistry and dietetics and perhaps biology may prove wholly illusory. Yet the tendency is marked, particularly west of the Alleghanies, to make provision in the high school for courses desired by a given number of pupils. With the growth in the teaching of household arts, chemistry and dietetics must receive a new emphasis. It may not be unreasonable to expect that the requirement of these subjects for entrance to the training schools might, within a reasonable period, be an added stimulus to the high schools to provide them.

Certainly, whether or not science is to be ultimately required for entrance, provision should be made in the meantime for giving credits to students entering with science courses and passing satisfactory examinations in them. With classes so mixed as in the school of nursing, its students ranging from college graduates to girls of less than high school education, it is clearly unreasonable not to discriminate between them, so far as possible. While, as already stated, girls entering with chemistry and dietetics would need supplementary instruction from the nursing point of view, an appreciable saving of time could be effected by excusing them from the present elementary courses in those subjects. The time saved might be used to enlarge and enrich the education of these specially prepared students by special training not available to others. With a good grounding, the special applications to nursing can be made, and indeed inevitably recur and are reinforced throughout the training, in the later teaching of drugs and solutions, of materia medica, of diet in disease, and in the later professional lectures and clinics on medical and surgical diseases.

THE TEACHING OF PRELIMINARY SUBJECTS OUTSIDE THE TRAINING SCHOOL

Whatever the possibilities of the future in relieving the present congestion of the training school program by requiring elementary science for entrance, some effort must evidently be made in the meantime to standardize the widely variant scientific instruction now offered during training. The expense of suitable equipment, the scarcity of adequate teachers, are at present serious obstacles in the way of a standard science training at the smaller hospitals. There seems to be but one way of insuring a uniform level of efficient teaching, and this way has been already blazed by the training schools. It is significant to find them in many places trying to meet their difficulties by recourse to science teaching outside the hospital. In some towns and cities they have turned to the high school or to the normal or vocational school; in other places to the junior college.

In order to obtain some idea of the types of such outside instruction a questionnaire was sent to the official board of nurse-examiners or to nursing associations in a number of states. From the replies received, inquiries were addressed to a selected list of training schools in which arrangements for outside teaching were said to be in effect. Data obtained from these inquiries and from other sources of information covered 40 schools availing themselves of outside instruction for their students in one or more subjects. Nearly half of these (18) sent students to high schools or vocational schools or to a normal school. A quarter (11) sent students to the junior college; two schools sent their students for dietetics to the Y. W. C. A. Nine schools made use of a neighboring college, university, or medical school. Arrangements for courses in the last group are included in a subsequent chapter on university schools of nursing and are not treated here.

USE OF THE HIGH SCHOOL OR THE VOCATIONAL SCHOOL

Of the training schools which availed themselves of high school or vocational school instruction for their students, the largest number (10) sent their students for instruction in chemistry; 9 sent their students for instruction in dietetics. The hours in chemistry ranged from 8 to 48 hours; in dietetics from 20 to 50 hours. Two schools sent students for instruction in materia medica; one school respectively for biology, for bacteriology, and for pathology. Some of these courses, such as materia medica and pathology, it is readily evident, deal with subjects manifestly unsuitable for the preliminary term, before the students have had acquaintance with actual disease.

The cost of these courses is usually borne by the hospital; in some instances it is provided free by the educational authorities for the student nurses as for their regular students. While these high school courses are undoubtedly in many instances better than corresponding instruction given in the training school, they are open to objection for students actually in training except as a more or less temporary expedient. The aim of the school of nursing is to give professional training based on the completion of high school. The science teaching in the school should therefore be of higher than high school grade.

We have already discussed the probability that the small high school will find it difficult if not impossible to offer laboratory branches. Yet it is true that the increasing ease of motor transportation may make it possible for students of training schools in small communities to take advantage of the educational facilities of neighboring cities or towns.

USE OF THE JUNIOR COLLEGE

More promising than high school courses in the preliminary term has been the increasing use of the junior college for centralized scientific training. In such affiliations some disadvantages of the high school courses are obviated. The instruction is of post-high school grade, and special classes have in some cases been organized with nurse instructors to provide the needed connection with specific hospital problems. Valuable experiments in providing central instruction for students from several hospitals have been made in two mid-western cities, Grand Rapids, Michigan, and Kansas City, Missouri. In the former city students from three training schools, and in the latter from eight are sent for several hours daily to central courses at the junior college for instruction in preliminary subjects. At Grand Rapids the basic sciences are thus taught, together with dietetics and materia medica; at Kansas City most of the subjects usually given during the preliminary term, and in addition ethics and history of nursing.

Yet while these science courses unquestionably mark a great advance over the science teaching offered at the individual training schools they are handicapped, as are those in the schools, by the utterly inadequate amount of time allowed. In other subjects, moreover, the equipment is not always equal to the standard college facilities supplied for science teaching.

Another difficulty to which the junior college is subject is that of relating the work in these courses closely enough to the nurse's practical training. In nursing subjects correlation with hospital training may indeed be guaranteed by the provision of nurse instructors. College instructors giving expert instruction in science, on the other hand, are naturally not equipped to apply their subjects to the special problems of the nurse. Still worse is the situation where the college instructor is expected to teach the special nursing subject. Thus the teaching of materia medica must be *in vacuo* when the instructor is unable to connect it with the use of medication in the hospital or its effects on diseased conditions. Again, in dietetics, the instructor who gives only theoretical work in nutrition, leaving all practical teaching of cookery to be done at the hospitals, without opportunity to follow up or supervise her students in diet kitchen or on the wards, must be admitted to have left the main problem of her subject unsolved.

But these difficulties, incident to a new project, will in large part create their own remedies. Better equipment in nursing subjects will be provided; some plan will be worked out for providing the needed application of the branches taught to the special ends of nursing; even the scanty time allowance cannot in central courses be forced so low as it may be at individual hospital schools.

EXPERIMENTS IN CENTRAL TEACHING

A larger recent experiment in centralized teaching is that initiated during the war emergency in the city of Toronto. The shortage of physicians, the necessity of conserving the instructors' time, the inability of the smaller schools in the crisis to meet the standard requirements [37] unaided, all pointed to the centralization of training school instruction as a piece of immediate practical wisdom and economy. The plan is still in operation. All the eleven training schools of the city enter their students for a joint course in chemistry arranged and given by the Central Technical School. Here large and small schools alike share the advantages of instruction and laboratory facilities better than any single school could furnish. Nine of the 11 schools, moreover, send their students to the centralized course given at the University

[37] The curriculum of the Graduate Nurses' Association of Ontario.

of Toronto [38] and taught by instructors appointed by the medical faculty of the university. This central course includes lectures in bacteriology in the first year, as well as in all of the so-called professional subjects throughout the course.

The advantages of this plan of central teaching are obvious. Prominent among them are better instruction and equipment. Of prime importance also is the uniformity of teaching and the standardization of the training school curriculum secured by the centralized course. Not less desirable is the further standardization of the nursing diploma assured by the adoption of the uniform examination and the appointment of a central committee for the grading of the papers.

On the other hand, two drawbacks to the Toronto plan must not be ignored. The didactic instruction in disease given without clinics or quizzes is totally lacking in concrete application. Moreover, the standardization, valuable as it is for the smaller and weaker school, is of questionable benefit for the leaders.

A LATER EXPERIMENT

An enterprise in central teaching of decided promise which has been launched in the current year in Philadelphia is the Central School for the Teaching of Preliminary Courses in Nursing Education. The school has been organized by the Philadelphia Hospital Association and the League of Nursing Education, and financed by these organizations as an educational experiment without charge to the individual hospitals benefiting by it, except for the car-fare and laboratory material of the students attending the courses. The best teachers from the city training schools were secured for the experiment, rooms and laboratory facilities were arranged for at the Drexel Institute, the Girls' Normal School, and the University of Pennsylvania, and the school was opened at the midyear (February, 1922) with 66 students representing 11 schools of nursing. All preliminary subjects were taught except nursing practice, for which in this first semester no facilities were available.

It is planned by the committee in charge to carry the school as a demonstration through a full academic year, after which it is hoped that the several hospital boards will recognize its value

[38] These schools have no direct affiliation with the university which extends to them, however, the courtesy of placing a classroom at their disposal and permitting its medical faculty unofficially to plan the teaching of the centralized course.

by financing it for their respective students. Further plans look toward an ultimate affiliation with the University of Pennsylvania, the appointment of a director who shall be a graduate registered nurse, and a staff of paid instructors, all of whom as well as the director shall measure up to such educational standards as will make them eligible to membership on the University faculty. A notable indication of the wisdom of the present management of the undertaking is evident in the projected division of the students' time between school and hospital. This division, which is to provide for definite study periods and ward work not to exceed two hours daily during five days in the week, leaves the students unusually free for study during their term of attendance at the school.

But this system of centralized teaching is in effect transitional to the plan already in practice in a number of university centers by which the training school becomes an integral part of the university. This highest development of standardized central teaching as shown in university schools of nursing connected with one or more hospitals, forms the subject of a separate chapter.

8. Practical Training

WARD TRAINING

In a previous chapter we have indicated that immediately following the preliminary term, or earlier in schools having no such term, the student's training is continued by service on the wards.

We have already seen in the teaching of nursing procedures the diverse methods of various schools in transferring practice from demonstration rooms to the wards. We are next to analyse the details of ward training which, in the course of three years, is designed to transform the raw student into the competent nurse, or at least the nurse so far trained in the school of experience that she is safe to send out into the community.

Training on the wards varies widely in the different schools, ranging from carefully planned educational systems to service totally haphazard and without educational value. Indeed, even in a single hospital, to the amazement of the investigator, the training in different departments may be superlative, commonplace, or so deficient as to be even dangerous, alike for patients and students. Thus an invaluable surgical service, illuminated by clinics and carefully supervised, may coexist with a medical service in which probationers have charge of erysipelas cases, practically unsupervised; or a fine medical service may be under the same roof with diet kitchen or dispensary duty wholly wasteful, indistinguishable from mere maid's service, and continuing months on end. Even in the leading schools there lingers pure apprenticeship or, worse, the uninstructed "picking-up" of experience, miscalled training. On the whole, the various types of ward training fall into two more or less distinct categories, that is, graded and ungraded training.

THE GRADATION OF TRAINING

It would appear a mere matter of course that the new students who have had opportunity to practice only simple nursing procedures should on assuming full ward duty be allowed to care for only the least sick patients, that is, convalescents, chronics, etc., or should, to begin with, merely assist more experienced students in the care of sicker patients. As the beginner progresses and becomes capable of assuming greater responsibility, she would naturally herself be given charge of more seriously ill patients, gradually taking on in addition to the minor nursing duties all the items of care, such as treatments, medication, charting, etc. Such carefully graded procedure is indeed more or less closely followed at many hospitals, and the assignment of patients is planned so as to afford the student a genuinely educational gradation of clinical experience.

But unfortunately this system does not obtain in all hospitals. Due on the one hand to the overcrowding and pressure "to get the work done" at many large institutions, particularly the municipal, due on the other hand to the desire for intensive training in special phases of nursing, a system of excessive specialization and subdivision of functions has grown up. In order to make clear the fundamental differences between the two types of training we must describe them in some detail.

EXAMPLES OF GRADED TRAINING

Thus, for instance, in a large school at a general hospital of high standing where the teaching of nursing procedures is excellent according to the standards laid down in Section 5, the further ward training is admirably adapted to developing perfection of nursing care, increasing accuracy of observation and a sense of responsibility in the students. Each nurse on the wards, except the probationers, has complete charge of a small number of patients, giving all treatments and keeping the charts. Medication only is excepted, which is given out by the senior nurse to the entire ward,—a custom on which we shall presently comment.

Each student by relieving the nurse next above her in seniority during the daily hours off duty, is slowly day by day initiated into acquaintance with increasingly serious types of cases and into correspondingly greater responsibility.

On the day of our visit to this hospital, in the men's medical ward having 27 patients the staff consisted of a graduate head nurse, 5 students, 2 orderlies, a maid, and a cleaning woman shared by two wards. The work of the ward was planned to give over the care of patients to students in accordance with their degree of experience, under the supervision of the responsible graduate head nurse. Accordingly the fifth nurse, a probationer of 3 months' standing, who was having her first ward duty, had 7 convalescent patients assigned to her who, being out of bed most of the day, needed a minimum of nursing care. In relieving the nurse next above her when off duty, whose 5 patients in their turn were more seriously ill than the probationer's though not acute cases, she began her actual care of the sick, but she was not allowed to give any treatments, except under the careful supervision of head nurse, supervisor, or instructor.

Much of the probationer's time was spent in housekeeping duties, such as dusting and cleaning the wards, and also the broom closet, maid's closet, wheel chairs, locker tops, insides of lockers, bathroom, etc. "Cleaning of bathrooms," comments our investigator, "might well be eliminated." Indeed, the fact that much of the cleaning in this men's ward was done by the 2 orderlies "if they are so inclined," shows that the large amount of cleaning done by nurses in the women's ward where there are no orderlies might with no educational loss be otherwise cared for. But we shall postpone to a later section the full discussion of time wasted in excessive housekeeping duties.

The fourth nurse, next in order of seniority to the probationer, was on the day of our visit a student of 8 months' standing. The cases assigned to her (chronic mastoiditis, cerebro-spinal lues, etc.) though not acutely ill, needed considerable nursing to be kept comfortable, especially care of their mouths and backs, and afforded the student opportunity for new experience in treatments and charting suitable to her stage of training. Certain specific housekeeping duties of no particular educational value, such as folding and putting away blankets, cleaning and dusting supply and workrooms, were assigned to her. Again, in her hours of relieving the third nurse, she entered upon the next stage of her training.

The third nurse in her turn had been in the school a year. Two of her 6 patients were out of bed, pneumonia convalescents. The 4 others were not acutely ill (acute inflammatory rheumatism, chronic nephritis, chronic arthritis), but needed special diets. This involved more advanced training than this young woman had yet had in exactness in noting orders, in observation of patients, and in recording. Her manual duties were also more responsible than those of the two younger students, being care of the treatment trays, which gives familiarity with assembling the instruments and articles needed for various procedures, and special emphasis to sterile procedure. The chief responsibility of the third nurse, however, was the assumption of the duties of her immediate senior, the second nurse, when the latter was off duty.

For the second nurse, a student towards the end of her second year, by a somewhat curious but common division of duties, had charge of the sickest patients on the ward. Three at least of her 5 patients were acutely ill with pneumonia and pernicious anæmia. With several cases so serious to care for, the planning of her work required not a little executive ability. The actual nursing required skill in handling the very sick, and a further advance in observing and reporting symptoms and results of treatments. Her special manual assignment, aside from dusting and cleaning her own patients' beds and stands, consisted in the responsible duty of caring for the typhoid stand and closet with its utensils. In daily relieving the senior or first nurse, she assumed administrative duties, becoming responsible for the conduct of the ward.

Now, if the second nurse, near the end of her second year, can thus be entrusted with the care of the sickest patients and can also gain administrative experience, the question inevitably arises as to what ward duties are left the first or senior nurse in her third year. So far as concerns the medical ward under consideration, the second nurse had in effect at the end of her second year finished the training which should be basic for all nurses. For the senior nurse was having no further training in the care of the sick, but was purposely assigned patients who, again, were not acutely ill, in order to have time primarily for training in the executive duties of ward management, making rounds with physicians, etc.

The Use of Seniors as Head Nurses

Invaluable as this experience indubitably is, it is as plainly experience in a nursing specialty, and at that, a graduate specialty. It is abundantly evident that without devoting to it a material proportion of the third year, the student's executive ability can be sufficiently developed by responsibility thrown on her in the progressive gradation of duties, in night duty, in relieving the head nurse during her daily hours and half-days off duty. Early in the student's career this assumption of responsibility begins. The head nurse and senior may both be absent, one on her half-day off duty, the other at a meal or classes. On the day of our visit to Hospital No. 10, for instance, the second nurse (1 year and 8 months in the school) was according to her time slip alone on a male surgical ward of 28 patients from 1:30 to 3:30 p. m., and in charge until the senior's return at 4:30. In this instance the graduate head nurse was off duty through illness.

Instead of the present system of keeping students in training a third year often to use them as head nurses and thus save the expense of employing graduates, the administration of wards, head nurseships, should be paid graduate work, to training in which students wishing to specialize in administration might devote a third year, after graduation from the basic clinical course. We comment later on the fallacy of having students hold the position of head nurse, since it involves teaching as well as administration.

How frequent this employment is of students as head nurses is shown by statistics of the hospital experience of students from 100 different training schools studied in the course of this investigation. Half of the students had served as head nurses at least 1 month; one-fourth of the group approximately 3 months or more.[39]

Omissions in General Care

Besides the time devoted to head nurseships in the graded training described above, another undesirable but common pro-

*See page 190 for method of obtaining these figures.

cedure is the assignment of all medication of the ward to the senior nurse. The younger nurses thus lose one important experience in the care of their patients. That this is unnecessary is proved by the inclusion, at some hospitals visited, of medication as well as all other duties in the student's general care of patients.

A practical objection sometimes raised against so including medication is that as several students have to give out medicine at the same time, the situation may lead to confusion, especially in large wards, and that responsibility for medicines is more safely centered in one person. If we admit that the performance of this duty by one person is safer and more time-saving, we may yet suggest that it can be assigned to different students in rotation. One can, for instance, give out medicine in the morning to all patients including her own, a second at noon, and a third at night. Some rotation is today practically in effect during the seniors' weekly afternoons and daily hours off duty. It is, indeed, regularly instituted in some hospitals so that different students, while giving out medication for the whole ward during a short period, at the same time give it to their own patients instead of missing this experience. At one hospital visited medicines were assigned for a week at a time to different nurses in turn.

The disadvantage of centering sole responsibility for medication in the senior was well shown at a large municipal hospital. Here on the day of our observation of a mixed ward for men, the senior finished giving 1:00 o'clock medicines at 2:40 p. m. The graduate head nurse being off duty for the afternoon, the senior had had to assume so many pressing duties that medication was delayed.

"The amount to be given out was moderate," says our investigator, "but no one had been able to start it before she returned from dinner at 1:00 o'clock."

In some hospitals giving a graded training, by a less desirable arrangement, temperatures or charting are like medication assigned to the senior nurse. The failure to include these duties in the student's general care is a serious omission. Even when, as at various hospitals, all the older students ultimately have these experiences, the failure to require nurses from the start to take the temperatures and chart the condition of their own patients is, from the educational point of view, disintegrating and mistaken.

"It inevitably tends," notes one of our investigators, "to make students less observant of symptoms in their patients and less observant of changes in their condition."

With the exception of medication and time devoted to head nurseships, the training described above in detail affords a genuinely educational gradation of experience. We must turn next to the ungraded type of training common to many schools.

EXAMPLES OF UNGRADED TRAINING

Under this plan the first or senior nurse not only gives all medication on the ward, takes all temperatures, and does all charting, but also gives all treatments, and helps to serve all diets. The younger nurses give merely the daily minor nursing care practically for 2 years, thus having the hardest work, while knowledge of their patients' condition, which gives point and enthusiasm to the service, is denied them. With no gradation of experience, all but the senior student performing about the same duties, they do not even have the incentive of ambition which a graded training affords. Thus on the day of our visit to a large municipal hospital, in a surgical ward of 28 patients, students at various stages of training, one of nearly 2 years' (1 year and 11 months) and another of 4 months' were performing identical duties. In this hospital there is no definite assignment of work to any student, except to seniors; the others give general care to as many patients as possible, "to get the work done."

In another large municipal hospital visited, different phases of daily care are assigned to each student under the senior, one having baths, another bed-making, a third care of backs, etc. But the experience is in no sense graded and, again, on the day of our visit students varying from 5 months' experience to one of 1 year and 8 months' were performing duties in no way differing in difficulty or responsibility. Can it be doubted that by the end of her second year a student so trained is wearied and dulled by monotonous repetition of routine?

Further, and even more damaging in the ungraded training, a third-year student, after serving as responsible senior or having other advanced training, is later again assigned to routine ward work under another senior. At one of the hospitals mentioned above, two students in their third year of training were with younger nurses on the staff of a large medical ward of 142 patients, mostly chronics. In the worst instance encountered, at another municipal hospital, in a male ward of 35 patients, a probationer of 2 to 3 months' training and a senior of 2 years and 6 months' training were performing similar duties. The probationer had 11 patients; the senior, 6.

"Judging from the diagnosis given," comments our investigator, "the patients assigned to the probationer require as expert care as those assigned to the senior. Each one is caring for a case of cerebral hemorrhage."

Certainly for these seniors such assignments have no further educational value, and as certainly would lead to the drop of interest and "staleness" which is a commonplace of the third year of training.

Staleness in the Third Year

This "waning enthusiasm" has been a matter of deep concern to thoughtful training school principals.

"Why does the interested active junior and intermediate develop into the indifferent, bored, and somewhat skeptical senior, who makes no effort to conceal that she is only waiting till her 'time is up'?" asked one such principal at a round table discussion of the League of Nursing Education.[40]

Various explanations were offered, among them lowered physical efficiency.

"Her physical powers have been greatly taxed, and her attitude is partly the result of continued fatigue. She has had too little time for mental recreation."

Another reason given was precisely the reassignment to routine ward work which we have described, with such an instance as "heavy operating room duty where continuous excitement reigned, followed by routine ward duty with which the nurse was familiar." Small wonder that "in the tired, relaxed state in which she came to this period, she had no special interest to stir her enthusiasm." The remedy proposed was "new interests and new activities" for the senior year.

We, on the contrary, shall propose a different remedy: such a reorganization of teaching during the first and second years that interest will be definitely sustained, and the entire abandonment of the last 8 months of training.

[40] National League of Nursing Education, Proceedings of the 23rd Annual Convention, 1917. Reports of Round Table Discussion. Page 275.

Disadvantages of Specialization

Before giving in detail our proposed reorganization of service, however, we have still to consider under the ungraded system the postponement to the third year, of training in various special phases of nursing care. As we have seen in some schools, medical and surgical treatments are all reserved for the senior. While the younger students give routine care, one senior, for instance, variously known as "surgical nurse" or "dressing room nurse" at different hospitals, gives all surgical treatments either on the ward or in the surgical dressing room to which patients are brought for treatment. It is assumed that all seniors will ultimately get this experience. Too often in the pressure of work, the student misses or has curtailed such a fundamental assignment, but even for those who obtain them all, this specialization is open to the gravest objections—it gives instead of a total clinical picture of the disease or condition treated, only a fragmentary and even misleading knowledge of the single duty performed.

Thus the senior as "dressing room nurse" gains indeed a large experience of wounds and surgical dressings, but without opportunity to relate them to the general condition of the patient. In effect, she is taught to treat the wound rather than the patient. But, unfortunately, the complexity of the human organism does not lend itself to such subdivision, and the nurse, who is ultimately to be responsible for specific patients, will find herself confronted with conditions which she has never been taught to meet. On the wards she has given only routine nursing care; as "dressing room nurse," she has learned surgical treatments; never in her training, either on the wards or in the dressing room, has she been taught to care for the surgical patient as a whole; to watch for and recognize later effects of treatment, the entire human reaction.

The exceptional nurse may indeed, by virtue of unusual memory and imagination, combine her various experiences so as to draw for herself a total clinical picture and gain an intelligent understanding of the whole case. As a system of instruction, such an extreme of specialization needs only to be described to be condemned.

In contrast to this system and valuable in illustrating the possibilities of better instruction is the practice of a large municipal hospital. Here the student as part of her surgical training is assigned to a period in the gynecological operating room, while on duty in the gynecological ward. She thus has the rare opportunity of directly associating operation and post-operative conditions.

Just as in the surgical service, the subdivision of duties is often carried to the extreme in other services: medical, pediatric, obstetrical. In all these types of service similar excessive specialization of nursing functions exists in great variety, involving the assignment to different nurses of different phases of care without opportunity of continuously observing the patients treated. In the study of the diet kitchen in some hospitals we shall see this specialization carried almost to a *reductio ad absurdum:* special diets not only being taught unrelated to specific patients, but not even taught *in toto;* i. e., one student preparing the hot food, another the cold, another the salt-free bread, etc., not one understanding or even seeing the entire meal but merely filling unrelated orders for certain specialties.

THE COMBINATION OF GRADED AND UNGRADED TRAINING

We have chosen, for illustration of graded and ungraded training, the simplest and most characteristic examples encountered in our study. But no hard and fast lines can be drawn, and under either system are found numberless variations of practice.

One strange aberration of method should be noted. In some hospitals offering a more or less graded training, seniority on the wards is not established by length of training, but by length of stay in a given ward. Thus on the day of our visit to a school of the first rank, two third-year students (both, 2 years and 8 months in the school) were subordinate to a younger girl (in the school 1 year and 8 months) who was "senior" in a men's medical ward of 21 patients.

"This means," says our investigator, "that the student upon whom the responsibility rests in the absence of the graduate head nurse, may be but a month or two past her probation period, and that students in their third year are under her direction."

The only reasons advanced for a practice so educationally indefensible is that the custom in some hospitals is long-established, and that it is supposed to make for flexibility on the part of the senior. None of the students questioned liked this arrangement. Harmony seemed to depend on the attitude of the young nurse who was senior. It would indeed appear that, if a student of 1 year and 8 months is able, not only to nurse often the sickest patients, but to attend to the ward management, the senior has no further need of experience in the department.

It is indeed practicable to combine a well-graded general service with the devotion of part of the time to special duties, affording a wider range of experience than is obtained by the care of a small number of patients. Thus, at a leading school, effort is made to assign patients according to the nurse's stage of experience. Students usually have the same patients for some time, giving them morning care and morning treatments. Twice thereafter during the day assignments of work for the ensuing hours are posted. Different students in rotation are appointed to give out medicines, give treatments, take temperatures, etc. These assignments differ daily, since hours of duty differ and class hours often intervene. Students must, moreover, know the condition of all patients in the ward since any morning an older nurse may find herself posted for the 7 to 11 p. m. hours of duty, when she is entirely responsible for the ward, giving medication and treatments, making rounds with doctors, etc. From 9 to 11 she is alone on the ward. She thus combines care of her own patients with special treatment of others.

Instances might be indefinitely multiplied in which combinations of training are successfully carried out. It must necessarily remain for the individual school of nursing, with its varying necessities, to work out whatever modifications may prove desirable. But from our observations and analysis it is clear that with whatever additions of special intensive experience, the quintessence of training lies in the care, as complete as possible, of a small number of patients, graded to the capacity of the student.

INSTRUCTION AND SUPERVISION ON THE WARDS

EXAMPLES OF SUCCESS

We have already described in detail the varying methods of instruction and supervision of probationers on the wards (see page 244) and need not comment again here on the danger of losing, through countenancing bad and slipshod work on the wards, all the advantages of good preliminary instruction. After the preliminary term, the ward teaching of students again varies as widely as that of the probationers,—in some schools there is actually none at all, in others there are excellent methods of guiding and checking up student progress.

Teaching and supervision on the wards after probation is, for the most part, in the hands of the head nurses or, as they are sometimes called, charge nurses. In large hospitals the head nurses are usually under the direction of the training school office or supervisors.

Realization of the head nurse's dual responsibilities as teacher as well as administrator is found in many good schools. We have already enumerated instances of successful co-operation in teaching between the instructor of practical nursing and the head nurse, and have described some excellent methods of keeping the two in touch (see pages 242, 243, and 248). We shall presently show how head nurses, chosen for their teaching qualities, can and do supplement on the wards the lectures and clinics of the physician-instructor (see page 372).

Good teaching by head nurses was noted in many instances by our field agents.

"During the hour and a half I was on the men's medical ward, approximately 30 minutes was spent by the head nurse supervising students," writes one, concerning a school noted for its excellent supervision. "Supervision is given by head nurses, instructor in practical nursing and assistant superintendent," writes another, of a university school of nursing. "The chief points seem to be a very efficient planning and supervision of the work."

In general, the best examples of ward teaching are naturally found in the special services, in which students can obviously not be trusted merely to "pick up" experience for themselves but must be actually taught.

Thus, for instance, at a famous private hospital there is specially good bedside instruction in the pediatric service. On coming to this department, during two weeks of the month spent on the infant ward, small groups of students are given practical instruction by the graduate head nurse, in procedures and treatments special to infants and young children. A similar practice of giving good bedside instruction prevails in the pediatric departments of other hospitals.

Again, at a large school maintained by a municipal hospital where teaching on the general wards is practically lacking, there is excellent bedside instruction in the 3 months' obstetrical service. Here there is a special "instructor in obstetrics" besides a graduate head nurse who is responsible for running the ward. The instructor in obstetrics has classes in practical demonstration, is in charge of the delivery room, and gives all bedside teaching. Other schools are likewise experimenting with the introduction of clinical instructors for ward teaching, particularly in the special services. Where administrative duties are heavy, it may be that such a division of duties is most promising.

With the aim of improving ward teaching and aiding head nurses to realize their responsibilities as teachers, some schools have conferences of the entire staff at regular intervals. Thus, for instance, of 21 schools visited from whom information on this point was received in our inquiry, 15 or over 70 per cent have meetings of part or all of the staff, some of them weekly, others monthly, 4 of them "irregularly." Six schools have no staff meetings of any kind. The best showing is made by a small private school in a hospital of 140 beds whose staff meets daily, and a large university school connected with a hospital of over 800 beds whose staff meets semi-weekly. Such conferences, if well conducted, should do much to integrate the training and to enlist the interest of the supervising staff in the general educational problems of the school.

But too often, as already noted, there is a marked division of sentiment between the teaching and supervisory staffs. The head nurse appreciates only the needs of running her ward, and views with jealousy what she regards as the encroachments of the instructor on the time of the students. On the other hand, the teaching staff, including the principal, too often refuse to include the head nurses as co-workers in educational policies and relegate them to the narrow interests of a single ward, with results which might be foreseen.

Clearly, in the interest of good training the head nurses must not be so overburdened with work as to lack all appreciation of their responsibilities to the students as well as to patients, and must themselves, moreover, by staff conferences or any other educational means, be made to feel sharers in a common and compelling educational enterprise. Unfortunately their own equipment, in many instances, has not fitted them to become teachers, as will become clear in a later section on this special topic. No more cogent reason exists for the prompt establishment of university schools of nursing, able to give a high order of training, than the dearth of well-fitted supervisors and head nurses.

EXAMPLES OF FAILURE

Too often the pressure of "getting the work done" removes any possibility of either good teaching or good supervision. It is naturally in the further instruction of students on full ward duty, that hospital pressure makes its greatest inroads. For the office staff or supervisors or head nurses whose business it is to supervise and give bedside instruction are themselves for the most part hard pressed by the business of running the ward, or even of giving routine care to patients, and have little time or energy left for anything else. This is a situation the evil of which is widely recognized by the nurses themselves.

"Nurses in this audience," said a leading superintendent of nurses at a recent meeting of the League of Nursing Education, "have as pupils chafed under the arrangement whereby they were required to clean utensils, stack linen, and dust furniture day after day when their patients needed them. Nurses in this audience as graduate head nurses have done hours of this work themselves rather than take the pupils away from the actual care of the patients—these head nurses have in this work spent hours which they should have used actively supervising and teaching the pupils under them. . . . Ask the average pupil nurse what are the looked-for results of the treatments and medicines she is administering to her five patients? How intelligent will be her answers? Why are they not more intelligent?—because of lack of time of the charge nurse as well as the pupils." [41]

We have shown the chaos in the length of assignments to different departments of students in a single class. Even more fatal to the possibility of honest teaching is the understaffing of wards, the reliance upon student services for the total care of the great majority of patients. Here we see the practical outcome of the conflict between care of the sick and education of students described at the outset of our study. Here is the *impasse*, the impossible dual task of the heads of training schools, which they have never or rarely succeeded in effectually voicing to trustees or public; the inevitably resulting sacrifice of education in hospitals staffed by students.

Of this sacrifice of students, if more proof were needed, our inquiry gave abundant evidence. "Impossible to give anything

[41] National League of Nursing Education, Proceedings of the 26th Annual Convention, 1920. Report upon Readjustments in Practical Training of Student Nurses. Pages 106, 107.

but the most necessary care and that in the most rapid way possible," is the terse comment on the instruction given in a scandalously understaffed department of a large city hospital. This was a ward made up of several connecting rooms, for 58 patients, including 24 children and babies, "filled with cases of great clinical interest," says our agent, "venereal, alcoholic, erysipelas, septic surgery and gynecology, nerve cases, paralytic," and staffed by a graduate head nurse and 7 students—a service which the student must leave no wiser than when she entered it, and probably with the acquisition of bad habits due to hurried work.

At the opposite pole from the pediatric service described on page 308 as offering successful teaching is the pediatric service visited at a university school of nursing. This department was so understaffed that the head nurse herself was kept entirely occupied merely in routine care of the children. Here a student who had been 10 days on duty in the milk laboratory stated that the head nurse had been "too busy" to give her any instruction or supervision whatever. "Fortunately," as she put it, she had not had any difficult formulæ to prepare and so had "managed pretty well." Such was her practical instruction. What if she had had difficult formulæ? A day spent in observation on the ward confirmed her statement.

"No organization of the work and absolutely no supervision," comments our investigator. "The head nurse was busy making up beds and giving care to patients herself, giving some directions as to what was to be done by different nurses, but not in any way noting manner of doing. Evidently the children were fed well, but as to daily bathing, the usual routine for children's wards, it certainly was not done for the sickest patients, the empyemas probably needing it most, and such confusion prevailed that I am not prepared to say whether the other patients got such care or not. Do not believe the head nurse herself could check up the question."

In contrast with this picture of disorganization, is the milk room service in another school connected with a large private hospital in the middle west. Here supervision is careful; the milk room duty is given, as a rule, preceding a month in the nursery, because in the opinion of the school "students having had milk laboratory experience are much more intelligent as regards observation of cases in the nursery." This presupposes of course the real teaching of formulæ and their effects, instead of the mere "managing" with formulæ mentioned in the first instance.

Again, at a school connected with a university medical school, a rich opportunity for training is offered by the variety of cases grouped in the communicable disease department.

"The service in this department is so valuable," comments our investigator, "that it would seem justifiable to withdraw student nurses from other parts of the hospital and concentrate on their teaching here."

Yet in practice this department is so understaffed that one student nurse was assigned to 12 sick children, several of them diphtheria, and one a gonococcus eye case, needing hourly irrigations and cold compresses to be applied for 10 minutes every 2 hours. "I have seldom witnessed such confusion as existed, or such totally inadequate staffing for the care of such cases," continues our investigator. "The lack of supervision left the students to their own resources in situations where they needed much knowledge and skill to prevent cross-infections and protect themselves.

A cardinal point is touched on in the final comment:

"Students were totally lacking in appreciation of many aspects of interesting cases they were handling."

This, from the point of view of education, is the worst feature in the lack of ward teaching which we have been considering. Cases of extraordinary interest may be under the student's care, clinical opportunities not easily duplicated may be offered her, she may take part in unusual treatments or procedures, but without supervision or teaching, encouraged only to cover the utmost ground as quickly as possible, this wealth of experience will be in large part lost or meaningless.

EXAMPLES OF PREMATURE RESPONSIBILITY

The lack of time for supervision, so lamentably evident, the pressing into service of every possible student at the earliest possible moment, far earlier than safety permits, works injustice both to student and patient. The student is placed through no fault of her own in a false position; the public is offered inexpert and often untrustworthy service. Premature responsibility placed on students unprepared for it is unfortunately too common to excite remark.

We have already mentioned the assignment to a probationer

THE HOSPITAL SCHOOL OF NURSING 313

of 2 to 3 months' training in a municipal hospital, of 5 erysipelas patients among 11 cases. This girl was necessarily ignorant of the dangers of cross-infection; as certainly uninformed of the measures needed to protect herself as well as her patients from infection. In the same hospital disastrous possibilities were involved in the ignorance of a probationer appointed to take temperature, pulse, and respiration in a men's surgical ward of 28 patients. Her equipment consisted of two thermometers placed in a glass with a little cotton in the bottom and a small amount of solution, hardly covering the cotton or the tips. There was not even a pretense of wiping the thermometer between cases. It was placed in the glass after use by one patient and at once taken out and given to the next.

"There was no supervision of this process," states our field agent, "and the probationer was not at all embarrassed by being watched while she did it," having evidently no sense of sin in the performance.

In these examples of the failure of supervision, the head nurses were graduate nurses. In hospitals using students to run the wards, the chances of good teaching or supervising must evidently be even less, the chances of premature responsibility even greater. We have already quoted the simple admission of one school: "We rely on the students to supervise each other." Others less frank use the same method. In a well-known maternity hospital a small ward of 8 patients was, on the day of our visit, staffed by a senior (2 years and 8 months in the school) and a probationer of 3 months. Three of these cases required expert nursing, 3 were under observation, 2 needed knowledge of aseptic technique. A supervisor responsible for 3 floors made about 3 rounds a day. The senior gave all treatments and medication, ordered supplies, ran the ward, and supervised the probationer. The probationer was assigned to give douches, catheterizations, even bladder irrigation. When the senior was absent from the ward, she was in charge of all cases. The situation at this hospital is made worse by the fact that there is no classroom teaching of nursing procedures, and but little instruction on the wards during the first 3 months, and that often ward instruction is given by the older students instead of a responsible instructor.

Thus the young nurse is called upon for observation, knowledge, and judgment she has had no time to acquire. Whatever her errors, the responsibility for breaking faith with the public must be on the heads of the hospital authorities rather than on hers.

For with sufficient funds and under good management, it is proved that such conditions need not arise. Indeed in the very same hospital, under the same roof with the dangerously disorganized and student-exploiting medical service described above was an operating room in which the training was of a high order of excellence. A sufficiently large number of graduate nurses was employed to insure that no student should have undue responsibility and that no work should be required which was unnecessary for instruction.

LACK OF GOOD MANAGEMENT

In the instances cited, as in many others, confusion was due to the lack of any organization or specific assignments to students. Obviously, the greater the pressure, the greater the need of exactness and good supervision. If work to be done by each student is not only listed, but listed in the order of its importance—the most important treatments to be done first, the least important tasks last, such as folding linen, cleaning closets, etc.—such a list, if checked as work is performed, shows at a glance what has been perforce left undone.

"Such a system," notes another of our nurse agents, "makes for honesty and helps students to think in terms of the relative importance of various tasks. Moreover," she sensibly remarks, "it is good to have such records to present to superintendents of hospitals and trustees."

When temptations to bad or slipshod work are innumerable in the general urgency, it is clearly of first importance for the training of students as well as the safety of patients, to insist upon having some adequate record of student performance. To gauge the effectiveness of supervision in another way we may briefly review some methods in vogue at various hospitals.

METHODS OF RECORDING AND CHECKING WARD WORK

In almost every hospital visited, orders were carried out only at the written direction of the physician. The rules usually require that the orders be written by the doctor; in some instances they are written by the head nurse at his dictation and initialed by the physician. Many different methods of recording and checking the student's work were found. These are matters of administrative routine, the details of which it is obviously not the province of this report to treat. But it is essential, as we have said, to emphasize that alike for the nurse's training and the public safety there should be required some simple method of recording work by the student and checking the record by her superior.

In some hospitals this is done by having the student enter each item of care, when performed, on the patient's chart; in others, this is done only for the sickest patients, and for the other patients only temperature, pulse, and respiration are noted. Under a different system, each item of care is checked and initialed by the student when performed, in the doctor's order book; or again a daily list of duties for each student is made out from the order book by the head nurse and posted, or the students themselves copy their orders from this book, or, in a loose leaf system, orders are attached to the chart. Usually, then, the head nurse in making up her daily report at 5 p. m. or thereabouts, and stating the treatment and condition of patients, automatically checks up the students' records of their work.

Some written assignment of work and description of conditions is usually given the night nurse, and she, as she has less supervision than the day nurses, is usually expected to make a written record of the care of each patient at night. Often the night nurse makes a 24-hour summary of each chart. Special precautions are usually taken, by means of individual cards for each patient or some such device, to insure accuracy in giving medication.

It would appear self-evident that all schools must adopt such methods of record and check, or others answering the same purpose, to teach accuracy in carrying out orders and to provide means of detecting, as promptly as may be, any omission or errors. But such is not the case and, even in the superior group of hospitals studied, examples of flagrant mismanagement were met, jeopardizing patients and fatal to any system of instruction.

Thus for instance, in one large municipal hospital when a student goes off duty, she reports undone work orally to the head nurse, who must then assign it to some one else. "After the early morning," notes our investigator, "the head nurse must always carry in mind what is to be done, and find some one who is free to do it." As this is a hospital in which many wards are understaffed and work is done at high pressure, it may often be long before "some one" is found free, while the head nurse "carries in mind" what has been left undone. No comment is needed on so wasteful and dangerous a system.

In a well-known school maintained by a prominent general hospital where the training is excellently graded, the head nurse each morning posts the patients assigned to each nurse, and lists of treatments. No special form is used; it varies in different wards. Each student is supposed to consult this list and carry out treatments as listed. The charting of treatments is done by the head nurse or senior nurse. "But the nurse giving treatments," states our investigator, "is not required to make either verbal or written report. It is taken for granted that as the treatment is listed, the nurse carried it out." Obviously such extraordinary laxity may lead, as our investigator points out, to the charting of treatments which have never been given, since there is not even the pretense of a check on performance of duties.

Again, in a special hospital of high standing, charting is done only by the head nurse, who may or may not be a student. But in this hospital the chart has no record of medication or treatments given. It is merely a graphic chart, on which are plotted temperature, pulse, respiration, also fluid intake and output, and sometimes blood-pressure. Every day, or in some cases less frequently, the interne physician writes notes on the condition of patients and writes out the orders for treatment and medication. But except at night there is no system of checking the carrying out of these orders. A record is made by the day nurse of what is to be done at night and the night nurse records in writing what she has done during the night. Otherwise there is no recording by students either of the condition of patients, or of medication or treatment given.

Aside from the jeopardy to patients, it is self-evident that any school which countenances such methods has practically no gauge of its students' performances.

USE OF CASE RECORDS

Contrast with these chaotic conditions the possibilities inherent in the method of case study which should be an integral part of the ward training. In order that the nurse may appreciate the medical treatment and participate in it intelligently, without in any way impinging on the domain of the physician, it would appear that she should be acquainted with the patients' records, medical and social, so far as these are available, from diagnosis to end result, whatever it may be. Instead of the monotonous repetition of minor duties, now often continued long after skill has been acquired, there would be real, intensive teaching of a smaller number of cases. In point of fact, such use of case records on the part of nurses on the wards was found to be only occasional. Wherever it was even partly in effect, the intelligence of the nurse's care and interest was found to be notably augmented. Thus, for example, at a small hospital where the supervision of students on the wards is of unusual excellence and the student service is supplemented by an adequate graduate staff, case records are regularly used in teaching.

"I was much impressed," writes an investigator at this hospital, "by the students' intelligent knowledge of the patients. In stating the diagnosis the student gave a brief *résumé* of the treatment and general condition of each patient in a manner which showed her to be unusually well informed and interested in the clinical side of her experience."

The ward in question had only 24 beds but the types of cases showed much variety and were so acute as to give adequate training. The student discussed at length the treatments given and the results noted, such as the effect of thyroid extract on a child suffering from cretinism, formerly chronic, now acute; effects of treatment in empyema, acute nephritis, spastic paralysis, etc. A like intelligent interest was noted among all the students interviewed.

Again, in a university school of nursing, each student, as part of her ward assignment, is required to write up in full every fortnight certain case records, which are returned to her if necessary for criticism and discussion. Another valuable example of the use of case records in teaching nurses was observed in a psychiatric department of an eminent hospital. Here case records are a regular part of the clinic instruction. The nurse's intimate observation of the patient, peculiarly needed by the physician in treatment of psychiatric cases, may thus be guided by a knowledge of the total previous history of the case.

PRIVATE SERVICE

In connection with teaching and supervision in bedside care, it is important to point out the superior advantages of the wards over private service, the value of which in teaching has been often over-emphasized. In the private service, restricted experience of one or two cases is offered in place of the greater range and variety of opportunities provided by the open ward. Moreover, actual bedside instruction is for the most part impracticable in private service. The claim is sometimes made that refinement and delicacy of manner and service are better inculcated in this service than in the wards, where the standards of the patients are less exacting. But this is to admit differentiation in standards of nursing which can obviously not be endorsed by the authorities. Gentleness and considerateness are plainly prerequisites of any nursing training, and the greater refinements, such as for example of the meal service, in the private room may be acquired at the expense of a richer clinical experience.

The loss in opportunity for observation and study to the student who spends a long period of time in the private services is irreparable, and often deeply resented. The actual length of time spent in this educationally least valuable duty is shown by records of students of one class from each of four schools connected with hospitals having large private services. The median time varied from $3\frac{1}{4}$ to $7\frac{1}{4}$ months. In a larger group of about 200 students from 100 different schools, to whose records we had access, over half the students had nearly 4 months in the private service and one-quarter of them had over 6 months.

Hitherto in this chapter we have treated of what is known as the "practical" experience of the student, her bedside instruction in the actual care of patients. Before considering the instruction in theory which must interpret the diseases and conditions encountered, we will take up other phases of the student's practical experience, in the diet kitchen and the dispensary.

DIET KITCHEN

DIET IN DISEASE

We have already seen that in the preliminary course in dietetics students should be taught in classroom and laboratory the fundamental principles of nutrition and simple cookery, and should be given supplementary practice in a short assignment to the diet kitchen. The diet kitchen service proper, on the other hand, should be a specialized intensive training in the dietetic treatment of disease, with special reference to the diseases of metabolism and other conditions requiring special diets, and should be accompanied if not preceded by classroom instruction. The aims of this instruction are to apply the principles of nutrition and the cookery learned in the preliminary course to the dietetic treatment of disease; to teach students to translate diet orders into attractive and palatable meals, and finally to teach them how to make patients understand the purpose of their dietetic treatment in order that they may co-operate fully with the measures prescribed.

TRAINING IN INFANT FEEDING

In many training schools infant feeding is included as part of the general diet kitchen service. In others, by a better plan, service in the milk room is given as part of the obstetrical or pediatric training.

As we have seen in Part A, within the space of one generation the feeding of babies and young children has become a matter of scientific routine, governed by definite rules, and regulated by tests, according to which the content and quality of the child's nourishment is to be varied.

The proper preparation of milk formulæ is indeed the foundation of the baby's health. In sickness it is the condition of his cure. The nurse who is to be in contact with children either in private duty or as a public health nurse, or on the wards or in the dispensary of the hospital, is obviously in need of a thorough grounding in the principles and practice of infant feeding. She is not only herself to carry out the doctor's orders as to the baby's diet, but to teach mothers how to do so.

TIME ALLOTTED TO DIET KITCHEN SERVICE

In our survey of the various types of diet training offered to the student nurse, nothing points more sharply to the prevailingly unstandardized condition of this service than the wide variation of the allotted time. The extreme character of this variation is indicated by the range of assignments from about 18 hours to 2 months. Thirteen of the 19 hospitals affording information in the matter assign over 4 weeks. Five of these assign exactly or approximately 2 months. The median is 6 weeks. Moreover, in the individual hospitals the variation of actual experience is very wide. For a little more than half the class, according to actual experience records, in 7 hospitals, the length of assignment falls somewhat below the time planned.

INSTRUCTION AND SUPERVISION

At the 20 hospitals offering diet kitchen service, or, if we include those giving milk laboratory or babies' food room training only, 22, some information as to the instructors is afforded by all but 2. With few exceptions the service is, as it should be, in the hands of trained dietitians—a better showing than can be made for the rank and file of the country's training schools.

Exceptions are a university school where a student dietitian is in charge of the diet kitchen work; 2 schools where there are no resident dietitians; a maternity hospital where the milk laboratory to which the students are assigned for one or two weeks, is in charge of a sister, a graduate of a 15-months' course only; and another special hospital where there is no diet kitchen service and no dietitian, and where in the food room of the babies' ward to which students are sent for 2-weeks' service, the preparation of the feedings is presumably in the hands of the housekeeper and of lay assistants.

DIET KITCHEN EQUIPMENT

Diet kitchen training at the hospitals studied is carried on in the majority of cases under a considerable handicap from the point of view of plant and equipment. Out of the 14 hospitals affording information in the matter, only 4 have diet kitchens well equipped for teaching purposes; in a fifth the equipment is adequate and clean though somewhat old-fashioned. In more than half of the rest such standard equipment as the steam table or the dish sterilizer is lacking. In 2 of these less well-provided kitchens, the trays and tray equipment are noted as excellent. In one large municipal hospital, where plant and equipment are old and much run down in all respects, the tray service is so worn and poor that food, it is said, however good, cannot be appetizingly served. In one hospital, otherwise of high standards, the diet kitchen is far too small, and the equipment quite inadequate. Another has no separate diet kitchen, and must utilize the main kitchen of the hospital, without proper equipment for teaching.

At 2 hospitals the diet kitchens are open to criticism on the score of cleanliness.

CONDITIONS OF VALUABLE TRAINING

To realize the full value of the diet kitchen service, the student must have had sound instruction not only in the basic principles of nutrition but also in the dietary treatment of disease. She must also have had some experience in ward duty of the conditions of disease for which the diets she is to prepare are prescribed. The value of the service will be further greatly strengthened by opportunity to make application of her experience to the care of patients on the wards.

We shall find that, while excellences along one line or another are found in the diet kitchen services at many of the hospitals studied, the experience in others, so far from taking rank as a scientific training, is in effect almost wholly wasted in such duties as preparing salads and desserts for private patients, or in dishwashing and cleaning vegetables, or in general cookery, wholly unrelated to illness. If we examine in detail the various types of service offered we shall find their range of value very wide. At one end of the scale is an intensive professional training in infant formulæ and special diets, including the relation of diet to disease and the study of individual cases for whom the diets are prepared; at the other an assignment of cookery and housework equivalent to the merest maid service.

CLASSROOM INSTRUCTION IN DIET IN DISEASE

Instruction in diet in disease is far as yet from being an established part of the training school curriculum. Even where this important professional training is included, it is seen to hold as yet but a precarious position by the scanty numbers of hours allowed it in many hospitals.

Hours and Year When Given

Of the 23 hospitals studied, 2 give combined courses of diet in health and disease of 54 and 75 hours respectively; 9 other schools teach diet in disease in courses ranging from 30 to 8 hours. Seven schools teach this subject negligibly, either assigning a totally inadequate number of hours or teaching it incidentally in the diet kitchen; 3 schools give no instruction in the subject, and for 2 information is lacking.

Of 11 schools affording information, 4 place the work in diet in disease in the second year, 5 in the third year, 1 in the second and third years. Only 1 school places classroom instruction in diet in disease, where it should logically be, in the first year, following the basic course in nutrition and cookery on which it builds.

A conspicuous failure of the hospitals is to correlate diet kitchen service with classroom instruction in diet in disease. In many instances the diet service precedes any such instruction. A student's practical experience in feeding patients during her first or second year may have to await interpretation until towards the end of the third year she receives the instruction in diet in disease without which intelligent understanding of prescribed diets or appreciation of their effects is impossible.

At only a few of the 16 training schools giving advanced courses does there seem to be any attempt to correlate the diet service with class instruction. General standards of correlation are significantly indicated by our investigator's comment at a large municipal hospital where about half of the students having had diet kitchen experience at the time of her visit had previously had the course in diet in disease; this correlation, she remarked without irony, was "somewhat above the average." At one school only, a university school with a long and thorough course in dietetics, is there a satisfactory adjustment. Here the diet kitchen service follows the first-year course in cookery and is co-ordinate with the second-year course in nutrition and special diets.

NECESSITY FOR PRACTICAL EXPERIENCE WITH DISEASE

The diet kitchen assignment should also presuppose a fair amount at least of experience with actual disease and instruction relating to it. For in her preliminary course, the student is handicapped by a practical experience of disease, and an instruction in its nature and symptoms, too limited to enable her to get the best value from her diet kitchen experience. Thus at one eminent training school, the 6-weeks' service of the preliminary period, while correlated with the instruction in nutrition and cookery, precedes any experience of disease on the wards at all.[42] The diet training for students so ill prepared, as may be noted also at other hospitals giving the service in the preliminary term, tends to become a period of housework and routine rather than education.

On the other hand, a diet kitchen service placed late in the course in the interest of practical experience may be too widely

[42] It is possible that some probationers may have as much as 2 weeks' general ward service before assignment to the diet kitchen.

separated from the earlier instruction it is supposed to illustrate. Thus, at one of our leading eastern training schools, the theory of nutrition is taught in the preliminary period, but the students are not assigned to the diet kitchen until senior year, when after the interval of two years or more they are likely to have forgotten most of their instruction.

NEED OF CORRELATION WITH WARD CASES

For an intelligent understanding of the special diets which constitute so large a part of the work of the diet kitchen, it is necessary, furthermore, that their preparation should be supplemented by study of the special cases to which the diets prepared are applied. Obviously the service is largely deprived of interest as well as of educational value unless the student knows something of the condition of the patients for whom she is preparing special diets and has the opportunity of seeing their effects. While, clearly, it may not be possible for all students studying diet in disease to care continuously for patients for whom special diets are prepared, yet they may be given opportunity to study the effects of diets far more than is at present attempted. In point of fact such correlation is almost the exception instead of the rule.

By assigning students to the diet kitchen during part of the time while they are receiving general ward training, such correlation can often be effected. Examples of this practical application may be seen indeed at some of the hospitals studied.

SOME INSTANCES OF EFFECTIVE CORRELATION WITH WARD CASES

It is of interest to note that the hospital offering the best example of diet kitchen training also provides the only instance of a fairly complete correlation with ward work among the hospitals studied. During 4 weeks of their assignment the students themselves serve to the patients the diets they have prepared, thus having opportunity to observe them, consult their tastes, and weigh the food not eaten. During the remaining 2-weeks' service they observe the infants for whom they have prepared formulæ. Another leading hospital offering a valuable diet service relates the training in so far to ward cases that students are sent to the wards to serve diabetic diets and thus keep in touch with the patients for whom these diets are prescribed. One lecture, moreover, and one clinic a week on diabetics, to which students on diet kitchen duty are admitted, tend to emphasize this correlation with concrete cases. A small training school of good standing adopts the plan during diet kitchen service of devoting 2 or 3 hours daily to special diets and invalid cookery, and assigning the students to the wards for the rest of the 9-hour day. This arrangement insures at so small a hospital a fairly good correlation with ward cases and opportunity to see the effects of diets prescribed.

Elsewhere, parts if not all of the service show some attempt at practical application. Certain hospitals arrange correlation with ward cases not for the diet kitchen proper but for the floor kitchens or for the milk laboratory. Thus, one of our largest city hospitals makes no connection for students in the diet kitchen proper between diets ordered and patients prescribed for, but establishes an excellent correlation between the training in the milk laboratory in infant feeding and practical ward experience, students on this duty being assigned in the afternoons to the infants' ward. Unfortunately the value of this training is of limited application; at the time of our survey less than one-third of the senior students had been given the experience.

Three other hospitals which divide diet service into two terms make no connection with ward work during the first period spent in the diet kitchen, but in the second, on the ward floor kitchens, offer at least a partial correlation between patient and dietary.

There is no assurance, however, that assignment to the floor kitchens gives any opportunity for correlation with ward cases. At one of our highly reputed hospitals the division of the student's day between the diet kitchen and the wards suggests excellent possibilities of practical application and study. But these are rendered illusory by the entire absence of any effort to correlate the student's diet work with the ward cases. Washing bedside stands after each meal constitutes her sole opportunity for observing patients. On the private wards she has no opportunity at all; her duties, consisting of setting up trays, a limited amount of cooking, and serving from the steam-table, are confined entirely to the kitchen.

At least 8 of the hospitals studied make no provision whatever for correlation between diet kitchen training and the ward cases it serves.

EXAMPLES OF VALUABLE TRAINING IN THE DIET KITCHEN

Of the 22 hospitals offering diet kitchen experience to students, 3 may be instanced as giving a training of genuine and positive value for the student's education. We may indicate the ground covered and the emphasis given by a brief sketch of these special services.

We have already referred, in connection with its careful correlation with ward cases, to the best example of diet training offered at any of the hospitals studied. At the hospital in question the 6-weeks' assignment to the diet kitchen for the three students on duty is an intensive progressive training in the preparation of special diets and infant feeding, the former averaging about 25 daily. For the first 2 weeks the student weighs and cooks individual portions for all diets ordered; in the second fortnight she puts up infant formulæ and is taught to calculate diets by the senior student; [43] in the third she has general charge of the diet kitchen, makes out daily diets from doctors' orders (19 diets and 9 infant formulæ), calculates calories, proportions of proteins, etc., and orders all supplies. Thus, with its close connection throughout with ward cases, the service at this hospital offers a thoroughly rounded experience. The students progressively do all work that relates to diet in disease.

This admirably planned and thorough training in the diet kitchen is in sharp contrast to the slight and ill-correlated classroom instruction—20 hours of dietetics given in the preliminary course, from one to two years before the diet kitchen assignment, and 10 lectures on diet in disease in the senior year after most of the students have had their practical experience.

At one of the large city hospitals, the one student assigned at a time to the diet kitchen staff is given a comprehensive and professionally most valuable experience in the preparation of special diets. The service here is extremely active and various, from 40 to 90 special diets being sent out daily, 20 of which are for special metabolism cases. Two weeks of the student's assignment are devoted to general diets; two weeks to weighed diets, largely diabetic. This second period includes, moreover, calculations of amounts, figuring of food returns on functional test diets, planning of special diets, ordering, and instruction in costs. The training in the preparation of milk formulæ is at this hospital included not in the diet kitchen but in the obstetrical

* During this time students make all desserts and salads as well.

service, where it is given during the two-weeks' period spent in the nursery.

A third example of good training is seen in the diet service planned by a large private general hospital, already deservedly mentioned for its effort to bring students into contact with the ward cases whose diets they supply. The work assigned here to the three or four students on duty at a time seems somewhat less professionally concentrated than that in the services already described; the first of the three 10-day periods into which it is divided includes such non-educational duties as the preparation of vegetables. The second is devoted largely to the preparation of special diets, except diabetic; the third to diabetic diets, weighing and cooking portions, as worked out by the dietitian. In this final period the student learns also to work out diets for herself, and must be able to do so correctly before leaving the kitchen.

The preparation for this service consists of a dietetics course of only 48 hours given two or more years earlier, in the probation period. Thus the student is entirely dependent on the diet kitchen experience for training in diet in disease. Furthermore, since the diet service is selective, nurses graduate from the school quite without knowledge of this important professional subject. Of the class graduating in the year of our study, one-half had no diet kitchen service.

PROVISION OF KITCHEN HELP

In the diet kitchen services thus picked out as valuable, the crowded program of actual training given shows little chance for educational waste. Yet in no hospital department, it should be noted, is there a more constant temptation to use the students for hospital convenience and hospital economy, regardless of educational ends, than precisely in the diet kitchen. Against this temptation a standing safeguard is erected in at least 2 of the 3 services just described by the provision of maid service which relieves the students of non-nursing duties and of most routine work that is not educationally useful.

INSTANCES OF CONSPICUOUS FAILURE

At the other extreme from the essentially educational character of the diet services at these 3 hospitals, we find others offering absolutely no training in special diets or in the relation of diet to disease. At one hospital, for example, the so-called dietetic service consists in the preparation and serving of ordinary diets merely, the students doing much work elsewhere easily performed by competent maids. At a special hospital, again, the students' work consists in preparing menus for private patients. At still another hospital where special diets are served, the dietitian prepares them all, and what passes for student training consists again merely of kitchen service.

These hospitals and others like them illustrate all too plainly the use of the students' time in the diet kitchen rather for convenience and economy of service than for the benefit of their own training. The educational field such hospitals offer is admittedly poor. But other hospitals of higher standing afford similar examples of lost educational opportunity in the diet kitchen service. One leading institution offers an extreme instance of the waste of students' time and the exploitation of students' services. Here a group of probationers, after a short, very elementary, and badly taught course in dietetics unaccompanied by any laboratory work, are assigned for 6-weeks' duty in the diet kitchen, the ward kitchen, and the private patients' department, at work a large proportion of which could readily be carried by a competent maid service. The presence in this school of a high proportion of college graduates makes their assignment to non-educational tasks of preparing food and vegetables (one student spent three hours a day in washing lettuce!), cooking, and serving, all the more deplorable.

At this hospital some of these preliminary students are indeed assigned to work on special diets, but even for these an extreme specialization of duties defeats any possibility of intelligent appreciation of what they are doing. They work simply to fill orders, one preparing one detail of the meal, and one another, without ever seeing the entire meal to which their work contributes, let alone understanding its objectives in treatment or cure.

From the point of view of education, at least two-thirds of the 6 weeks allotted to this service, according to our observer's estimate, may be considered waste time. In point of fact, at this particular hospital the average waste is even greater, as the assignments tend greatly to exceed the periods planned.[44]

[44] Among 21 records of actual experience studied, the median girl spent 65 days, or over 9 weeks in the diet kitchen. A reliable student stated to the writer that in her first year she had spent 18 weeks in the two diet services.

328 NURSING AND NURSING EDUCATION

An additional 5-weeks' assignment is given to certain students
as diet nurse in the private patients' department later in the
course. But as this period, too, makes for efficiency of service
rather than benefit to education, it must be counted for the
most part as waste, the total time lost amounting with this added
period to a minimum of 2 months.

COMPROMISES BETWEEN EDUCATION AND SERVICE

Between these extremes of successful and worthless services,
other examples of diet kitchen training at the various hospitals
studied may be variously criticised and commended. We have
recommended in our discussion of dietetics that a short period
of diet kitchen practice be allotted in the preliminary term as a
supplement to the laboratory training in cookery, each student's
progress to be regularly checked and certified. At a number of
hospitals the practice of assigning two periods in the diet kitchen
in point of fact already prevails. This system where it exists,
however, is used too often not to provide a needed practice field
for the principles of cookery already taught in classroom and
laboratory, but again to furnish unpaid maid's service to the
hospitals.

Thus in 2 prominent hospitals studied the time devoted to
cooking and general maid's service in the diet kitchen is twice
and four times as long, respectively, as the time allotted to
special diets.

PERCENTAGE OF STUDENTS ADMITTED TO DIET KITCHEN SERVICE

Whatever the merits or defects of the various types of diet
kitchen training offered in the group of hospitals under our
examination, the diet kitchen service is an experience of basic
value to the nurse and should be available unquestionably to all
students in training. This is far from being the case. The
failure of the hospitals to provide equal opportunity to their
students to enter this basic training has already been made
sharply evident by a quoted example (page 326): that of the
large private hospital at which only 50 per cent of the graduating
class had been given experience in the diet kitchen.

At other large hospitals observed, the assignment of but one
or two students at a time to the diet kitchen staff indicates
clearly the restricted character of the service. It is obvious that
with large student classes the proportion of students to graduate
without this experience may easily be very much larger than

in the case mentioned. Thus, at a large training school offering a month's training of exceptional value in the diet kitchen, only one student at a time is assigned to the staff, making it possible for only 12 students a year to obtain this opportunity.

CONCLUSIONS

From the analyses of the different services studied, it is clear that the diet kitchen experience in most hospitals needs reorganization. Elimination of non-educational manual, work is a first need. No less necessary is the reorganizing of the curriculum, on which we have laid emphasis. Competent classroom and laboratory instruction in dietetics with accompanying practice of cookery in the diet kitchen is an indispensable preparation for a training in special diets of high educational grade. Such preliminary instruction is increasingly being given in good high schools and may well, at some future date, be required as a prerequisite for entrance to the training school.

Following such instruction, given during the preliminary term in the training school and supplemented by some practice of cookery in the diet kitchen, the diet kitchen service proper should be accompanied or preceded by classroom instruction in diet in disease. On this solid basis of preparation, the time may then be devoted to intensive training in the professional work of calculating, weighing, and preparing special diets. An important part of the training should be the student's study and observation of the cases served. As we have already suggested, this can in part be effected by assigning students to the diet kitchen during part of the time while they are receiving general ward training. Just as in various hospitals students are assigned to the milk laboratory in the mornings and help in the babies' wards in the afternoons, feeding cases for which they have prepared formulæ, so, to some extent at least, students can have actual care of patients for whom they are preparing special diets.

If the practical difficulties of such assignments should prove too great, students should in any case, under the guidance of the dietitian, be taken to the wards and allowed to study, if they do not actually have the personal care of, the patients for whom special diets are prepared.

If such concentrated, carefully planned, and correlated training were substituted for the present too commonly wasteful and planless diet kitchen experience, two to three weeks of part-time service while assigned to the general wards, together with two weeks' part-time service in the milk room while assigned to the obstetrical or pediatric departments, might be held ample to replace the present fantastic range of assignments.

A special point for emphasis, too often ignored, is to include instruction in the feeding of the well child as an essential part of the children's service.

THE DISPENSARY

Among the opportunities for student training in the hospital, none is richer or offers better facilities for teaching than the dispensary or out-patient department. A wealth of experience, available nowhere else in the hospital, irreplaceable for the nurse's professional training, is here offered at the very door of the training school. The more deplorable is the failure in most hospitals to use this teaching field so as to realize its essential value. Let us see wherein the importance of the dispensary for nursing education consists.

GREATER NUMBER AND RANGE OF CASES IN DISPENSARY THAN ON THE WARDS

As compared with the number and range of cases in the hospital wards, dispensary departments care for a much greater number of patients and a far wider range of cases.

Thus one of the hospitals visited, with a long-established out-patient department, accommodates about 450 patients in its wards and rooms, while over 14,000 visits are made to its clinics each month; another more recently established hospital with 250 beds, has a monthly dispensary attendance of over 3,500. We have in another connection referred to one hospital which, in the 31 years of its existence, had 132,589 patients in its wards and 2,000,000 attending its dispensary.

The differences in types of cases are equally striking, for while the great majority admitted to the wards are for the most part in acute or advanced condition, those treated in the clinics present other stages of disease—incipient, convalescent, and chronic—as well as disease groups which do not require bed care in any stage. Here, then, the student may broaden her study of the cycle of disease by the convalescent cases discharged from the hospital but still needing care and advice to confirm their cure; and may learn how chronic conditions may be checked or at least alleviated.

PREVENTING SICKNESS THROUGH THE DISPENSARY

In addition to caring for actual sickness, hospitals are more and more using their dispensaries for the prevention of sickness. The tendency in this direction is shown in the establishment of clinics such as we have already examined in our public health study: clinics for well babies, concerned with keeping babies well and teaching mothers; nutrition classes for school children; prenatal clinics, with supervision planned to give prospective mothers a safe maternity; venereal clinics, with their examination and safe-guarding of the families of patients—these are but a few of the means by which some hospitals, through their dispensaries, are entering the field of preventive medicine.

Moreover, here in the dispensary are congregated those "minor ills," nowhere else to be observed in the hospital, which, unless prevented, will later fill hospital wards, and which are among the most fertile causes of social as well as physical disaster. Here, the student may learn the significance of minor symptoms, the importance of early physical examination and diagnosis; she may gain an insight into the new emphasis on checking disease in its incipient stages before it has advanced too far for cure, and of inculcating the laws of hygienic living before bad habits on the part of the patient have crystallized.

SOCIAL PROBLEMS IN THE DISPENSARY

Not less important for the future work of the student nurse is the prominence of community and social problems in the dispensary. Nowhere else in the hospital does the medico-social problem so inevitably compel attention. Here individual family problems such as the difficulties of the working mother, the man needing care so that he can hold his job, the wayward girl, the unmarried mother—these, and a long chain of similar problems, are immediate and cannot be ignored. These patients, most of them leading their usual busy lives, coming direct from their homes or work, dramatize the complex medical and social problem, as the ward patients, for the most part, cannot do. Dispensaries are no longer used only by the poor. The practice of charging small fees and the growing popularity of special pay clinics have removed the former taint of charity, with the result that wage earners in large numbers are attending them.

Contact with all these different types of cases cannot fail to give the student a more sympathetic understanding of her future professional opportunity and a keener realization of the close interdependence of medical and social work.

EVOLUTION OF THE DISPENSARY

The dispensary is one of the latest departments of the hospital to be organized, and is still naturally enough in a formative stage as to function and policy. Its development has been an individual evolution at individual hospitals, according to local conditions and needs. Hence the field today presents a great variety of types, differing widely as to organization, standards of care, number and character of clinics, and participation in community health activities.

"The dispensary has too often been treated," says the recent report of a comprehensive study of New York dispensaries made by the Public Health Committee of the New York Academy of Medicine, "as a Cinderella in the hospital household—neither sufficient funds nor sufficient thought have been given to its organization and work.

"The problems encountered in dispensary administration are probably more complex and more difficult than are the problems arising in the management of a hospital, yet the majority of institutions lack a definite policy with regard to dispensary work, and the administrative supervision is in too many instances purely perfunctory." [45]

Only recently have efforts been initiated to reorganize the whole organization and management of out-patient departments, and to make them over into the invaluable adjuncts to health as well as places for cure that they may be.

In view of their history and present condition, it is not surprising that the rare opportunities for training student nurses offered by the dispensary should have been hitherto largely neglected or indeed unrecognized. Many training schools are connected with hospitals which have no dispensary department. In many others the dispensary is staffed with graduate nurses, and students are not admitted to the service. In still others, as we shall see, students are assigned to duty in some of the least valuable clinics.

* The Dispensary Situation in New York City. E. H. Lewinski-Corwin, Ph.D., Executive Secretary of the Public Health Committee, New York Academy of Medicine. The Medical Record, Jan. 31, 1920. Page 182.
See also publications of the Committee on Dispensary Development, New York City.

DISPENSARIES STUDIED

Of the 23 hospitals studied, 17 had dispensary departments,[*] varying from those with a limited service of one or two clinics, to those with highly organized schedules of 11 to 14 clinics handling a wide range of curative and preventive work and employing better undergraduate and graduate nurses.

In addition to the general study made of student assignments and duties in the 17 schools, a detailed study was made of 4 of the leading dispensaries to observe both the extent to which they were being used for teaching and the specific duties of the students in the different clinics.

LENGTH OF ASSIGNMENTS

The length of time for which students are assigned to the dispensary in the hospitals visited varies, according to the hospital plans, from 3 weeks to 3 months, the average school having a service of 2 months. This service may be given in the first, second, or third year, may be one straight period of service or may be broken up into two or three periods of a varying number of weeks. Fifteen of the 17 schools plan a term of dispensary service for each student, the remaining 2 offer a selective service for a limited number of students.

But just as we have already seen in other services, the facts do not always correspond to the plan. Thus, in one school planning a 2-months' service for all students, the records of seven seniors in the school for 34 months or more showed that some students had no dispensary experience, while others had either less or more than the amount planned. Four of these seniors had not as yet had any time in the clinics, one had had less than 3 weeks, one had had 1 month, and one 2½ months— exceeding by 2 weeks the time planned for each student.

Our studies of the student nurse in the dispensaries yielded two salient facts: (1) the almost total loss of the great educational opportunities for training offered by the dispensary, and (2) the corresponding waste of the students' time in routine duties.

[*] In view of the similarity of duties in certain emergency departments they have been included in the number of dispensaries. Two schools obtain dispensary experience by affiliation.

The failure of the training school to use the dispensary as a teaching field for students, either to enlarge the range of their nursing and medical knowledge or to give them an insight into the social and community problems available here for study, is reflected clearly in:

The lack of correlation between dispensary assignments, previous class instruction, and ward duty;
The absence of planned dispensary instruction;
The assignments to clinics of no educational value;
The failure to encourage study of cases by the reading of case records.

Correlation between Clinics and Ward Experience

Since the chief work of the dispensary deals with cases in other than the acute stages, the student nurse has the chance to round out her ward experience by experience in the earlier and later stages of the diseases she has already cared for in the acute stages on the wards. To enable her to make the connection between these different stages, the assignments to the individual clinics should be preceded by class work on the clinic's specialty and should accompany, if possible, assignments to corresponding wards where she may have the opportunity to observe or care for the cases or types of cases seen in the clinics.

Thus, for instance, at a university school of nursing the student has 2 months in the dispensary.

"During this time," say our investigator, "she is moved about several times. She does not get all lines of work, since graduate nurses alone are used in a few. Her service in pediatrics is particularly good. There she sees and works in all rooms:—skin, genito-urinary, nervous, heart, feeding, two rooms for general and new cases. . . . Her service in this department supplements some of the weaker sides of the hospital work, notably skin and genito-urinary for children."

The experience in the children's clinic of another hospital of high standard is singled out by our investigator for praise in its supplementing of ward experience. During their service in the pediatric department, the students assist every morning from 8:30 to 1:00 o'clock, during two weeks, in the children's clinic.

"The clinic experience," says our field agent, "adds very much to the value of the service, as they must become familiar with the early signs of disease in children, the various rashes, etc., indicating the acute exanthemata, as well as conditions only seen in the clinic or not admitted to the wards."

Again, in a large municipal hospital, planned correlation was shown in the assignment of students to a recently established venereal clinic during their six-weeks' experience in a gynecological and women's venereal ward. Another instance was the assignment of the student on service in the orthopedic clinic to duty in the orthopedic ward where she cared for the cases seen in the clinic. The student in this case was a five-year student who had had two college years and was in her first year of hospital training. She pointed out the clinic cases she had previously cared for in the ward and said that the combination of the two services was the only thing that made the clinic experience worth while.

But these are unfortunately isolated examples of good correlation between ward and dispensary training. The importance of such correlation has been recognized in but few schools. While students in surgical clinics may serve in surgical wards before and after clinic hours, as already described, and others in medical wards, while assigned to medical clinics, the connection is too often one in name only, for the ward duty bears no relation to the clinic experience. Instead of following cases admitted through the clinics, the students make beds, give baths, serve as "dish nurse," or are "generally useful" in miscellaneous odd jobs about the ward during part of the day.

Correlation with Class Teaching

A still graver lack of correlation exists between class work and dispensary assignments. Students are assigned to important services without any previous instruction in the cases and conditions they will meet in the clinics. Weeks and months may elapse after seeing groups of cases in the clinics, before the student has any instruction as to their cause, symptoms, and treatment.

The result of such an educational policy was shown in a school of high standing, in the case of a second-year student who was serving in a clinic where only salvarsan treatments were given. She had no knowledge of syphilis except a vague idea as to its infectiousness—in her own words she had "heard the doctors talk about it." On inquiry it appeared that the head of the nursing service in the dispensary "did not know" whether the student had had any lectures on venereal diseases. In this school the instruction in communicable disease (including venereal) is given in the second year, but students assigned to this clinic may or may not have had such lectures.

That such instances are not unusual is shown by the case of a second-year student in another hospital, serving in a genito-urinary clinic without any previous lectures on venereal diseases, though constantly in touch with syphilitic conditions; by the case, again, of an affiliated student in her third year, on duty in an eye clinic where she took the vision of old and new cases both with and without glasses, assisted at examinations when needed, chaperoned patients, and kept the examining chairs filled. She had had no lectures on the anatomy of the eye or on eye diseases, either at her own or this affiliating school.

In fact, case after case might be cited, all pointing to the same lack of educational planning: of the student, for example, assigned to a gynecological clinic who had had no instruction in the anatomy of the generative system or of gynecological disorders; or of the student assigned to a nerve clinic treating many patients with late manifestations of syphilis, who had had no previous class work in syphilis and its significance in mental cases.

Absence of Planned Dispensary Instruction

According to the prevailing system, students in most dispensaries receive practically no professional instruction, except in the routine duties of individual clinics. Not even at our leading schools has any rounded program as yet been developed for the use of the dispensary as a teaching field. Training schools do not have special instructors for the dispensary nor is any other effective provision made for the instruction of student nurses on duty in the clinics.

The heads of nursing services in dispensaries, and the head nurses in charge of different clinics and special sections, were unanimous in saying that the pressure of their own work left them no time for teaching. The general sentiment among them seemed to be that students can learn by observation, by asking questions and by listening to doctors. The instruction they give, if any, is confined to matters related to the running of the clinics —setting up tables, cleaning instruments, handling of numbers of patients, etc. This focussing of attention on the machinery of the clinics is quite natural, for under the present system the student nurse is used largely in attending to the smooth running of the dispensary, the quick handling of numerous patients, the efficient management of a thousand indispensable details.

How much the student learns during her dispensary service in the direction of her professional training, seems to depend almost wholly upon herself, and the chance good-will of the doctors. The students' own statements are illuminating. "The amount a nurse learns," says one, "depends upon the questions she asks." Others expressed the feeling that they should be taught more about the cases and given more time for reference reading and study. In a syphilitic clinic it was "almost tragic," a senior student felt, that the nurses should learn so little. On the other hand, in a genito-urinary clinic also caring for gonorrhea patients, the service was considered valuable "because the doctors explained so much about the cases," this being the only instruction received by the students except in the routine work of the clinic.

The quite accidental character of any professional knowledge gained in the clinics is well illustrated in the case of a school which gives no lectures in skin diseases. Students assigned to the skin clinic at the dispensary are present at the clinics and demonstrations held for postgraduate and undergraduate medical students. The medical head of the clinic happens to take the view that the student nurses are also there to learn, and expects them to observe, express opinions, and ask questions. Here, then, thanks to the physician's chance interest in nursing education, the students fortunate enough to be assigned to his clinic obtain real instruction in skin diseases.

But the instruction obtained in an exceptional clinic, thanks to the liberal attitude of the physician in charge, cannot obscure the general fact that the clinics have no educational intention so far as the student nurses are concerned. Students, moreover, are fast coming to realize, not without resentment, that in spite of the wealth of educational opportunity offered by the dispensary, the only teaching they are for the most part receiving relates to the mechanics of the clinics and not to their real work.

Certain benefits may indeed be derived by an alert student from hearing cases discussed by the doctors, "listening in" at clinics and demonstrations for medical students, or the occasional instruction of a physician; but these cannot take the place of intelligently planned direction and teaching. A certain amount may undoubtedly be learned through observation of cases and participation in treatments, but such chance gleaning of information and experience is of limited value, because young students have not the necessary background to separate the important from the non-important.

Assignment to Clinics of no Educational Value

Equally striking in the student assignments to dispensary service is the evident and complete absence of educational design in the choice of clinics. To a marked extent students were found to be serving in the clinics of least value educationally, such as the surgical.

An illustration of the valueless experience offered by such assignments may be seen in the case of a third-year student on duty in a surgical clinic. It is safe to assume, especially in view of the over-emphasis of the surgical service already noted at most hospitals, that a senior student has had sufficient experience in surgical procedure, such as making surgical dressings, assisting at dressings, and the like, not to require special assignments to the dispensary for further practice. As a matter of fact, study of her assignments shows that her experience in the dispensary was limited to the repetition of surgical routine.

During the first two hours of the morning, before reporting at the dispensary, she was assigned to duty in a surgical ward. But her work there consisted merely of "being generally useful," making beds, assisting with dressings, etc. During the morning at the surgical clinic she dusted bottles and ointment jars, and set up the clinic rooms and dressing trays. During the clinic she cut down bandages, waited on doctors and medical students, assisted with minor dressings, got histories from the files, and, after the clinic, cleaned up. In the afternoon she was at the eye and throat clinic where she again prepared the rooms, assisted at examinations and cleaned up after the clinic was over. A day more barren of educational content for a student in her last year of training could not well be devised. While the student in this case liked the clinics, especially during the holidays when the medical students were away and she "got a chance to do dressings," the professional value of even this chance bit of experience is doubtful.

In contrast with this barren surgical dispensary service, merely duplicating earlier ward work, the enrichment of student training through good dispensary service may be illustrated by a two-months' assignment to an obstetrical clinic in a different hospital. One month is spent here in outdoor duty, visiting patients in their homes, and the other in the clinic. In this thoroughly educational plan, the students' work in all the different phases of prenatal supervision, home care of mothers and babies, etc., is supervised by a graduate nurse. It is of interest in this connection that probationers in about their fourth week are sent out with the prenatal nurse to observe and to receive some idea of nursing care in the homes of patients. This early initiation into home conditions of patients and the outdoor work of the hospital is a valuable background to the regular dispensary service received later in training.

Too often, however, the student nurse is deliberately excluded from such clinics of major interest and importance, which are staffed exclusively by graduate nurses. In a training school connected with a medical school, for instance, no students have any service in the notably live and interesting pediatric clinic. The clinic is directed by a member of the teaching staff of the medical school assisted by 6 outside doctors, an interne, and 16 third-year medical students. Children are referred to it from other clinics, a health center, and the local school nursing service. The variety of experience is shown by the diagnoses of cases under treatment on the day the clinic was visited by us:

Tonsillitis.	Two feeding cases.
Whooping-cough, two cases.	Frequent urination.
Chicken-pox.	Chronic bronchitis.
Enlarged tonsils and earache.	Thrush.
Enlarged tonsils and heart disease.	Rickets.
Acute otitis, two cases.	Inflamed nasal passages.

It is doubly regrettable that students have no service in this clinic, for, in addition to the range of cases treated, the standards as to physical examinations, medical records, laboratory examinations, medical and social follow-up work, etc., are illustrative of the best type of dispensary work.

In the obstetrical and gynecological clinic of this hospital, too, no student nurses were found. Here they might have had opportunities of training in the various branches of maternity service equal or superior to that described above. Through the records of the social service department the student nurses preparing for a profession so intimately concerned with community problems, might have been taught at first hand the grave social aspects of many of the cases admitted to the clinics and the social and civic agencies that deal with them.

Failure to Use Case Records

We have already commented on the importance of instruction in case records, medical and social, in ward training (see page 312), and on the failure to encourage even the reading of these records by the student nurses. In the dispensary the prominence of social problems and the fact that the social histories of patients are more often available than those of ward patients makes the neglect of the records for teaching all the more deplorable.

On the day of our visit, for instance, to the obstetrical clinic just mentioned, adequate explanation of a single case whose admirably complete records were, unused, on file in the social service department would have given the students genuine insight into the intricate medico-social problems involved in the history of an unmarried and defective young mother. The social service records portrayed concretely and vividly the constructive efforts made to deal with this unfortunate case. There was in black and white a history of several abortions, mental testing, recommendation of sterilization by the clinic doctors, attempts to place the children in institutions, and final resort to custodial care for the mother. But the student nurse observed on the day of our visit to the clinic, who might soon need to apply in her community work just such enlightenment as this history afforded, was as ignorant of these social facts and the agencies which dealt with them as though she were an inanimate mechanism in the room, or as though they had not been available in the filing-case for her instruction.

A second illustration of the educational loss from failure to use the available social history of a patient may be cited from a medical clinic. Here on the day of our visit was a cardiac case, a young girl long under the supervision both of the clinic doctors and the workers in the social service department of the hospital. The medical history of the case was of no special significance. But the social history of the patient showed that she was unhappy at home, at odds with a brother upon whom she was dependent, and that her periodic heart attacks were coincident with outbreaks of friction in the family. The wise and patient counsel of the hospital social worker had helped to re-educate patient and family. These facts, directly bearing on the patient's medical condition and necessary for proper medical understanding of the case, did not appear on the medical record. The social record would have brought home forcibly to the student the dependence of the patient's improvement upon social and mental adjustments, the helplessness of medical skill when home conditions block recovery, and the legitimate influence of the wise health worker in improving home conditions once she has gained the confidence of the family.

In a genito-urinary clinic in which gonorrhea cases are also treated, where there were two student nurses, two social workers, and a paid secretary whose salary was covered by a state appropriation for venereal work, the social workers stated that any knowledge of social problems or social work on the part of the student nurses was purely accidental. Here, where the importance of the cases was emphasized by the personnel, and by the concern of the state itself in supplying a paid worker, the student nurses sit and make cotton balls and swabs between cases.

These significant cases were cited from among many seen in the clinics where the social histories revealed difficult problems of human relations as well as simpler instances of ignorance and thoughtlessness, and where social readjustments were indicated as the necessary preliminary to any lasting medical benefit. Without knowledge of these social readjustments, the student's clinic service was indeed barren.

Yet in clinic after clinic visited the same statement was made: the students had "no time to read histories." Many individual students expressed their dissatisfaction with this state of affairs. One who said she had "no time to read medical histories and certainly no time for social problems" had nearly completed training and was serving in a clinic caring only for syphilitic cases. She spent an hour and a half daily getting ready for treatments, gave the treatments intravenously for an hour, and then was kept busy waiting on the doctors. Of the significance and social importance of the cases treated she can have had only the most casual conception.

"If there is any time, I read the medical histories, but this rarely happens," said another student, an affiliate, in a prenatal and gynecological clinic, who spent the major portion of her time in setting up tables for examinations. Another said that she occasionally got a chance to read the patients' dispensary cards but not their histories. Still another had ample opportunity to grow familiar with the medical records, but only because she had been assigned to work usually done by the medical students, namely, that of writing up the case histories.

Instead, now, of assigning a limited number of senior students to training in the social service department of the hospital, it is in our opinion urgent, as will be indicated at greater length in a subsequent chapter on the Social Aspects of Disease and Its Prevention, that all students should be instructed so far as possible in the medical and social histories of their patients, both on the wards and in the dispensary.

It is indeed small wonder if intelligent young women resent the hours spent daily in routine duties and housework when no time is available for the study which would teach the true inwardness of their cases. How the time is consumed in non-educational duties, and how a better educational scheme may be inaugurated, we are next to consider.

TIME WASTED IN NON-EDUCATIONAL DUTIES

That the student nurse in the dispensary is traditionally regarded as a "pair of hands and feet" and not an intelligence in training, becomes abundantly clear in the light of a study, however brief, of how she spends her time in the clinics.

For it is very evident that the great bulk of student time in the dispensary is not spent in acquiring any new knowledge or nursing experience, it is not devoted as might be expected to giving personal service to patients, but is given over mostly to a variety of routine manual duties for which little or no nursing skill or knowledge is required. Such duties are cleaning, dusting, setting up tables and arranging clinic rooms, sterilizing and cleaning instruments, making supplies, chaperoning patients, mending rubber gloves, doing errands, waiting on doctors and medical students, listing supplies, copying records, and the like. Students must act the parts in alternation with attendants, maids, clerks, and messengers, because hospitals have as yet devised no plan for using lay assistants to carry on the routine operation of the dispensary.

Perhaps nothing shows more clearly the unquestioned acceptance as student duty of the routine dispensary work which is properly paid service, than the detailed schedules of work for students drawn up at various training schools. These schedules contain careful and minute directions as to tables, desks, closets, shelves, supplies, listing and checking hospital property, articles and arrangements preferred by the different doctors, etc., in endless detail.

In one school the chief of the dispensary nursing service instructs the students serving in the different clinics in the details of their routine work from carefully compiled lists prepared for the purpose. The students study these lists and also receive oral instruction in their duties during the half-hour preceding the clinics. This is the only teaching given, except that each afternoon the head nurse "checks up the condition in which each clinic has been left and calls the attention of the students to any mistakes the following morning."

This detailed planning shows that the training schools are actually and chiefly concerned with preserving the established routine of the different clinics. While it is undoubtedly necessary both for the well-being of the patients and the best work of the doctors that routine procedures should go forward smoothly, the waste of students' time in such routine operation need hardly be argued.

Administrative and Clerical Duties

In addition to running the mechanism of the clinics, students are frequently expected to fill purely administrative or clerical positions. In one dispensary with a daily attendance of about 600 patients, students assigned as admitting nurse must handle all cases needing special attention, such as isolation cases, workmen's compensation cases, cases referred to or from other institutions, all of which require a great deal of clerical work and special adjustment. At another, the students in one clinic spend fully an hour and a half a day in purely clerical work, filing medical record cards and medical histories.

Miscellaneous Duties

In a nose and throat clinic visited much of the students' time was spent in accompanying post-operative cases to a recovery ward, a distance of 275 feet and a three-story trip in an elevator, and in making dressings between trips. In a dental clinic the work done in most offices by attendants was performed by student nurses. As maids and scrub-women their services are constantly taken for granted,—witness the not unusual assignment of students who spend three hours daily cleaning clinic rooms, and the hours of student service devoted to dusting, cleaning instruments, and—most of all resented—the interminable task of mending rubber gloves.

Some of these varied activities are clearly not legitimate student functions; others are repetitive routine duties which, once learned, can add nothing to the student's nursing equipment.

Delegation of Non-Educational Work to a Permanent Staff

Some hospital managements, it is true, form an honorable exception to the rule of thus exploiting the time of students in the dispensary, and have made a definite effort to assign such routine work to maids, attendants, and other workers, but these exceptions are as rare as they are honorable. Indeed, even in those dispensaries in which lay service has been to some extent introduced, the substitution has not been extended to all the clinics. In the same dispensary the students in some clinics are largely relieved of non-educational work, while in others they are still assigned day after day to repetitive duties adding nothing to their nursing knowledge or skill.

In one of these dispensaries an attendant makes supplies, prepares and cleans clinic rooms, cleans instruments, mends gloves, assists with etherizing in nose and throat operations, etc., and a maid assists in the dental clinic. Yet the students still spend hours in cleaning, replenishing supplies, and checking needed articles. In another clinic the student on duty spends one whole afternoon a week in cleaning the shelves, lockers, closets, and drawers in a laboratory, and in checking up and replenishing supplies of drugs, stains, acids, stationery, culture outfits, etc.

This is not an isolated instance. Another hospital in which it was repeatedly stated that the students in the dispensary had been relieved of all house-keeping duties showed similar inconsistencies of policy and practice. While in one clinic an intelligent maid did cleaning, made supplies, sterilized and cleaned instruments, and even assisted with operations, in another clinic a student performed practically identical duties.

Nevertheless, in the face of the long-established tradition regarding the student's place in the dispensary, it would be shortsighted indeed not to recognize the importance and significance of these genuine efforts towards a change. The substitutions already made are new departures in hospital management and carry additional weight from the fact that the hospitals acting as pioneers in the movement are among those with the highest medical and nursing standards.

To make real use of the dispensary as a teaching field, it is evident that definite reorganizations are needed. These are, first, reorganization of the school curriculum in order to provide teaching in the dispensary and to correlate class work and ward experience with the clinic service; and, second, reorganization of the mechanism of the dispensary by providing a staff of paid workers to do the routine work now being done by the students.

Length and Content of Student Assignments

At what point in the student's training dispensary service should be assigned, and what should be the definite instruction in the different clinics must be left to the judgment of individual schools. The details of a dispensary schedule and teaching program must plainly be affected by the type of hospital and the organization of the dispensary department in question, the size, number, and character of the clinics, as well as by matters more closely connected with the training school.

The length of dispensary assignments in the different clinics should be determined by the educational content of the experience offered in each clinic. Thus, as the dental clinic offers small opportunity for nursing experience and teaching, it would not justify more than a short assignment, while another clinic, such as the pediatric, may offer so much of educational value as to justify a long assignment. So far as possible, students while on ward duty should be assigned to corresponding dispensary services for part of the time, so as to have opportunity of observing different stages of the diseases cared for on the wards.

In our proposed curriculum approximately three months are allotted to the dispensary service, divided between the medical, the surgical, and the children's clinics. In the medical, as wide an experience as possible is advocated, including tuberculosis, skin, and venereal. In the surgical, experience in the specialties, eye, ear, nose, and throat, is advocated. In connection with the children's clinic, some experience with fairly normal children should be given with special emphasis on the feeding of the well child.

It is desirable that during the preliminary period, probationers should have the opportunity of observing at least major clinics, and following up some of the patients at home, under supervision. They may thus gain a view of dispensary activities, and learn to see their ward experience in a truer perspective as but one phase of caring for the sick.

Need of Dispensary Instructors·

Clearly, the educational opportunities of the dispensary will continue to be lost to the students unless a responsible instructor is provided. In the selection of a dispensary instructor, schools should be guided in the main by the number and character of the clinics and the character of the attendance. Thus a dispensary in a manufacturing district with an industrial attendance will need an instructor with experience in industrial nursing and also knowledge as to the related subjects of industrial diseases, hazards, protection of workers, compensation, etc.; while another located in a crowded city section, in teaching the medical aspects of such conditions as poverty, malnutrition, poor sanitation, etc., will need a teacher experienced in city conditions and with a good working knowledge of private and civic agencies which may be counted on for co-operation.

The dispensary instructor should be a specialist in teaching, unburdened with executive or administrative responsibilities. She should teach methods of giving personal care to clinic cases, but she should do far more than this. She should help students to make the connection between the conditions seen in the clinics and on the ward, pointing out the different stages of the same disease and the medical and nursing care associated with each stage. She should make full use of the medical and social histories of patients. She should make clear the recent developments in preventive medicine and public health work, the social and economic significance of disease, and the relation between the hospital and the work of outside agencies.

CONCLUSIONS

In planning the necessary changes in dispensary personnel, it will be seen that two types of workers may be used, salaried and volunteer. A budget to cover paid workers should include a sufficient number of graduate nurses to handle all details of management, such as admissions, transfers, payments, supervision of maids, orderlies, attendants, etc., connected with the routine operation of dispensary departments. Additional workers such as history clerks or secretaries, messengers, chaperones, helpers in special clinics, persons to make supplies and dressings, may be paid or volunteer,—as was the case during the war, and as is the established policy in some of our hospitals which lead in institutional administration and vision.

When hospital boards come clearly to distinguish between work needed to run their dispensaries and work needed to equip their students, readjustments of duty on an educational basis will be made consistent and uniform, and the students will fit into the dispensary routine as students. As in the wards of the most enlightened hospitals, where cleaning, sweeping, dusting, dishwashing, setting of trays, etc., go on irrespective of the changes in student personnel, so eventually in the clinics, the cleaning, dusting, setting up of tables, cleaning of instruments, making of supplies, and mending the gloves, etc., will be done by paid and volunteer workers.

But the solution of these problems, it must be finally emphasized, depends not so much upon budgets, paid or volunteer workers, or any external thing, as upon the realization of hospital authorities that present-day nursing education demands planned teaching in the dispensary no less than in other departments of the hospital, and that it is not given under present conditions.

On the present disposition of student nurses in the dispensary, the facts assembled leave room but for one verdict: that of an educational wastefulness scarcely possible to over-emphasize. The priceless opportunities offered by the dispensary, are educationally lost. Student nurses leave this unique service scarcely wiser either in knowledge of disease or of social health problems than they entered it. Graver, moreover, than the individual loss to the student is the ultimate loss to the public. For the modern demands made upon the nursing profession for constructive community work cannot be met by the trained nurse, however experienced in bedside nursing, who comes from her hospital experience with her mind unawakened to the medico-social problems of today; those problems which in the dispensary even more sharply than in hospital wards confront both doctor and nurse.

TIME WASTED IN NON-NURSING DUTIES

We have seen in some detail in the dispensary and diet kitchen and more generally in other departments the signal waste of students' time in household and manual service. In this section

we shall seek to make a brief statistical showing, as accurate
as it was possible to obtain, of the time so wasted by the
student during her three-years' course, or during the part of
the three years of which we have authentic record.
Our records of waste time consist, on the one hand, of the
observations of our field agents in certain training schools
checked by their superintendents, and on the other, of estimates
made by other schools on the basis of detailed reports from
their students. From these varied data a striking general agreement emerges, a consensus of opinion that by conservative estimates between a fifth and a quarter of the student's time is
spent fruitlessly for her training on work other than nursing.
While these figures are more or less rough, they represent as
close an approximation to accuracy as is possible to obtain
without an exact scientific time study. If they err, it is on the
side of understatement rather than overstatement. This formidable amount of non-nursing service is so entrenched by
tradition in the routine of the student, so placidly accepted by
hospitals and public alike, that the extent of its encroachment
on genuine training must be amazing to everyone but the members of the nursing profession themselves. Let us see of what
these extraneous duties consist.

To make the situation clear, we shall first attempt to give a
general view of the non-nursing duties assigned to students at
the various hospitals studied; we shall then consider their incidence in the day's work of individual nurses; and shall finally
present as the result of a special study a well-defined picture of
the total time wasted at representative hospitals.

Before entering upon this description, let us state bluntly the
attitude of this report, the ground of our objecting to the assignment of the student to non-nursing duties beyond the minimum
necessary for her training. It is emphatically not that these,
whatever form they take, are lowering to her dignity, distasteful
to her feelings, beyond her strength: it is simply that she has
more important use to make of her time if she is to become the
trained and efficient public servant she is expected to be. She
must of course dust and sweep, cook and clean, wash and mend,
make supplies, run the sterilizer, and all the rest, until there can
be no question of her doing these things deftly and efficiently.
More than this, she must do enough of certain tasks, naturally
perhaps distasteful or repulsive, to get finally rid of whatever
inhibitions or repugnances she may feel towards them. The

nurse must have no shrinking nerves, no repugnances, no inhibitions; if she retains them she had better seek her vocation elsewhere. We raise no objection to disinfecting bedpans and washing stained linen because it is unpleasant; she will doubtless have many such tasks in her professional life. But the shortsighted economy by which the nurse in training spends an hour, say, washing diapers, when she has no time to learn her physiology lesson, cries for change.

These considerations are reinforced by the clinching fact that the training school's best plans, the instructor's best efforts for a genuine educational program are defeated because the one and one-half to two hours a day needed to realize it are devoted to dusting, cleaning, serving meals, and all the rest of the countless unskilled manual duties now relegated by tradition to the student nurse.

If devoted to instruction, this hour and a half to two hours each day would just suffice for the added hours of instruction indispensable in our opinion to interpret and illuminate the student's practical experience.

NON-NURSING DUTIES ON GENERAL WARDS

Cleaning, Dusting, and Putting in Order

While the so-called heavy cleaning is supposed in practically all hospitals to be done by paid workers, it is an accepted part of the student's duties to do the dusting, cleaning, and sweeping for the patients under her care. These general cleaning duties require in different hospitals from half an hour to an hour and a half daily, or even longer. The student also at many hospitals cleans the lavatory, bathroom, and other service rooms, and in some cases disinfects and cares for the bedpans and other utensils. The time spent in cleaning the lavatory one school reports at 35 or 40 minutes; another states that a first-year student spends an hour a day in cleaning service rooms. At the discharge of a patient, the student nurse must disinfect and clean the patient's bed, a process taking perhaps half an hour.

She is responsible, furthermore, for putting away linen and blankets in quantity, for the condition of the linen closet, the blanket closet, the closet or lockers in which the patients' clothing is kept, and the care of the clothing itself. Time required for such duties as these is difficult to gauge. The single item of folding and putting away linen occupies at several hospitals from half an hour to an hour a day, and in the case of one student on night duty rose actually to 2½ hours.

Meal Service

Moreover, in most hospitals the student spends much time in connection with the meal service, in setting and carrying trays, feeding appropriate patients, and at some schools washing her own patients' dishes. She is generally responsible as well for cleaning the ice-chest in the ward pantry. Of these duties connected with the meal service, setting and carrying trays alone is estimated to take from half an hour to an hour and a quarter of the student's time.

Of all these duties the part of the student's routine most nearly standardized at all hospitals, namely, the early morning dusting and cleaning for her own patients and the carrying of food trays, takes from 1½ to 2 hours daily.

DUTIES ON SPECIAL SERVICES

Operating Room

On special services more rather than less time is spent on non-educational duties. In the operating room, according to our observer's estimate at one hospital, a third of the student's time might be saved by more paid help; at another the training time "could well be reduced by half." Merely cleaning the room after operations, putting away equipment, and scrubbing furniture, is estimated at one hospital to take an hour and a half. Especially time-consuming among operating room duties is the cleaning of large numbers of instruments and the constant washing and mending of rubber gloves. In three well-known hospitals, these duties occupy each student in the service for an average of about 1 hour daily; at another they take 2 hours. At one of these until recently the total time wasted in instrument cleaning in the main operating room was 5 to 6 hours; the total time wasted in cleaning and mending gloves, 4 to 5 hours. Students in this service, moreover, are expected to assist so far as they can in the preparation and sterilizing of surgical supplies, and in many cases spend long hours in sorting and folding linen and putting it up in packages for sterilizing.

Obstetrical Department

A similar waste of time, though less excessive in amount, is seen in the obstetrical service. In this department the required sweeping and dusting, with the preparation and sterilizing of supplies, make up generally a heavy schedule of housekeeping and non-nursing duties. In addition to these, special duties often expected of the students are the washing of stained linen and diapers, washing and pulling of gauze, etc. Such assignments are not a matter of a single institution. On the obstetrical ward of a good-sized municipal hospital, the student is required to wash out all linen after deliveries, and often to wash out diapers as well. In the maternity department of a smaller hospital students are expected to wash out all stained gauze, at another small hospital to rinse out all diapers before sending them to the laundry. Such duties are frequently a part of the accepted routine not only in the obstetrical ward, but also in the children's and contagious wards. One student's assignment in an isolation ward included an hour at washing diapers.

Surgical Supply Room

In the surgical supply room the waste of time for student training and the provision of unpaid labor for the hospital reached its extreme in the long, educationally profitless hours of making supplies, pulling gauze, sorting, inspecting, and folding laundry, and putting it in packages for sterilizing, and in the constant running of the sterilizer. At one highly reputed private hospital distinguished for its modern standards, all sterilizing for the entire plant including the operating room is performed in the surgical supply room. Here in the sterilizing room two probationers spend 6 hours a day in running the sterilizer and checking incoming and outgoing supplies. Nor is the loss of time in this assignment compensated for by training of any value to the student during the rest of her time in the surgical supply room. Our investigator estimates that the 8-weeks' service could be cut to one week without losing any training or experience of educational value. At another hospital, of the 6½ hours spent daily by probationers in their assignment to the surgical supply room, according to our observer's estimate, 4½ hours was educationally wasted.

MISCELLANEOUS DUTIES: ERRANDS

There is also a long list of duties associated with no special service for which students in many hospitals are called on, and which add considerably to their hours of non-educational work. Many of these may be grouped under the head of *errands*. One of the most time-absorbing special types of errand is that of accompanying patients to the x-ray or operating rooms and bringing them back to their wards. Such an errand, especially if the hospital arrangements are old-fashioned and inconvenient, may take from an hour and a half to two hours. Other errands are taking empty bottles to the dispensary to be filled, carrying specimens to the laboratory, taking records to the office, fetching clean linen from the laundry, etc. In some hospitals students are assigned to telephone duty; in others to answer the door-bell.

DUTIES OF DAILY CARE

To the time spent in all these household and manual duties connected with the smooth running of the hospital service should be added as educational waste much time now spent by students in minor daily duties in the wards for women and children, which on the male wards are performed in well-ordered hospitals by orderlies.

A certain amount of waiting on and caring for patients not acutely sick may be safely entrusted, as it already is at many hospitals, to paid attendants. Among duties of this type may be instanced the patient's morning toilet and preparation for the night, giving drinks of water, serving meals, passing basins and mouth-wash, passing bedpans and urinals, helping dispensary patients to dress and undress, etc., and many others. Such duties, useful as they may be for the probationer, should not be allowed to take the time of the more advanced student to the detriment of her genuine professional study and training.

WASTE TIME IN INDIVIDUAL ASSIGNMENTS

In the preceding paragraphs we have attempted to give a general view of time educationally wasted in student training in a selected group of hospitals. Manifestly no one student performs the entire list of duties given, at any one time. Hence to visualize the actual incidence of waste time in a typical day's work we shall next consider the experience of individual students assigned to certain services in a given hospital.

Let us take for example the non-nursing duties performed by certain students on the obstetrical ward of a well-known general hospital (see Table 4). These duties, it should be remembered, with the time demanded by each one, were set down from the personal observation of our field agent or the statements of the students themselves, and checked in each case by the

superintendent of the training school. On this ward the time
wasted in non-educational work amounted for four students on
duty (not including the delivery nurse) to an average of 2 hours
and 11 minutes per day.

TABLE 4

TIME SPENT PER DAY IN NON-NURSING DUTIES

OBSTETRICAL WARD

Day Staff: 5 Students *⎰3 Third-Year
⎱2 Affiliating

Nursery Nurse	Minutes
Carrying babies to and from mothers (3 times daily) †	60
Washing soiled diapers	30
	90

General Duty Nurse ‡

Dusting in private and semi-private rooms	30
Washing babies' diapers	15
Setting up food trays	10
Washing out soiled sheets and gowns	10
Tidying linen cupboard	5
Serving dinner	20
	90

General Duty Nurse

Washing stained linen	10
Washing nourishment glasses	5
Cleaning medicine cupboard	25
Setting trays for private rooms⎫ Straightening up workroom⎰	15
Serving private trays and ward trays	30
Carrying all trays to diet kitchen (on floor below)	15
Cleaning workroom ⎱ Setting private and ward trays for morning ⎰	60
	160

General Duty Nurse

Dusting tables, etc., in ward	30
Washing out stained linen	10
Washing water glasses	10
Setting up trays for dinner	10
Cleaning utility room	20
Serving and carrying dinners	25
Dusting clothes room, washing bedpans	30
Making surgical dressings	50
Setting up all trays for supper	10
	195

* Delivery nurse not included in table.
† Many other duties done in intervals which could be very well done by a
nursery maid. No estimate of time thus wasted.
‡ General duty includes care of mothers, etc.

In the same hospital almost as bad a showing is made in the children's ward, with an average waste for the three students on duty whose time was analysed of approximately two hours (117 minutes). Here the largest items of waste time were in connection with serving the meals and feeding the children (more than an hour in one student's case), and in dusting, cleaning, and tidying (more than an hour in two students' cases), while one student spent nearly half an hour in preparing sheets and supplies for sterilization, and another a quarter of an hour in counting soiled linen. It is noticeable that on this ward the time educationally wasted is greater for the senior, the best equipped student, than for either of the younger students.

Similar conditions were found true of other wards of the hospital.

Night Duty

On the 12-hour night shift, according to the student's own records accepted by the training school authorities, the waste of time mounts to even greater extremes. The maximum is found in the case of a junior student on the male emergency surgical ward who spent on the night of the record actually more than half of the total hours of night duty—6 hours and 45 minutes—on non-nursing duties. For over 3½ hours of this time she made supplies or prepared gloves for the operating room.

The assignment of an intermediate nurse on the isolation ward was perhaps even worse in view of her more advanced training. Of 5 hours and 25 minutes lost time from the educational viewpoint, this student spent 2½ hours in putting away linen, some hour and a half in cleaning, and a further hour in making supplies. In several other assignments (3) the non-nursing duties ran above 3 hours; in 4 more, above 2. The minimum waste among the 13 students reporting on night duty assignments was an hour and a quarter. As especially wasteful assignments should be noted that of a senior on the maternity ward who spent nearly an hour (50 minutes) in washing soiled linen and diapers, and an intermediate student on the children's ward who spent half an hour in rinsing soiled linen.

While this time spent in non-nursing duties is of course not entirely consecutive, there is no doubt that there are sufficiently long intervals between calls for active nursing service which might be put to some use for study instead of being wasted on purely mechanical work. Indeed individual ambitious students have stated to the writer that they have found the intervals between active duty at night of great value for studying case records, on their own initiative.

EXAMPLES FROM ANOTHER HOSPITAL

The foregoing examples of student assignments on day duty are by no means extreme instances of time educationally lost in hospital service. Much more serious waste of student time may be noted at another prominent hospital where on the women's medical and surgical wards the average time per student spent in non-educational duties mounts up to 3½ hours a day. Lists of such duties performed by three students on women's surgical ward duty are given below together with the time requirement for each. It is highly significant, as we shall presently see, that on the corresponding male ward less than half as much of the students' time is wasted in non-nursing duties.

TABLE 5

TIME SPENT PER DAY IN NON-NURSING DUTIES
WOMEN'S SURGICAL WARD

Senior Nurse	Hours
Dusting	1
Folding linen	½
Carrying trays	½
Making surgical supplies	1
	3
Second-Year Student	
Dusting	1
Folding linen	½
Making supplies	1
Cleaning instruments	½
Washing gloves, etc.	½
	3½
First-Year Student	
Dusting	1
Cleaning service rooms	1
Carrying trays	½
Making supplies	1
Errands	1
	4½

ASSIGNMENT OF SENIORS TO NON-NURSING DUTIES

It might well be supposed that in the three years of the training course the time required of students for non-nursing duties might be longest in the period of probation, decreasing steadily with the student's advancement until in senior year it should leave her time as free as possible to be absorbed in her professional training. It is true, of course, that the manual and household duties are generally most time-consuming in the case of the probationer, and that an effort is certainly made at some hospitals to safeguard the older students' education by reducing their non-nursing assignments. That this effort often does not go far is indicated by the comparison of the duties of students of different years at the two hospitals just instanced. The time for housekeeping duties assigned to the senior in the women's surgical ward at one hospital is only half an hour less than the average time for the three students on the ward (3½ hours); in the children's ward at the other, the senior's assignment of non-nursing work is heavier, as we have already noticed, than those of the other students. On the obstetrical ward, again, the waste of student time is aggravated by the fact that in the case of three at least of the four students on duty it is seniors' time that is wasted.

Head Nurseships

But even at schools where the senior is largely released from ordinary household duties, her release is frequently in the interest not of a basic nursing course, but of clerical, executive, or administrative work in the hospital service. Cases in point are the assignments in many hospitals of head nurseships to students in their senior year. In such positions the seniors' time is filled with making rounds with doctors, assignment and supervision of students' work, direction of maids and cleaning women, requisition of supplies, keeping of records, and all the countless details of ward management,—special training valuable indeed for future executive work, but wholly out of place in a basic course.

TOTAL TIME WASTED AT A REPRESENTATIVE HOSPITAL

In the preceding pages we have made an effort to convey some realization of the many-sided aspects, the scope and variety of the non-educational service still required by the hospitals and still generally accepted as inevitably incident to student training. We have also illustrated at certain hospitals the waste time involved in the concrete ward assignments of individual students. It remains for us now to sum up as the result of an intensive study and present in tabular form the total picture of time wasted at a representative hospital.

Table 6 shows for this hospital the student's average daily waste of time in major services, her average total assignment to each service, and the percentage of this assignment spent in non-nursing duties, as well as the percentage so spent of her total training.

TABLE 6

AVERAGE TIME SPENT IN MAJOR SERVICES COMPARED WITH AVERAGE TIME SPENT IN NON-NURSING DUTIES BY STUDENTS OF ONE CLASS DURING 18 MONTHS OF SERVICE IN AN 8-HOUR HOSPITAL

Services	Average of Daily Hours Spent per Student in Non-nursing Duties in Each Service	Average Days Spent per Student		Percentage of Time Spent in Each Service in Non-Nursing Duties
		In Each Service	In Non-Nursing Duties in Each Service	
1	2	3	4	5
Day Duty				
Medical	1¼	95	15	15.6
Surgical	1¼	162	25	15.6
Mixed	1¼	67	10	15.6
Children's	1¼	27	4	15.6
Orthopedic	1¼	22	3	15.6
Skin	1¼	21	3	15.6
Operating Room	2	39	10	25.0
All Services	..	434	71	16.4
Night Duty	4	106	42	40.0
Average for all Services * .... (Day and Night)		540	114	21.1

* Excluded from this table is the time spent in the above services during the preliminary term, in an affiliated obstetric service, in dispensary and private services, elective work in services other than those included above, and vacations.

At the hospital here in question, our observer's estimate of 1¼ hours as the average daily waste per student on each ward was arrived at by her own direct observation of housekeeping service and of the average time required. This estimate was checked by the superintendent of the school and accepted as typical of all wards. Waste time in the operating room was estimated by the school superintendent. The figure of 4 hours for waste time in the night shift was also accepted on the authority of the school. This figure was calculated on the basis of the students' own records of time spent in non-nursing duties, carefully kept at the request of the superintendent.

Exclusion of Probationers from the Table

It is often held that during probation the employment of students in non-nursing manual duties is necessary for their education and hence cannot be held waste of time. In our opinion probationers are often kept at manual work far longer than is desirable either for their training or *morale*. In the figures and calculations of the table, however, in order to avoid any controversial question, we have totally excluded all time spent by probationers on the wards. In hospitals in which excessive manual work is required in the first months, the total waste of student time during the entire course would therefore be greater than is here shown.

Explanation of the Table

Column 2 is obtained by observation and student record as described on page 357.

Column 3 is obtained by dividing the *total* student days spent in each service by total number of students to show average days spent per student in each service.

Column 4 is obtained by multiplying the total student days in each service by the average daily waste for the service in question, then dividing by eight to reduce to eight-hour days, and finally dividing once more by the total number of students to show the average number of days spent per student in non-nursing duties in each service.

Column 5 represents the percentage of daily and total time spent in each service in non-nursing duties.

On the basis of these figures, at this prominent private hospital maintaining a training school of high reputation, the waste time, ranging from 15.6 per cent of total time on the wards to 25 per cent in the operating room and 40 per cent on night duty, averages for all services 21.1 per cent or more than one-fifth of the student's total time. The inclusion of time wasted in the private service, the dispensary, and the diet kitchen would have raised this average somewhat higher. For various reasons, it was not possible to include these items.

TOTAL TIME WASTED AT OTHER HOSPITALS

To serve as a check on the findings of this special study similar figures of waste time were obtained for two other hospitals of comparable type and standing.

At one of these, after careful analysis and calculation based largely on figures furnished by the school authorities, the percentage of waste time in total student service was found on the hospital's own showing to be about 21 per cent. At the other, where the figures used for daily time wasted were based, as in Table 6, on our actual observation, the percentage of waste time in total service, with the important omission of night duty, was 22.5 per cent. Of night duty, in which the percentage of time wasted is especially high, no study was made here and no figures were obtained. As the hospital's own data in the first case are not likely to exaggerate waste time, and as the figure in the second is disproportionately lowered by the exclusion of night duty, it is fair to conclude that the findings of Table 6 are conservative. In most hospitals the average waste of time would therefore be more than one-fifth of the student's total course.

THE SOLUTION: A PERMANENT STAFF

More than one-fifth of the student's time, then, is absorbed in duties unrelated to her training. That is, for a time amounting to 7 months and more of her nursing course she may fill the rôles, as we have seen, of cleaning woman, maid, cook, waitress, laundress, messenger, clerk, head nurse, and many others. For some two hours daily, or somewhat less at the 8-hour schools, her service is educationally profitless. She is frankly used "to get the work done."

Meantime the training school curriculum is complained of as overburdened; lectures and lessons, crowded in with long hours of ward duty, are offered to students too tired to take advantage of them. On the side of practical training the reaction is no less disastrous than on that of classroom instruction and study. Experience in important services is skimped or omitted, in order that a student may for a few weeks longer run the sterilizer, make supplies, wash vegetables, or cook for private patients. The situation is patently anomalous.

There is but one way out of this *impasse*, one solution of the problem, as urgent as it is obvious: the development of a permanent staff, which by assuming the burden of non-educational, non-nursing duties, shall release the time of the student nurse for her real business as a student, her professional education.

"The hospital nursing organizations of the future," said the director of a prominent hospital in a recent discussion of nursing education, "cannot and should not be wholly or mainly an organization of pupils in training. On the contrary, there should be a permanent staff of paid workers—trained nurses and others. . . . It is obvious that the needs of the hospital must be met, for the sick cannot be neglected; but it by no means follows that pupil nurses must be sacrificed to this end." [47]

Employment of Graduate Nurses

To enable student nurses to complete training within the minimum time needed for their education, undoubtedly more graduate nurses will be needed not only for administrative work as head nurses, but for the care of acute sickness. With the reduction of the three-years' course to two hospital years following four months of preliminary training, as later suggested in this report, young graduates who desire additional time in special branches, such as operating room service, work with children, communicable diseases, etc., will be more available than ever before.

Employment of Other Paid Workers

Besides these graduates, a permanent force of other paid workers must be provided, if the students' educational interests are to be safeguarded, larger or smaller according to the requirements of the hospital, and consisting of such assistant workers as cleaners, ward helpers, maids, attendants, orderlies, and clerks.

The effect of having permanent employees is strikingly illustrated at a well-known hospital already described (page 355). Here the daily waste of student time on the women's medical and surgical wards mounts up to an average of 3½ hours. On the corresponding male wards the waste of time in the same services comes only on the average to 1½ hours per student. What accounts for this extraordinary difference? The fact, simply, that the male wards have an orderly service. On each of these wards two orderlies give the minor nursing care and do

[47] Publicity and Progress in Nursing Education. S. S. Goldwater, M.D., Director, Mt. Sinai Hospital, New York. The Modern Hospital, February, 1921. Page 106.

the non-nursing work which might equally well in the women's wards be performed by paid attendants, maids, or cleaners. In the absence of these, 2 extra hours of the student's time are educationally wasted.

Another case in point is offered by the night service at one of our foremost eastern hospitals. On the men's medical ward the student on duty spent about 2½ hours on non-educational work; on the women's surgical ward two students spent respectively 4 hours and 6 minutes and 4½ hours on non-nursing duties. Once more the contrast is explained by the employment of orderlies on the male wards.

Status of the Movement: Municipal Hospitals

Let us see how far educational waste has been reduced among the 23 hospitals of our special study. The establishment of a permanent staff has in general gone furthest at the municipal hospitals, where it has been brought about as a deliberate hospital policy, chiefly because the greater shortage of nurses at many of these hospitals has made it imperative to conserve all possible student time for the execution of genuine nursing duties. Unfortunately this does not imply the release of student time for education; as pointed out in earlier sections, unnecessary repetition of nursing care, while better than maid service, becomes profitless routine. In only one of the 4 city hospitals studied, however, has the lay service effectively replaced student duty in manual and household work.

Here, according to our observer, "an outstanding feature of the training is the elimination of the really non-nursing duties." This is made possible in part by the employment of regular paid help, but in the main by the large amount of service furnished by chronic or convalescent patients, by men and women committed by the courts, or sometimes by ex-patients incapable of regular work who are kept on at a low wage by the hospital. In the maternity department, "waiting patients" supply all needed labor for housekeeping duties. By all these means the student is almost wholly relieved throughout the hospital of sweeping, dusting, cleaning, meal service, care of the linen room, care of soiled linen, and many other tasks of no value for training. In planning to reorganize this supplementary service on a more purely commercial basis, the minimum amount of help considered necessary by the authorities was two maids per women's ward and one man and one orderly per men's wards.

At another large city hospital, the management's policy provides liberally for a permanent staff, consisting for every ward of the following lay assistants:

1 ward helper ....for cleaning, sweeping, dusting, care of lavatory, etc.

1 ward maid .....for pantry work.

1 cleaner ....for general cleaning, two or three times weekly.

Transfer porters...as needed, to take patients to and from x-ray room, operating room, etc.

(2 male nurses on each male ward.)

In point of fact, the success of this plan was frustrated during the year of our study by the failure to secure sufficient women as ward helpers; the few in the service must be sent from ward to ward and the bulk of their work still fell on the students.

Improper Use of Attendants

In some instances attendants are used to perform duties for which they are not fitted. The employment of these workers must be carefully regulated if the patients, on the one hand, are to be safeguarded from inexpert care, and the students, on the other hand, are to have the benefit of all opportunities for essential training.

At one of the city hospitals of our group, in the children's department, for example, an attendant was in charge of a 6-bed ward, and responsible for the entire nursing care of 6 children, more or less acutely ill. An attendant in the surgical dressing room was assisting the doctor in making a lumbar puncture, while two third-year students on the same floor, losing this opportunity for practice in a rather infrequent procedure, were engaged in giving routine morning care. At this hospital, moreover, the responsibility for diets, even weighed diets, including their charting, is carried by attendants. The impropriety, to say nothing of the danger, of letting such duties pass into untrained hands needs no comment.

While such misdirection of the permanent staff must be condemned, the use of attendants at this hospital for minor nursing duties, such as waiting on patients, giving baths, shampoos, etc., is thoroughly commendable, as is the assignment to them of errands, and the relief of students by maids in the routine meal service.

Private Hospitals

In another hospital of our group connected with a university where student training is definitely influenced by academic standards, lay help for housekeeping duties is extensively employed. In private hospitals, on the other hand, the employment of a permanent staff has made comparatively little headway. Aside from the provision for heavy cleaning made at practically all hospitals, such a staff is established in few instances through the wards. Two private hospitals in the group of our study and one special hospital employ a certain amount of paid assistance on the wards. Five others provide some form of attendant service in certain departments.

Use of Paid Help on the Wards

At one of the private general hospitals of our study, the partial introduction of lay help on the wards has had excellent results. Here attendants are employed for an 8-hour day to relieve the students of housekeeping duties on private floors where, as is well known, the waste of student time is generally heavy. They are responsible for dusting, care of flowers, answering the telephone, and for most of the meal service, and in free hours for making surgical supplies. For 4 months of the year, during the vacation period, attendants are likewise employed on the general wards to supplement the student staff, but the superintendent fears to prolong such a service throughout the year lest the probationer should not obtain sufficient practice in hospital housekeeping.

At a smaller hospital, high school girls are employed as "nurse helpers" on the wards during the afternoons in various accessory services.

Use of Paid Help in Special Services or Duties
Economy of Student Time

At other hospitals permanent employees are found in certain special services where the pressure of routine work is heaviest, though not on the wards.

Thus in the main operating room of a distinguished hospital, a 16-year-old colored girl now does all the routine cleaning of instruments which used to demand from 5 to 6 hours of student time. At 4 other hospitals a woman is employed to clean instruments; in one case she also relieves students from one of the most wearisome tasks of the service—the mending of rubber gloves; in another, she assists in making surgical supplies; in still another, two attendants clean utensils as well as instruments and fold and put away linen into the bargain.

In the surgical supply room, a special stronghold of waste time, there are signs too of a breach in the traditional use of students for routine service. Three hospitals at least of our special group employ one or more paid helpers here in addition to student labor in making supplies. In one the students are released from the work altogether. In another probationers are said to be given a little experience in making dressings so as to become familiar with them, while no work of the kind is done by advanced students. At a school where, of the 8-weeks' duty in the surgical supply room, 7 weeks is estimated by our observer to be waste time, an entering wedge may be noted in the fact that the gauze, formerly all pulled by the probationers, is now pulled by a single young colored girl.

One or two hospitals make provision for taking off the students' hands the time-consuming and educationally profitless job of sterilizing. At one of them an orderly does all sterilizing of ward and operating room supplies; at another a like attendant is responsible for sterilizing all dressings in the operating room.

An example of another great economy of student time is the employment in one municipal hospital of a so-called "linen man" for the entire plant. This man collects and counts soiled linen from all wards, and on the basis of his report to the head nurse the proper amount of fresh linen for each ward is ordered from the central linen room.

Efficiency and Economy Combined

Such concentration of work traditionally done by students in the hands of a paid employee often serves the ends of efficiency as well as economy. A striking case in point is the accepted assignment as routine of the duty of washing or rinsing out soiled linen on different wards where such service is needed. Conveniences for the purpose are often primitive or inadequate, as in one instance where the only available place to do such washing was the slop hopper in which the bedpans were emptied. In contrast with such very casual and primitive methods is the efficient system adopted at many hospitals by which a paid and usually well-paid employee, in a separate room assigned for the purpose, washes out all stained linen before it is sent to the laundry.

Finally, one of the most glaring instances of the need of replacing student or nurse service by regular paid assistance is in the matter of clerical help in the various departments and especially in the training school offices. No comment on existing conditions could be more revealing than the difficulty experienced in the course of this study in obtaining precise information for the present report. In spite of every desire on the part of the schools to facilitate our work, the data, whether about curricula or records of practical experience, in almost every instance showed every mark of having been compiled by an already overburdened office staff, so that repeated verification of almost every detail was needed to insure their trustworthiness. The employment of efficient clerical assistance would not only release a large amount of nurse and student time but would revolutionize the record keeping of the training schools.

No better proof could be given of the value of such a change than the unique efficiency of service developed in the training school office of one of our municipal hospitals. Here the number of nurses employed in the office is reduced to a minimum and their places are taken by a trained lay staff consisting of bookkeeper, office clerk, stenographer, and information desk clerk. The employment of this paid and trained assistance instead of the amateurish record keeping of persons unused to office methods not only insures accuracy of detail but makes it possible to have needed information summarized and ready for reference at any time in the planning of assignments, classes, or lectures.

COST OF A PERMANENT STAFF

From the foregoing examples, it is evident that the employment of a permanent staff for the non-nursing duties of the hospital is already an existing system, a policy established by many managements, yielding excellent results and needing only extension and right development to insure the release of a considerable fraction of student time for the demands of genuine training. It should indeed be borne in mind that the movement towards the employment of permanent employees, well advanced in a few hospitals, but in its infancy or not yet begun in more, is beset by practical difficulties and must everywhere fight its way against the fear of expense. Yet this expense must be frankly faced if the training school is to make good its undertaking as an educational institution.

The establishment and steady increase of a permanent staff, initiated by war conditions and the shortage of students, is not to be turned backward. At the prominent hospital where hours of student time once spent in pulling gauze and cleaning instruments have been released by the employment of young colored maids, it is not likely that this educational waste will again be tolerated. The city hospital which wisely relieves the students on operating room duty by the use of graduates for all work after regular hours will not go back to the reckless overtime demanded of students for emergency service in some other hospitals. Nor will the time-consuming tasks of making supplies, mending gloves, running the sterilizer, and answering telephones, when once, as at some hospitals, they have been given over to paid helpers, be allowed again to encroach upon student training. These replacements of student service will suggest and indeed enforce other substitutions not less practicable and urgent.

A Fixed Charge on the Training School

One of the fixed charges upon any training school, which hospital boards and the public must alike learn to reckon with, should be the employment of a sufficient permanent staff to release student time from non-educational duties to study and instruction. It will be a short-sighted economy to set this charge too low. During the war and immediately afterwards, the dearth of domestic help was undoubtedly great, owing largely to the competition of high-paying industries. Yet, aside from this special shortage, the difficulty so often complained of by the hospitals of getting trustworthy and sufficient paid service has been largely, as a glance at their wage schedules will show, a matter of wages so low as to make it impossible for them to compete in the open market for the better grades of help. The permanent service in the hospital must clearly be put on a financial basis equal at least to that of domestic service, if it is to give the satisfaction of which it is capable.

"Hospital wages before the war," writes the eminent hospital authority already quoted in favor of the permanent staff, "were far below those prevailing in industry and domestic service. . . . The wage scale that prevailed in most hospitals before the war was morally indefensible. It is to be hoped that instead of attempting to follow in the footsteps of industrial enterprises that have recently reduced wages, hospitals will make an effort to maintain, as a rule, the wage scale established during the war. In order to do this, hospitals must of course have the moral and financial support of the community. Let us hope that this support will be ungrudgingly given when the actual conditions are understood." [48]

It is to the hope of enlisting this support as well as the more active interest of hospital boards in establishing the permanent staff that the present section is addressed.

9. Theoretical Instruction

Having now completed our review of the student's practical training and of some of the problems incident thereto, we turn next to the theoretical instruction which is to interpret for her the cases and conditions which she encounters. We have already covered the teaching of the basic sciences and of the theory and practice of nursing. In order to discuss in a brief compass the remaining contents of the curricula, and the methods of teaching which were observed by our investigators, it is obviously necessary to group under some general heads the various subjects composing the course of study. Without attempting to lay down any dogmatic classification of subjects, we have for this purpose roughly divided them under three general heads, that is, the different forms of disease and their treatment; social aspects of disease and its prevention; general nursing subjects dealing with ideals in work and their background.

DIFFERENT FORMS OF DISEASE AND THEIR TREATMENT

THE PHYSICIAN-INSTRUCTOR

Almost without exception in the hospitals studied, instruction in the different forms of disease and their treatment—medical, surgical, obstetrical, etc.—is given by physicians, either those of the regular hospital staff, outside specialists, or professors in affiliated medical schools. [49]

[48] Hospital Administration in 1920. S. S. Goldwater, M.D., Director, Mt. Sinai Hospital, New York. The Modern Hospital, March, 1921. Page 220.
[49] Two cases only are exceptions to this custom: one class in pediatrics, of seven reported, which is taught by the resident theoretical instructor, a woman; and the only course in anæsthesia reported, which is taught by the hospital anæsthetist, a woman graduate nurse.

The advantages of this plan of instruction by physicians present themselves obviously. If the right physicians are available, the student has the inspiration of contact with men and women of high training who speak with an authority that comes from wide experience in their chosen calling. Individuals of a quality to have achieved distinction in their special lines of work are likely, moreover, to be of convincing personality and to have developed a large capacity for human understanding. The opportunity of classroom association with professional men and women of this sort cannot fail to be stimulating and to give to the student a larger vision of her work.

The importance of care in the choice of the physician lecturer cannot, however, be too strongly emphasized. Unfortunately, eminence as a surgeon or physician does not necessarily insure pedagogical skill. That the two are as a matter of fact frequently found together is happily proved by the observation of numerous classes taught by physicians, whose method has been found generally excellent in choice of subject matter and in clearness and effectiveness of presentation, and whose personality has been such as to inspire respect and hold the intelligent interest of the class. A sincere devotion to the interests of the nurses characterizes most of these men and women, who as a class are pressed by many other urgent demands on their care and thought. To them a debt of gratitude is due from all those who have nursing education at heart.

But lamentable exceptions to this rule have been noted. Men little suited to the work are occasionally found holding appointments. One superintendent of nurses thinks that, since the policy has been adopted in her hospital of paying staff physicians for their services, those holding certain positions have been appointed without sufficient regard for their teaching ability. On the other hand, the superintendent of nurses in a hospital associated with a medical school of high standing said that a certain physician lecturing with great brilliancy was the only head of a department who had been invited to lecture to the nurses, since in her judgment the others were not good teachers.

That this wise discrimination is not always exercised was evident in another training school, where a course in nervous and mental diseases is conducted by a specialist of standing. A lecture on general paresis took the form of a "rambling, unconstructed talk without outline." The lecturer's method of presentation was miserable, "his voice indistinct and low, dropping into an inaudible monotone after the first three or four words of every sentence." His style was "utterly lacking in vigor and clearness," and he used a "highly technical vocabulary entirely over the heads of the class." No wonder that the observer comments: "One-third of the class was asleep. Most of the others seemed to be thinking of other things."

A serious disadvantage which in some measure offsets the privilege of depending for class work on physicians with pressing outside interests is the laxity they sometimes show in being prompt and regular for their appointments. Some complaint on this score is made in certain hospitals, and the custom of paying physicians for their teaching services is doubtless an attempt to increase their sense of obligation to the school as well as to remunerate them. Failure of the physician to keep his appointments regularly works great inconvenience to the students, who have no leeway of time for their engagements, and also seriously affects their *morale*. It is of the utmost importance that physicians in assuming teaching responsibilities should recognize the necessity for strict adherence to the class schedule, and deference on the part of the school authorities to their professional standing should not excuse laxity on their part in the keeping of definite engagements.

FAILURE TO STRESS PREVENTION OF DISEASE

Broadly speaking, the chief weakness of the physician-instructor is his stress upon curative medicine to the detriment or total ignoring of preventive medicine. Even in the care of children, where today the prevention of sickness through proper feeding, hygiene, and the creation of right habits is beginning to make headway, the teaching of the nurse still remains almost wholly instruction in the diseases of childhood.

This limitation, typical of her whole curriculum, is one of the most serious handicaps in the training of the nurse. For nurses, pre-eminently those in public health work, are to be engaged primarily in the prevention of sickness; nay more, they are to have the more difficult office of *teaching* the prevention of sickness in people's homes. This is, as we have seen, their special function. It is therefore of the first importance that they should be equipped not only to recognize symptoms of disease and learn methods of cure, but that they should be more fundamentally equipped to recognize symptoms and conditions antecedent to disease and learn the means of combating these before disease appears. It is, then, surely an anomaly that their training should deal so largely with cure alone.

Curative medicine has, however, until recently so wholly taken precedence over prevention that it is perhaps unreasonable to expect of the physician-instructor an emphasis scarcely yet found in medical practice, new indeed even to the medical school, and almost wholly lacking in the organization of the nurse's course. Yet this new emphasis on something greater than pill and bottle, this stress upon the now well-established principles of hygiene and prevention is perhaps the cardinal need in the nurse's didactic instruction. This means not a single course in preventive medicine but instruction throughout the curriculum from the standpoint of advanced medical science, including for instance in pediatrics the feeding of the well child, and the normal hygiene of childhood; including in obstetrics instruction in prenatal care; including in communicable disease instruction in the wide principles of hygienic living which alone of therapeutic measures can successfully combat tuberculosis, and the like.

METHODS OF TEACHING

Correlation with Ward Training

The physician, to be successful in the teaching of nurses, must bear in mind the special object of such instruction. He must realize that it differs essentially from that given to medical students in needing stress pre-eminently on the significance and meaning of symptoms manifesting themselves in the patient. A nurse must be taught, above all else, what to look for, both in recognizing symptoms of disease, and in noting the effect of a given treatment. It is, therefore, clearly essential to have the classroom instruction closely connected with the observation of ward cases. This may be accomplished through co-operation of the head nurses, by whom appropriate cases can be pointed out to students during their ward service. The intelligent co-operation of these head nurses is furthered by the practice found in some hospitals of having them attend the lectures covering their particular branches, thus enabling them to keep track of their subject matter, or of having the outline of lectures posted so that they may know each week which cases in their charge are of timely interest to the students on their wards.

This practice has been introduced, for instance, at a prominent New England training school, which states in its last report:

"This year the graduates in charge of the medical wards are attending the lectures and clinics and conducting the quizzes on medical nursing; the graduate in charge of the children's department is doing the same with the teaching of pediatric nursing. This means that the nurse who is in daily contact with medical patients is teaching medical nursing, and the graduate in daily contact with sick children is teaching the care of sick children. This scheme also emphasizes the dual responsibility of the head nurse,—that of teacher as well as of administrator." [50]

A close correlation between class instruction by the physician and the student's ward experience is also in some places assured by the custom of having the topical outline of the physician's course, with the time assigned to each subject, made out by the resident instructor in charge of the student's practical work. Physicians are said to like this plan where it is put into practice, as it is difficult for them without knowledge of the student's ward duties to co-ordinate their lectures with the practical training.

The Bedside Clinic

But the correlation of class instruction with the study of ward cases is best accomplished when the course is conducted by the physician in the form of "rounds" or bedside clinics, in which the students have the opportunity of having the subject of the lesson actually demonstrated at the bedside of the patients. Unfortunately, the system of ward clinics is found as yet in only a few hospitals. It is in successful operation for the courses in medical and surgical diseases in one of the country's most famous training schools, where a class in medical diseases was observed. In this round, cases had as usual been chosen beforehand and were presented in sequence to fit the talk. The physician led the group from bed to bed for discussion of the cases. Students were asked to comment on the patient and to answer and ask questions. Each case was discussed simply, with some exposition of history and symptoms, in addition to those which could be observed, treatment, and, in some cases, the probable outcome. Additional opportunity for questions is given in the quiz hour held by the theoretical instructor on the day following each round, and advanced nursing demonstrations are held contemporaneously in the course of practical nursing.

[50] Massachusetts General Hospital. Extract of Graduation Report, January, 1921.

Admirable as was the teaching in this ward clinic, the course in question is to some extent handicapped by the lack of classroom work supplementing the ward demonstration. The need of lectures relating the special cases studied to a wider range of material than can be given at the bedside is obvious. The eminent success of the laboratory method in the rounds seems to have obscured here the essential desirability of classroom instruction in furnishing background and weaving the special case or experience into the general fabric of the theory of disease. The course in surgical diseases given at the same training school is more ideally planned in that it consists of lectures and rounds in alternation. The distinction of this clinic teaching and the eminence of the school throws into all the sharper relief the disparity of the time allowed with the importance of the subjects treated. Thus the course in medicine consists but of 10 rounds; the course in surgery of 10 rounds and 5 lectures! Each course is supplemented indeed by quizzes conducted by the theoretical instructor, 10 in the medical and 5 in the surgical course; but these reviews, while making the most of the actual instruction, cannot change the deplorable scantiness of its amount.

At another large and distinguished general hospital clinic teaching by a physician-instructor is also in successful operation. Here the desirability of supplementing the bedside demonstration by some more formal presentation has been better met. In the study of surgical diseases, 16 bedside clinics are supplemented by 32 classroom lectures, and 16 oral quizzes by the theoretical instructor. In the study of medical diseases there are 8 bedside clinics, 16 lectures, and 16 quizzes.

In another training school, where classroom demonstration and an occasional ward clinic is provided, the value of the work is greatly lessened by the fact that no preparation is required of the student and no opportunity is given to ask questions at either demonstration or clinic.

The Use of Quizzes

A strong reinforcement to the instruction given by physicians, either in lecture room or clinic, is the separate quiz hour which in many hospitals is conducted by a nurse-instructor. Twenty-four such quiz classes are reported in connection with 48 classes held by physicians. In 20 cases these review quizzes are held by the theoretical instructor of the training school; in the remaining 4 by head nurses acting as assistant instructors.

The advantage of this system of quizzes is that it gives opportunity for fuller review and explanation than could be offered in the time given by busy visiting physicians, and further, that it assures that the material shall be emphasized and amplified from the point of view of the nurse. It is in these classes, also, that much of the correlation with ward cases can be advantageously demonstrated and advanced nursing procedures taught or reviewed coincidently with the lectures on various diseases.

We have already spoken, in connection with the ward clinics described, of the supplementary quizzes conducted by the theoretical instructor at a well-known training school. In another school allied with a university, the correlation between class instruction and ward experience has been developed with great success by means of quiz classes in charge of the head nurses in the various departments.

These classes correspond in number to the lectures given by different doctors, who are specialists in their respective fields. In these classes the physician's lecture is reviewed and case reports from the wards are given by students and discussed by the instructor and the class. This system of case reports has been carefully worked out by the assistant superintendent of nurses, who feels very keenly the value of student participation, and who has spent much effort in training the younger head nurses to an understanding of the work. The head nurses at this hospital are selected for their teaching ability as well as for their other characteristics. Quiz classes are held in connection with the work in surgical diseases, medical diseases, pediatrics, obstetrics, and skin and venereal diseases, for which material for study comes mainly from the dispensary.

In the medical quiz class observed, notes on the recent lecture were read and questions answered. References were made to points in anatomy which might have been forgotten. Reports were made by students of certain cases with full discussion of history, symptoms, treatment, and present condition. The instructor added further explanation and brought out other points by questions. For one case an x-ray plate was shown and discussed briefly. One patient was brought in and the members of the class all had an opportunity to listen to his very pronounced heart murmur.

Similar procedure was observed in the class following the lecture on obstetrics. Two patients were brought in from the wards—one to demonstrate several points mentioned in the lecture; the other, who had been all but dead, to illustrate the effects of certain treatments. The draping needed for one of these treatments was demonstrated on the doll by a student. In this demonstration use was made of all hospital facilities, but students were told how to utilize makeshifts as might be necessary in home delivery and care.

In the surgical class there was a discussion and quiz on hemorrhage, following a recent lecture on the subject, with demonstrations of several procedures in the adjustment of different styles of tourniquets, the giving of a hypodermoclysis, and an intravenous injection. The students helped in demonstration and asked and answered many questions. On another day an interne did two types of dressing in demonstration before the class—one the removal of stitches from a gall bladder case 10 days after operation; the other, the dressing of a nephrectomy in which there was much pus, calling for the use of Dakin tubes. Both patients were brought to the classroom and the members of the class gathered where they could see best. The interne explained the cases briefly and the dressings were done just as usual, though more slowly to allow time for the class to see and ask questions.

The value of thus bringing together the physician's lecture, the student's study of cases on the wards, and the comments of the experienced nurse, was very marked in the opinion of our observer, herself a teacher of experience.

A similar use of the head nurse as instructor is seen in the pediatric service of another well-known hospital. Lectures given by physicians are accompanied by quiz and nursing classes conducted by the very able nurse in charge of the department. Students receive all their practical instruction in this branch of nursing while actually working among the children on the wards. Successive small groups of students are sent to the department and, following their entrance into the service, are met daily by the head nurse in half-hour appointments for a week for instruction in the simple procedures which they will need at once and in which methods necessarily differ from those in use in other departments. Lists are carefully kept of the procedures and treatments taught to each nurse, and she must show that she understands by being able to do in the presence of the instructor the things she has been taught. The more complex treatments are explained and illustrated later to larger groups.

The program of the nursing class is as follows: discussion and quiz on one or two preceding lectures, discussion of assigned brief reference in Holt, demonstration of treatments and condition of babies, with one written question occupying the last 5 minutes of the hour. The scope of this plan shows clearly the valuable contribution which the teaching head nurse can make.

Failure to Correlate with Ward Training

The rich opportunity for students just described is in shining contrast to that shown at a neighboring large hospital, where lectures in pediatrics are given by the resident nurse-instructor with practically no correlation with ward service. Some of the class have had experience in the department and some not. The lecture heard followed the textbook assignment with some amplification. Students were unprepared for quiz questions and seemed not to remember much about their previous work in medicine. There were few allusions to cases on the wards and the visitor felt doubtful whether the class got much more than from a perfunctory reading of the book. The hour is reported as being "poor as medicine and with little of real nursing in it."

Such a failure to take advantage of the concrete opportunities offered by ward service is unfortunately not an isolated instance. The value of close connection between the lecturer's work and the student's daily experience on the wards seems too self-evident to need stress, and yet any attempt to connect the two is conspicuously lacking in many hospitals. One very large municipal hospital, for instance, where the wards offer rich material for study, has a course in gynecology consisting entirely of formal lectures. The students take notes which are not inspected, and no quizzes are held. A lecture on ovarian tumors, which was given on the day of our visit by a woman specialist of high standing, was one of remarkable excellence. The subject was simply and effectively presented, and the talk was skilfully illustrated with diagrams and drawings made on the blackboard with colored chalks, and by descriptions of specific cases quoted from time to time. The students took no part in the lesson, but showed the keenest interest throughout. The detachment of the subject matter, however, from their own experience was complete, as the physician is not a member of the hospital staff, had no service in its wards and, therefore, in citing cases for illustration, could refer only to those in her own private practice. It is plain that much is lost to these students in not having, in connection with this theoretical presentation, an opportunity for close study and discussion of the cases in their own hospital, with which they have themselves come in contact.

Another large municipal hospital of high standing shows the same disregard for the correlation of class instruction with the study of ward cases. Medical, surgical, and other professional lectures are given without accompanying quiz classes, or other means of interpretation in terms of the students' experience. No demonstration of ward cases is planned to illustrate them and make them concretely intelligible.

This hospital has a surgical dressing room attached to the surgical wards, where all cases are taken for needed dressings. A whole section of a class could be taken to this room to see any dressings that might be useful as demonstrations, but as a matter of fact only the nurse on special dressing room duty gets whatever experience comes in her brief service in that department. The excellent facilities are not used for teaching at all.

PSYCHOLOGY

In addition to her instruction in nursing in the various forms of disease, the study of psychology as an aid in her approach to all disease is highly important for enlightened future work on the part of the student nurse. Both to aid her own adjustment to a new and difficult way of life, and to lend insight into the mental and nervous disturbances which accompany in one form or another so large a proportion of all illnesses, some psychological training is invaluable. A good grasp of the essentials of normal psychology is moreover a much needed introduction to the abnormalities of mental disease with which she is later to be brought in contact in her instruction in the nursing of nervous and mental cases. For the nurse's education in the patience, sympathy, and tact essential in meeting helpfully the apparently unreasonable demands, desires, and fears of nervous patients, so baffling to the layman, the value of this study can scarcely be over-estimated. Yet in only 9 of the 22 training schools whose curricula were studied is psychology a part of the curricula.

It is lacking in 3 out of 4 schools connected with municipal hospitals, where large groups of nurses are trained; also in the 4 largest of the private general hospitals, as well as in 6 smaller hospitals, where the omission of this subject might be more readily expected. Its omission is doubtless due to the fact that the results of such training are intangible and less obviously valuable for practical application; it is therefore a subject easily neglected in a curriculum already difficult to find time for. But the lack of psychological training is frequently evident in the students. For example, in one of the large municipal hospitals, where psychology is not taught at all, clinics for mental testing are held in connection with certain lectures on nervous and mental diseases. Obviously, as a background for such a course, some knowledge of normal as well as abnormal psychology is a prerequisite. On the day of our visit the questions put by the doctors to subjects in the clinics could have no significance for the students because of their lack of understanding of the simplest principles of psychology.

In another important training school the students themselves felt the lack of psychological equipment and asked that a course be given them. Such a course was arranged, and they were enthusiastic over a series of lectures being given at the time of our visit by a woman physician of the psychiatric department.

Another valuable course illuminating problems encountered by the nurse in the course of her work is given at a university school of nursing. The class meets in the regular psychology classroom and is conducted by the head of the department of psychology. On the day of our visit there was first a general discussion of the phenomenon of "multiple personality" and its causes, with illustrations drawn from the students' experience. The last half of the hour was given over to a demonstration of the application of psychology to backward and delinquent children. This part of the course was given by the director of the Juvenile Court psychopathic clinic, who brought as a "case" a boy of 8½ years, who took Binet and other tests before the class.

The course is one of the most popular at the school in question and individual nurses were all emphatic in pronouncing it one of the most helpful and illuminating they had ever had. The instructor on his part said that the nurses' constant dealing with "humans" made them quick to see connections and gave wide range for illustration.

TIME ALLOWED TO THE TEACHING OF DIFFERENT FORMS OF
DISEASE AND THEIR TREATMENT IN 22 SCHOOLS [51]

Time devoted in the 22 schools studied to instruction in the
different forms of disease and their treatment ranges from 137
to 324 hours. That the time allowances in the majority of the
schools tend toward the minimum rather than the maximum may
be seen by the average for all schools of 210. Most striking is
the relatively low time allowance assigned to the main body of
professional instruction by most of the training schools. According to the following table, half of the schools studied allowed
less than 200 hours.

DIFFERENT FORMS OF DISEASE AND THEIR TREATMENT

Number of Hours	Number of Schools
100-149	3
150-199	8
200-249	6
250-299	4
300-349	1
	22

SOCIAL ASPECTS OF DISEASE AND ITS PREVENTION

It is in connection with teaching the social aspects of disease,
and the social interpretation of medical problems, that our
recommendations will break away most sharply from existing
practice in the training of nurses.

Within recent years short periods of experience have been
offered to a limited number of students designed to give them
some insight and practical experience in the two comparatively
new fields of hospital social service and public health nursing.
Besides this, special series of lectures are usually given on
general social and health topics, sometimes related to one another
in a more or less integrated course, sometimes singly and wholly
unrelated to one another. In all of the 22 hospitals studied,
for instance, lectures were given on one or more of the three
subjects of social problems, public health, and sanitation, the
last being properly a part of public health but in training school
practice often treated as a separate and distinct subject.

[51] Including general medical diseases, pediatrics, communicable, venereal
and skin; general surgical diseases, gynecology, orthopedics, operating
room, eye, ear, nose, and throat; obstetrics; special branches; materia
medica, pathology, clinical analysis; mental and nervous diseases, psychology, occupational therapy.

Before describing briefly the instruction and experience of students in these general community subjects as at present conducted, it will be clarifying to state the fundamental reorganization which, in our opinion, is needed. Instead of attempting to teach in a basic course of training, to a comparatively small proportion of the senior class what should be graduate nursing specialities, the school of nursing should give to every student in classroom and ward that minimum of social interpretation and instruction in the social aspects and prevention of sickness which is indispensable in the modern treatment of disease. That this desideratum is not impossible, and that it can be accomplished without undue extension of the curriculum we shall seek to make plain in our subsequent discussion.

HOURS AND YEAR WHEN GIVEN

In the 22 schools of our group, the total number of teaching hours devoted to these subjects ranged from 7 to 90 hours, or if we exclude this isolated maximum, at a university school giving a 60-hour course in sociology, from 7 to 58 hours.

Lectures on public health are given in the senior year, in all but two cases, where they are placed in the second. Sanitation on the other hand, including such topics as water purification, sewage disposal, etc., is often given in a separate course, generally in the third year, but in some few cases in the second, the first, or even in the preliminary period. It is noteworthy, moreover, that the subject is sometimes treated in the elementary course on personal hygiene, given at many schools in the preliminary period. Social service lectures generally given in the student's third year, are also in several cases (3) given in the preliminary period, and the 60-hour course in sociology already mentioned is also given at this time as a background for the student's further social experience.

INSTRUCTORS

The teaching in these several groups of community problems is arranged for in whatever way local conditions make expedient. The success of the teaching, therefore, is peculiarly dependent on the personal qualifications of lecturers available for the work. In some instances, lectures in sanitation, as almost always those in hygiene, are in charge of the resident nurse-instructor; and short periods of training in social service are in several hospitals under the head workers in charge of the hospital social service work. But the general lectures are usually given by persons connected with outside social agencies—social service workers, probation officers, public health directors, clergymen, etc. In some cases the lectures are given outside the hospital and are attended jointly with other nursing schools.

Among the lectures heard by our investigator were several of genuinely stimulating and enlightening quality. One such was on the modern development of mental hygiene and the value of this knowledge in the equipment of the public health nurse or social worker. The history of the movement, with its vast attendant change in the attitude of physicians and society towards the mental patient, the work of the State Society for Mental Hygiene, and the aid which such an agency stands ready to give, the restoration to normal of patients who would formerly have been committed to institutions for life, were all made vivid by abundant illustrative material, and closely connected with the nurse's field of work and probable personal experience.

Another enlightening lecture—one of a series on the work of the juvenile court—dealt with the functions of the probation officer and was given by the chief probation officer of the court. The problems with which the probation officer comes in contact were discussed in their relation to the public health nurse, and with emphasis on certain physical causes of delinquency as a subject with which nurses are particularly concerned.

Aside from the fact that the lecture was interesting and informative in itself, two things were noticeable in its preparation: it was evident that the lecturer had consulted closely with the director of the social service department in adapting his material to the nurses' needs; and that he had taken care not to encroach on phases of the subject which presumably would be dealt with by other lecturers in the course. Such a carefully adapted lecture suggests how the co-operation of the lecturer with an able director may synthesize and unify a course given by a series of different speakers.

There is, of course, great danger in these outside courses that even able lecturers, who are unfamiliar or unconcerned with hospital training, may fail to make their talks directly applicable to the special needs of nurses. For instance, one lecture by a clergyman of standing on the social service work of the church was a sufficiently interesting and eloquent presentation of the need for reform in certain social conditions,—race relationship, sex hygiene, child welfare, etc. But as the speaker gave no concrete facts on the work of the churches nor any suggestions as to the nurse's possible rôle in these reforms, the lecture was of insignificant value as a contribution to practical training.

TRAINING IN PUBLIC HEALTH NURSING IN 22 SCHOOLS

In addition to the lecture courses described, training in public health nursing is offered in 15 schools. Eleven schools offer the course as an elective to a limited number of students ranging from 5 per cent to 50 per cent of the senior class. Two university schools offer public health nursing to all senior students. Two small schools with clinical and teaching facilities too limited to offer a good basic training, by a mistaken policy *require* students to take the course in public health nursing. In all, the training is available for about one-quarter or 27 per cent (179) of the total number of students (665) enrolled in the senior classes for 1919-1920 in the 22 schools of our study.

Seven schools offer no training at all in this subject.

The length of the time allotted ranges from 1½ months to 4 months in the different schools, with the single exception of one school which offers to two students a combined course of 8 months in public health nursing and social service.

Disadvantages of Undergraduate Training

The quality of the practical training received at the various hospitals in this branch of nursing depends on local conditions, as it is necessary in most instances to make arrangements with some outside agency doing public health nursing, such as visiting nurse associations, infant welfare societies, etc. Through these agencies the students receive their instruction in the field.

The objections to this arrangement are in our opinion twofold: the lack in many instances of adequate teaching and supervision in the field and the wholly inadequate time which can, under the best circumstances, be allotted to this subject during a basic undergraduate course of 2 years and 4 months.

Lack of Teaching and Supervision

Our study of modern public health nursing as it has developed and achieved its best results in the United States has made it clear that for this new profession for women, with its manifold demands on skill in nursing and teaching, its dependence on adequate social training and case work with persons of many different nationalities and racial customs, a special professional training is requisite.

In our subsequent study of special schools or courses for public health nursing, the essentials of training both theoretical and practical are discussed at length. Here it suffices to point out that no more than in the hospital can students in the field "pick up" the necessary technique. They must be taught and supervised. Yet in many instances busy staff nurses of public health nursing organizations to which the students are sent for instruction have neither time nor equipment to teach. The weakness inherent in the relation between training school and hospital may easily be duplicated in these courses; they may easily be conducted merely as an apprenticeship, for the convenience of the organization in question, without an ordered educational program.

Inadequate Time

Even when training schools are able to make connections with public health nursing agencies genuinely equipped for teaching and capable of giving students the expert direction which is the *sine qua non* of an honest educational enterprise, the time allowed for such training in any undergraduate curriculum is wholly insufficient. Even in the superior schools of our study the length of the training ranged from only 1½ to 4 months.

In view of the recency of any special training for public health nursing and the successful work of many nurses in the field who have learned only by experience, by the method of trial and error, it is sometimes urged that any training is better than none. But this is clearly no defense from the educational point of view. The slightness of the professional value of some of these undergraduate courses is indicated by the fact that in at least one of the best schools of public health nursing the 2 months of training given to undergraduate nurses are not even credited towards the school's diploma.

Undoubtedly some of the longer 4-months' courses to which undergraduates are admitted do afford them a short practical experience of stimulating value, with a certain amount of concurrent theoretical instruction. But educational authorities agree that for a properly balanced program a full academic year of 8 to 9 months is indispensable. The 4 months' courses still being given are regarded as emergency measures to meet the unprecedented demand for public health nurses which should be superseded as soon as possible by the full course.

The short undergraduate training in public health nursing is sometimes further defended as at best an introduction to a new field. But too often it proves difficult or impossible for the student to supplement this initial experience; and considering herself sufficiently prepared by this small experience, she is misled into joining the number of ill-equipped public health nurses who later obtain their training, if at all, at the expense of the families and communities which they are serving.

One and one-half to 4 months' training in public health nursing has no logical or legitimate place in a basic training course of 2 years and 4 months and should be replaced by a new stress on prevention and health teaching in the training of all students, both on the wards and in the dispensary assignments.

In our proposed curriculum, instead of inadequate field work for a fraction of the senior class, adequate class instruction for all students with visits of observation in the field under competent direction is recommended under the inclusive title of the Social Aspects of Disease and Its Prevention. We shall consider somewhat further the scope of such a course after outlining the present undergraduate training in hospital social service.

TRAINING IN HOSPITAL SOCIAL SERVICE IN 22 SCHOOLS

Of the 22 schools of our study, 9 schools offer some experience in hospital social service. Six schools offer it to a limited number of students, ranging from 9 per cent to 45 per cent of the senior class. One school offers it as an elective for all students. In 2 schools it is a required course. Thirteen schools offer no courses at all in the subject.

In all, the service is available, by the most liberal estimate, for about one-third (218), or 32 per cent, of the total number of students (665) enrolled in the senior classes for 1919-1920 in the 22 schools of our study. The length of time allotted ranges from 2 weeks to 4 months.

The conclusion that under present conditions experience in this service is entirely lacking to a large majority of each year's graduating nurses is corroborated by the findings of an investigation made by a Committee on Hospital Social Service, appointed in 1920 by the American Hospital Association.[52] This

° Report of the Field Secretary on the Survey of Hospital Social Service. Hospital Social Service, January, 1921. Page 35. Supplemented by information from the Secretary.

investigation covered 61 hospitals, 39 of which had training schools connected with them.   In 7 of these the social service department was so little developed that it would have been of no advantage to nurses to serve in it; but in the 32 remaining, conditions were favorable for student training.   Nevertheless experience was found to be offered in but 12 [53] of the 32 hospitals, and in only 2 was it available for all.

The survey of this Committee showed that of the 3,000 non-proprietary hospitals of the country, about one in ten has a social service department.   The primary function of hospital social service, as defined by the Committee, is case-work with individual patients.   This case-work should afford the relevant medical and social facts needed for the diagnosis of the disease or social problem involved and for making a program of treatment.   It should also assist in carrying out the treatment.   Among the primary duties of social service in hospital or dispensary the following are singled out for mention: reporting to the physician facts regarding the patient's personality or environment which relate to his physical condition; arranging for supplementary medical care or diagnosis when suggested by the physician; overcoming obstacles to treatment, such as lack of medical supplies, clothing, food, and improper environment or employment; influencing the patient to co-operate with the doctor's program.

A second function of hospital social service is the performance of certain administrative activities within the institution in which social relations are important, such as the admission of patients to hospital or dispensary; interpreting for foreign-speaking patients; aiding in the management of clinics; furnishing information on medical resources to individuals or social agencies for cases which cannot be admitted to hospital or dispensary, etc.; performing friendly services such as escorting patients or arranging for transportation.

The Committee on Hospital Social Service found that work carried on by social service departments was largely unstandardized, including in its scope a wide range of activities.   Almost 100 diverse activities were found in operation, from buying railroad tickets for patients to educating colored orphans.

Hospital social service is clearly itself in process of experiment and definition.   A second committee of the American Hospital Association appointed in 1921 to report on the training of hospital social workers says:

[*] Of these 12 hospitals 6 are among those also studied by this committee.

"Social work as a whole, and hospital social work especially, is yet young and undeveloped; it has as yet no universally accepted and applied standards."

The committee then expands the definition of hospital social work cited above to emphasize the central importance of its social aspects and continues:

"To summarize, hospital social work is the application to the uses of a medical institution of a method of adjustment of environmental relationships, which is being developed in the field of social work. Its purpose is to contribute to improvement of individual and public health through study of and influence upon social behaviour. Through study of the patient's experience, social work should aid in medical diagnosis; through teaching and through changes made in home and work, it should aid in medical treatment; and it should help the administration of the hospital through a special knowledge of neighborhood characteristics, needs, and resources. The specialization of the social functions of the hospital should make possible research into the social elements of physical and mental health."

More important than the number of students admitted to social service departments is the type and quality of the experience at present available. Training for hospital social work has hitherto received some attention in the schools of social work in New York, Boston, Philadelphia, Chicago, etc., as well as in the social service departments of hospitals. So far as nurses are concerned, they have naturally, for the most part, received their experience as undergraduates in hospitals, and before proceeding further we may briefly describe some examples of the best services that the hospital system has to offer.

Some Examples of Present Training

Of the 11 hospitals of our study giving social service periods to students, 2 or 3 offer an experience valuable enough to be worth quoting in some detail. Unfortunately, the excellent opportunities offered by these courses are open only to a handful of students.

Thus, at a well-known special hospital with a highly organized social service department, but one student at a time is admitted to an elective course of 3 months. The training is therefore available to only four students a year.

The course here opens with an introductory survey under the head of the department, which includes the relation of social service to the several departments of the hospital, a study of its organization throughout the wards and in the dispensary, an introduction to office technique emphasizing the use of social and medical records, and a discussion of the common social situations which block effectual medical treatment.

After this introduction the student begins on the practical case work offered both in the medical and surgical wards and in the medical and surgical clinics of the out-patient department. The work in the wards and clinics includes the study of types of cases handled and the practical handling, under guidance, of new cases assigned. In connection with this case practice the student makes special visits to other institutions and attends weekly case and policy conferences of the staff, special conferences with the head of the department, and the medical teaching clinics. Reference readings are also assigned.

Of the many problems presenting themselves we may cite some typical cases chosen as specially educational in student training: cases involving public health problems, such as tuberculosis or syphilis; long range cases involving correspondence with local social or medical agencies; cases unknown to other agencies involving original investigation; foreign families, especially non-English-speaking and needing an interpreter; cases in which other members of the family need treatment for related or unrelated difficulty; cases of broken family with problem of public or private aid; cases needing school arrangement; cases involving mental defect besides crippled condition.

Besides the practice in adjusting under supervision such new cases as these, one or two visits are made with the worker on cases of long standing showing results of treatment in similar or contrasting situations to those which the student is handling. Stress is laid throughout the period of service on conferences with the student, consulting about and discussing cases under the student's care, and on visits to other agencies likely to be called upon for co-operation.

Similar training is given in a large private general hospital where the social service department is very highly developed. Here also this valuable experience is available for only four students each year—between 1.5 per cent and 2 per cent of the entire senior class.

The course is planned to give the student an introductory

bird's-eye view of the out-patient department and of the social service organization throughout the hospital. With the history of its origin, growth, and purpose, a study is made of the work of the various agencies which social workers need to connect with, and the best methods of making such contacts as are necessary. Throughout the course, use of the library is encouraged, certain reference readings are required, visits are made to various co-operating institutions, and the student is assigned a definite number of cases to care for under the guidance of an experienced social worker. Two months of the training time are spent in district case work in connection with out-patient clinics, one month on cases in the hospital wards.

In addition to this course, 8 lectures given to probationers by the head of the social service department are planned to interpret the social aspects of the hospital, the community from which the patient comes, and the service the department is prepared to render. In connection with these lectures probationers are taken in groups to factories, a tuberculosis sanitarium, and other places of social interest.

Need of Special Postgraduate Training

Such, then, are some examples of experience in social service as conducted at present. It must at once be evident that certain aspects of this training, especially the new accent on the background, home conditions, and social welfare of the patient, are factors which must profoundly modify the student's whole approach to her work. It is this new accent on the social and preventable aspects of disease that we seek to make available, in the course of their ward and dispensary service, to all students, instead of confining such instruction, so far as it is given, to the fraction of the senior class admitted to the hospital social service department or the public health course.

As preparation for the special field of hospital social work such a brief undergraduate term in the social service department is plainly insufficient. Neither in allotment of time nor in amount or quality of teaching, nor in the usual preliminary equipment of the students can it approximate to the needs of this service, whose future, in the opinion of the Committee on Training of Hospital Social Workers, "depends largely on the judgment, imagination and initiative of those who enter its field now," requiring persons able to do more than routine work, who are mature and capable of leadership. The Committee accordingly unites in recommending a special training course of 2 years, and as preliminary education for entrance it recommends 3 years of study after graduation from high school, allowing thus for college work, nurse's training, or other systematic education.[54]

NEED OF GENERAL SOCIAL INTERPRETATION FOR ALL STUDENTS

So far as concerns the basic undergraduate course we recommend, as we have already suggested, in place of the present limited training in public health nursing and hospital social service, inadequate in time, scope and number of students reached, required courses in what may be termed the prevention of disease, with special reference to its social aspects. A total of 60 hours is allotted to these courses: 15 hours in the preliminary term on social aspects of disease, 15 hours later in training continuing the course, and 30 hours on preventive medicine and public health.

The course on social aspects of disease would include an introduction to modern social problems and the agencies which deal with them, with special consideration of public health nursing and hospital social work. The lectures on preventive medicine would include, besides the application in nursing of modern methods of prevention, instruction in public hygiene and sanitation. Closely bound up with this part of the curriculum dealing with the interrelated social aspects of disease would be the instruction in case records medical and social, on which we have already laid stress, from the patient's entrance to the hospital to the end result of treatment.

In our discussion of the dispensary (see page 340) we have given concrete instances of what the study of social case histories might add to the insight and experience of the student. Such study is limited at present by the incompleteness of the social records, but this is a lack which is being increasingly remedied every year.

With such a general grounding of all students in the medicosocial causes of disability and sickness, the later graduate instruction in the specialties of public health nursing and hospital social service would be greatly strengthened. These graduate courses could go further, for they would have a far better foundation to build on. In the proposed course of the Committee

[54] For curriculum see Report of the Committee on the Training of Hospital Social Workers, of the American Hospital Association. September, 1922.

on Training of Hospital Social Workers, credit is to be allowed to nurses and persons other than nurses for certain previous instruction. The student nurse, instead of coming from her hospital course having learned to care for her patient only as a single isolated individual, would from the first gain some understanding of the individual's family and social and economic conditions and the often determining part they play in health and in sickness.

TIME ALLOWED TO THE TEACHING OF SOCIAL ASPECTS OF DISEASE AND ITS PREVENTION IN 22 SCHOOLS [55]

The general allowance of some time at least in all schools studied to the teaching of community subjects which we have included under the general title of the Social Aspects of Disease and Its Prevention, shows conscious if sometimes limited recognition of the importance of social interpretation and the social point of view to the student of nursing. Yet the average, 24 hours, to say nothing of the absurdly low minima offered by some of the inferior schools, shows that the majority do not yet realize the significance of these subjects in the training course. A single school only exceeds the allotment of hours suggested in our proposed curriculum.

SOCIAL ASPECTS OF DISEASE AND ITS PREVENTION

Number of Hours	Number of Schools
5-14	4
15-24	13
25-34	3
35-44	..
45-54	..
55-64	1
65-74	..
75-84	..
85-94	1
	22

TEACHING OF GENERAL NURSING SUBJECTS

As a background for her practical and theoretical training, there is a certain group of subjects instruction in which is designed to develop the nurse's personality and point of view and to give her an introduction to the duties and etiquette of her calling. These courses are also to set her future profession be-

* Including sociology, social service, sanitation, and public health.

fore her in historical perspective, relating the part it has played under successive civilizations in man's long march from prehistoric days, and introducing her to the great leaders who have established its traditions and ideals.

History of nursing, ethics, and various topics which fall under the general head of professional problems are sometimes presented as separate courses. This is the case in 5 hospitals, but in most schools the subject matter is variously combined, under one name or another, into two courses, or even one, for the general discussion of professional problems and etiquette. Classes touching these subjects are found in some form in all but one of the 22 hospitals whose curricula have been studied. Whatever combination of topics is made, these courses are with few exceptions taught by resident nurse-instructors or by the superintendent of nurses herself.

HISTORY OF NURSING

In 8 hospitals the history of nursing is given as a separate course with hours ranging from 8 to 22. The general method of presentation in the classes visited was by informal lecture with quizzing over previous work, and reports by students on topics for which reference readings had been assigned. Some use of lantern slides which was greatly appreciated by the class, might be developed to great advantage. The latter part of the course in all the schools naturally centers in the life of Florence Nightingale.

As an inspiration to the young nurse in her chosen career and as a background against which to see the nursing activities of the modern world, these courses may be of immense value. If ably and sympathetically conducted they should serve as a powerful professional incentive and, in contrast to the routine that plays so large a part in the nurse's day, make real to her the ideal phases of the profession. The course is worth making much of as the one purely cultural subject presented in the nurse's training and capable of broad treatment.

ETHICS

Of the general nursing subjects ethics is the one most nearly universally included in the curriculum. A course under that name is given in 20 of the 22 hospitals. In 13 of these schools, professional problems are dealt with in a separate course. In others, whatever problems of this type are discussed are regarded as an integral part of nursing ethics and are covered in the same course.

The contents of these courses and the methods of conducting them vary somewhat, but in practically all, the ethical principles discussed are applied concretely to the interest and duties of the special nursing group.

The success of the work necessarily depends on the personality and teaching ability of the instructor. Where the head of the school herself conducts the course, a valuable opportunity is offered of bringing the students into close intercourse with their chief, in discussing questions of vital interest and importance to both. In a life filled to crowding with matters of routine and necessarily formal relations, the chance of friendly intimate contact with their superior tends to vitalize and rationalize the student's interest in her life and daily duties. Such opportunity for friendly intercourse if well used would tend to make impossible the well-founded complaint of a student in one hospital, "We never see the superintendent except when we are blamed." On the other hand the course in the hands of a superintendent or other instructor, overworked and harassed by excessive administrative or teaching responsibilities, may be purely perfunctory and not serve its best purpose in the least.

For one reason or another the desirable spontaneity was felt to be lacking in some of the classes visited. For example, in one class the work is presented in the form of a lecture on which the students take notes, and little is done in the way of requiring reading or of encouraging discussion as a means of developing initiative in thinking. The lecture visited was "clear, definite, calm, and forceful," but there was nothing sympathetic or inspiring in the talk and it was entirely lacking in the always stimulating illustration from personal hospital experience of the students. It is possible that the superintendent purposely avoids this; she expressed herself as feeling it "a difficult subject on which to quiz, because of the tendency of the students to be personal in their replies." Yet the expression of personal opinion, the opportunity to drop for an hour the military rigidity of intercourse is precisely the end to be aimed at.

In another hospital the series of talks to seniors is less formally conducted, some of the students sewing or making supplies during the class hour. The topics presented in the class visited were such as should be of distinct interest and importance to students, such as Helps to Nurses after Graduation, the Journal of Nursing, Funds Available for Scholarships and Other Aid, etc. The material was in good form and well arranged. But here, too, the talk was given from a platform and the visitor felt a certain constraint between the students and superintendent. There was no discussion by the class, although two or three went to the platform to ask questions at the end. It is probable that an easy relationship between student nurses and their chief is often difficult to begin on account of the long-established tradition of military subordination and "suitable respect." But the question must be faced by all heads of institutions whether the world has not outgrown this system and whether finer results without loss of necessary discipline cannot be obtained by a more democratic spirit. Students from this school expressed freely to the writer their eager desire for greater opportunity for expression and exchange of ideas with their instructors and superiors.

The interest of the students was more marked and discussion more spontaneous in a third class, in which the members asked intelligent questions and were evidently troubled about many things. The criticism of this course lies rather against its content than the method by which it was conducted. After some discussion of their efficiency records, which the students had just received, the lecture consisted of a statement of the ideals of the nurse's calling. The ideals presented were closely associated with the rules of the school and many of them were the ideals of twenty years ago, now obsolete. There were no broad principles laid before the class and no stimulus to thinking offered. For example, one of the matters discussed was friendship and the choice of friends, especially the "harmfulness of forming friendships outside one's own class." It seems worse than folly to waste valuable time in the discussion of so limited a topic, so little calculated to widen or deepen a young woman's outlook on her profession.

TIME ALLOWED TO THE TEACHING OF GENERAL SUBJECTS RELATED TO NURSING IN 22 SCHOOLS [56]

This group of subjects related to nursing, its history, ethics, and etiquette, and designed to furnish a general background, correct point of view, and ideals of the profession for the student, is afforded time as follows in the 22 schools of our study.

[56] Including ethics, history of nursing, professional problems.

GENERAL NURSING SUBJECTS

Number of Hours	Number of Schools
Under 9	1
10-19	4
20-29	5
30-39	5
40-49	5
50-59	..
60-69	1
	21 *

* For the 22nd hospital of the group no data are available.

TABLE 7

TIME ALLOWED IN 22 SCHOOLS TO INSTRUCTION IN THE SEVERAL GROUPS OF SUBJECTS AND IN ALL SUBJECTS

Preliminary Sciences *	Different Forms of Diseases and Their Treatment †	Theory and Practice of Nursing, and General Nursing Subjects ‡	Social Aspects of Disease and Its Prevention §	All Subjects
52	137	70	7	365
88	137	83	10	365
94	143	92	12	371
102	155	120	12	439
118	160	120	15	468
140	166	127	15	472
144	169	140	16	489
145	187	144	16	493
146	189	147	17	505
148	193	162	18	530
155	194	164	19	569
166	211	172	20	572
169	218	172	20	579
170	222	177	22	598
176	236	190	22	609
182	240	192	22	655
186	248	212	22	662
208	253	216	30	672
209	270	230	30	745
320	278	232	32	746
338	293	264	58	820
510	324	266	90	994
Average 180	210.1	168	24	578

* Including anatomy and physiology, bacteriology, chemistry, dietetics, and hygiene.
† Including general medical diseases, pediatrics, communicable, venereal, and skin; general surgical diseases, gynecology, orthopedics, operating room, eye, ear, nose, and throat; obstetrics; special branches; materia medica, pathology, clinical analysis; mental and nervous diseases, psychology, occupational therapy.
‡ Including bandaging, massage, hospital housekeeping, ethics, history of nursing, professional problems.
§ Including sociology, social service, sanitation, and public health.

Following our discussion of the teaching of the various subjects and groups of subjects composing the curricula, we show in Table 7 (page 393), for each of the 22 schools studied, the hours of instruction allowed for each group of subjects, ranged in each column from lowest to highest, and in the final column, similarly ranged, the total hours of instruction in each school. At the foot of each column representing a group of subjects is given the average number of hours devoted to this group, and at the foot of the total column, the average total hours. In our final conclusions (see page 470) we compare these total hours with those recommended in our proposed curriculum.[57]

10.   The Correlation of Class Teaching and Ward Work

We have already seen in the teaching of nursing procedures and of professional subjects examples of success and of failure in the application of teaching to ward experience. We have shown the reciprocal enrichment of both teaching and ward work from good correlation between the two. We have still to discuss the general time relation of the student's class instruction to her practical experience, that is, whether it precedes, accompanies, or follows ward training.

It would appear only in consonance with elementary principles of education that in any professional school, instruction should precede if it does not accompany its practical application. Yet in practice, under present conditions while students still are responsible for staffing the wards, this elementary principle is extremely difficult of application, indeed "an impossible thing," as an able and thoughtful superintendent of nurses expressed herself to the writer.

To insure the dismissal of students from the wards of their classes at stated hours means, of course, not only careful management, but also a sufficiently large and stable body of graduate nurses who shall be available during the students' absences. That such conditions are not impossible to provide is once more proved by the schools which have successfully demonstrated the possibility in various services. In the operating room, for instance, dismissal of students might appear particularly difficult, in view of the practically continuous nature of the service. Yet even in the operating room students are regularly dismissed for

[57] It should be noted that, since each of the first four columns represents for its respective group, the hours of instruction in each school, *ranged from lowest to highest,* the final total column is obviously not the sum of the four other columns.

class in certain hospitals because graduate nurses are permanently employed to relieve them.

But at most hospitals the major services, medical, surgical, obstetrical, pediatric, communicable, are staffed by students too often without teaching as to the diseases or conditions of patients committed to their care, except such as is given by the practical instructor in teaching nursing procedures. Instead of an ordered sequence of direct instruction in disease and practical application, we find too often a disconnection between these two closely related aspects of the student's training as complete as if they were wholly irrelevant. The class instruction in theory needed for intelligent understanding and even adequate mechanical performance of the duties of a certain service precedes, accompanies, or, as is more frequently the case, follows the service in question at haphazard.

Correlation in the First Year

It is practically inevitable that the student's first-year experience shall include some months of the main hospital services, the medical, surgical, or both. This being the case, clearly medical and surgical lectures and clinics should be given in the first year also, accompanying, if they cannot be arranged to precede, the experience in the corresponding services. How far from the actual case such correlation is, may best be seen by the following summary which shows the year in which medical and surgical theory is taught in each of the 22 hospitals visited:

  5 schools give surgical and medical theory in the first year;
  2 schools give medical in the first year and surgical theory in the second year.

But on the other hand,

  14 schools give surgical and medical theory in the second year;
  1 school gives medical and surgical theory in the third year.

Thus of the 22 schools, 7, or approximately one-third, give their students instruction at the time when it either precedes or accompanies their ward services, while twice as many, 15, assign their first-year students to a number of months of service whose rich potential value is largely unrealized in default of adequate means of interpreting it.

How much of the first-year course this merely routine service may cover is shown by the number of days actually spent by students in services in which no theory had been studied. Thus it appears from the training school records that, in a prominent university school which gives medical and surgical theory in the second year, a class of first-year students spent from 36 to 143 days (a maximum of nearly 5 months with a median of nearly 3 months or 86 days) in the medical wards; and an even greater range of time (29 to 147 days with a median of 92) in the surgical wards.

Another large and widely-known training school is in even worse case in respect to the surgical service. Here, where surgical theory is taught also in the second year, a class of first-year students was assigned to the surgical wards for service ranging from 2 months actually to 7 months (61 to 211 days) with a median period of 5 months (145 days).

Other professional subjects show the same lack of correlation. Pediatrics, assigned as ward service in the first year at 4 prominent hospitals, is not taught at any of the 4 until the second, or even in one case the third year. Two hospitals detailing first-year students to obstetrical duty give no theoretical instruction in obstetrics until the third year.

CORRELATION AFTER THE FIRST YEAR

While the disparity between actual experience and theory is at its worst in the student's first year, examples of it are not wanting later in the course. One very large municipal hospital which wisely arranges ior surgical and medical instruction in the first year, offers eye, ear, nose, and throat, and nervous and mental disease lectures to all students only in their third year, but allows their ward experience in these services to be practically completed in the first and second years—before, that is, they are able to realize its value. An eminent private hospital assigns students to communicable disease service in their second year while it postpones theoretical instruction till the third.

Instances might be multiplied, but the foregoing, which are thoroughly typical, will serve to suggest at least the educational waste involved in offering experience of high potential value to students mentally unprepared to take advantage of it for lack of proper instruction in theory. Such disregard of the first principles of education defeats the ends of the nurse's training. It robs the student of the essential interest and value of her experience; and in many cases exposes her to risks which she cannot in the existing limitations of her knowledge fully appreciate or guard against.

THE EDUCATIONAL LOSS

The loss on the first score is obvious. The young student assigned prematurely and without preparatory instruction to important services must of necessity act as an automaton, without understanding or appreciation of what she sees and does. At the very time when her interest is keenest, her curiosity most alive, they are inevitably blunted and deadened by a service in large part of unintelligible routine. Take, for example, the nervous and mental service. At one of our large municipal hospitals this service is of extreme interest and value to older students, both as a field for the development of their powers of observation and as an opportunity for special study of the results of congenital and acquired syphilis. To the junior student, however, assigned to these wards for some three months in her first year [58] without previous instruction or preparation this service seems to be largely the routine bodily care of a large number of trying and disagreeable patients. At the same training school, the admirable opportunities of ward experience in tuberculosis are practically lost to students assigned to this specialty for 2½ months in their first year.[59] While precautions are taken to insure that no girl with a tuberculosis history or symptoms should be detailed to this service, she is without the fundamental protection afforded by instruction in the nature of the disease, which is not given until the second year.

THE DANGER TO HEALTH

For beside the educational loss, the student herself is subject by the present system to unjustified hazards. It is generally conceded that the care of patients suffering, for example, from communicable diseases should come late in training after students have had experience in the medical and surgical wards as well as theoretical instruction in bacteriology, medical and surgical diseases, and communicable diseases. The actual case is very different. Ignorant often of the first principles of asepsis and disinfection, untrained in surgical cleanliness, which must for safety's sake have become second nature by practice as well as instruction, the student may be assigned to the communicable disease service and to the risks inseparable from it after her first

[58] According to the training school records, the median experience in a class of 31 students.
[59] According to the training school records, the median experience in a class of 31 students.

few months in the school. Thus a large and well-known municipal hospital makes a practice of staffing its contagious disease department entirely with very young students. Almost immediately after the probation period and after but 5 months in training, students are sent to the communicable disease wards for 4-months' duty which it is planned to extend to 6. Though some instruction in communicable diseases is given them in the department, they have previously had neither lectures nor experience in medical or surgical diseases and, as the observation of our field agent proves, have no knowledge or command of aseptic technique. It is obviously too early in training for them to have acquired it. A natural result of such unpreparedness, which might be expected, is the high illness record of the student staff. On the day of our investigator's visit the records showed that, whereas 18 students were on duty in the department, 7 students were ill with scarlet fever, a figure which speaks for itself.

At another training school students may be assigned to communicable diseases 5 months after entrance, though such appointments are said to be avoided as much as possible since classes in communicable diseases are not given until the second year. At the time of our visit, nevertheless, most of the students in the department, it was stated, had not had their lectures in communicable diseases. This difficulty is supposed to be met in the interests of safety by the presence of an "instructor in technique" in the isolation building. How insufficient a safeguard this has proved to be is shown by the examples of careless or faulty technique noted by our observer. Thus night nurses going off duty passed from the "infected room" to the "clean room" while still in isolation uniform and stood discussing work with one of the special nurses, and day nurses coming on duty passed carelessly from room to room. Gowns were changed according to regulation after each case, but the washing of hands was perfunctory, and breaks in aseptic technique were not infrequent.

At one of our most distinguished schools, the class instruction in communicable diseases is not given until the third year, while the student's ward experience is apparently assigned largely in the second. In point of fact the actual case is much worse. The bulk of communicable disease experience, not separately recorded, occurs at this hospital in the pediatric service, and to this most students are assigned directly after the preliminary term, before they have received instruction either in communicable diseases or in pediatrics.

11.   Nursing in Three Special Branches

Up to this point in our discussion of the training schools, we have made no distinctions between the general and special services.   The needs we have set forth for a genuine educational scheme, for the elimination of waste time, correlation of practice and theory, etc., are as germane to special services such as the pediatric, the obstetrical, the communicable, etc., as to general medical and surgical service.   In the concrete examples of good and bad practice given by way of illustration in the foregoing chapters, we have drawn from general and special services alike.

We devote no special discussion to the well-established special services, pediatrics and obstetrics, which are generally accepted as basic parts of the nurses' training, and for which, by requirement of state nurse practice acts, affiliations must be made if facilities for training are not adequate in the home hospital.   By growing practice, training in communicable disease, where available, is being offered as an elective if not a required special service.

Three special services in which the modern demands on nursing make training increasingly necessary, though it is as yet for the most part unprovided, call for special discussion.   These are training in tuberculosis, in venereal diseases, and in mental and nervous diseases.

It is of course true that every good general course of instruction in communicable disease sets forth a body of principles applicable in substantial measure to all communicable sickness. The nurse who has such a good general course therefore learns the principles which apply to the care of tuberculosis and venereal diseases as well as to other communicable disease. What is needed, however, is the expansion of such general principles into definite detailed instruction in the peculiar problems, above all in the underlying causes which are bound up with special communicable disorders such as tuberculosis and venereal disease.

Nursing in Tuberculosis

As we have seen in an earlier chapter, tuberculosis nursing plays a very large part in public health nursing.   It is generally accepted as true that of 100 average people, 90 have tuberculosis infection, 2 have active or arrested disease, 8 or 9 will probably die. Yet during the past decade great gains have been made in checking the advance of this terrible scourge. The tuberculosis rate has been almost cut in half, falling in 1921 to 115.1 per 100,000, a decrease of 48.8 per cent below the rate for 1911, "an unparalleled accomplishment in the history of public health." [60] In this decline, aside from social and economic factors, the earlier detection of incipient cases and contacts and their instruction in habits of hygienic living has been a determining factor. Of the nurse's part in the campaign against tuberculosis we have given varied examples in previous chapters. It is self-evident that to fortify her for this pre-eminently important field, effective training is needed. Yet in the past this special training has been very difficult to secure, owing to the lack of clinical facilities.

Every school of nursing can at least, however, give a thorough lecture course in tuberculosis, illustrated by such demonstration and clinics as the hospital may afford, and by visits of observation to near-by sanitaria or special tuberculosis hospitals. Such a course should consist of at least 10 or 15 lectures. A valuable outline of such a course with bibliography is published by the National Tuberculosis Association. It should cover a thorough discussion of tuberculosis infection, including bacteriological and pathological conception of the disease, characteristics of the germ, sources of infection, predisposing causes, etc.; a full description of the disease, with the appropriate anatomy, and symptoms; principles of treatment in detail, in institutions and at home. Equally important is a discussion of the organized campaign against tuberculosis, and the technique of prevention; its economic aspects and its influence on the whole social fabric; the large subject of industrial rehabilitation and placement.

Wherever possible, practical training should be given in special wards, or, if it can be arranged, in affiliated tuberculosis hospitals and sanitaria. Where tuberculosis patients are treated in general hospitals, they are as a rule at an advanced stage of the disease. In nursing these patients, students may effectively be taught curative and palliative measures; they are rarely taught the all-important measures of prevention and the education of patients which hold the hope of the future. These

[60] Metropolitan Life Insurance Company, Statistical Bulletin. January, 1922. Page 1.

measures are an integral part of the cure in all sanitaria of good standing.

Affiliations with such institutions have still to be worked out and put into effect. While there are many practical difficulties in the way, such as lack of living quarters for affiliating students and the shortness of the period during which such students from general hospitals would be available for affiliations, yet, with the necessary financial support, these difficulties do not appear to be insoluble. No determined continuous efforts to arrange such affiliations have yet been made. Tuberculosis sanitaria and hospitals have had great difficulties in securing adequate nursing service. Those which maintain schools of nursing have had difficulties in recruiting students. They accept, usually by preference, ex-patients in a quiescent stage of the disease. The nurse who has or has had tuberculosis, it is believed, enters more sympathetically into the physical and mental reactions of the patient; mutual confidence and sympathy is engendered. The fact that the nurse, by following the prescribed treatment, has been enabled to pursue a vocation, is a constant incentive and encouragement for the patient. On the other hand, only a small fraction, amounting at some institutions to not more than 10 per cent, of the student nurses are in physical condition to complete their course by additional training in an affiliated general hospital which is necessary to comply with most state nurse registration laws.

The training of such students is seriously open to question. How far is it justifiable to train nurses for a single specialty by a course which, owing to its restricted and special clinical field, is not recognized as adequate professional preparation and whose graduates are therefore necessarily debarred in most states from state registration? Some tuberculosis institutions send their students to general hospitals for a third year to obtain training in types of experience missing in the special institution. But even with an added third year, it is clear that the school of nursing as it at present exists in a tuberculosis institution offers a wholly unbalanced program, overweighted on the side of a specialty and unsuited for a basic undergraduate course. Moreover, in many tuberculosis hospitals, the institutionalism and atmosphere of almost custodial care robs the nursing of educational value.

The lack of teachers, teaching equipment, and supervision is even more marked than in general hospitals. Attendants or practical nurses who are often in charge of wards are clearly unsuited to teaching and supervision. Yet the large proportion of ambulatory patients can obviously be cared for by persons less highly trained than the fully prepared and registered nurse. In a subsequent chapter on the subsidiary nursing worker we shall point out that tuberculosis hospitals offer appropriate opportunities for training such workers, who are not destined to have the care of acute disease. But for the training of these nursing aides or attendants as well as for the training of student nurses, supervision by competent instructors is essential. In any system of affiliation, therefore, by which general hospitals might send students for a limited period to tuberculosis institutions, there must be some assurance that standards will be safeguarded by better educational methods than now for the most part prevail.

But, at its best, the experience of the student in sanitaria of high standing gives her a new insight into measures of prevention, into early recognition of treatment and symptoms, and into the gospel of courage and self-help, which is invaluable in the nursing of this disease.

The ultimate solution of the problem of nursing care in these institutions is, as in all others, dependent on financial considerations. For genuine education of students there is needed a permanent staff of graduate nurses and nursing attendants, supplemented by the services of students.

Nursing in Venereal Diseases

No discussion of nursing education can be complete without pointing to the imperious necessity of training in those communicable diseases now generally omitted, though more deadly and more fraught with menace than any others, that is, the venereal diseases. For the care of patients, for the protection of the nurse herself, and above all for preserving the physical integrity of the race, the causes, incidence, and treatment of these diseases should be explicitly taught and impressed with all possible stress upon the young nurse. With 10 per cent of the entire population affected with syphilis alone, with hereditary victims filling mental wards or at large with greater danger to the future, it is clear that the nurse should be enlisted as a better informed ally in the campaign against this racial menace.

While at present practical training in the care and prevention of these diseases may be slow in developing, yet it is essential that this should be made a part of the basic undergraduate course. And since patients suffering from these diseases at some stage or in some form are to be found in most hospitals, thorough instruction by lectures, demonstrations, and clinics should be required.

NURSING IN MENTAL AND NERVOUS DISEASES

We have already, in our discussion of the nurse's curriculum, touched on the importance of normal psychology as an introduction to the field of mental hygiene. We have also pointed out the increasing importance of nursing in mental and nervous diseases, owing to the startling incidence of these disorders. Moreover, the mental factors in all diseases, the need of reckoning, for physical as well as mental health, with humanity's instinctive reactions and cravings, is receiving a constantly growing medical recognition and emphasis. All the more necessary, therefore, has become the training of nurses in the mental and nervous field. Yet clinical facilities have been even more difficult to secure than for training in tuberculosis. Here a distinction must be made between the nervous and mental disorders. For the former there are no special hospitals. The mental, on the other hand, outnumber all special hospitals in number of beds. Few general hospitals except the municipal receive mental patients and these usually for detention and not for treatment. Training in this field has in most instances to be secured by affiliation. Comparatively few, again, of the special public hospitals for mental diseases have been in the past, or are today, of a calibre or equipment fit for the training of nurses.

Since care of mental cases has been and in many cases still is largely custodial, obviously attendants or persons less expert than fully trained nurses have sufficed for this type of work. Indeed, with so large a number of ambulatory patients not acutely sick, just as in tuberculosis hospitals, there is a legitimate place for nursing attendants in these institutions and genuine possibility of training them for the subsidiary nursing service on which we have laid stress in previous chapters.

But with the rapid development of psychiatry and mental hygiene in the last few years, nursing in these fields is also making rapid strides. The new medical emphasis on early diagnosis especially in childhood, the recognition of abnormalities of conduct, the new interpretations of old symptoms,—all these hold out the hope of alleviating, by re-education of the patient and his better relation to his environment, the mental maladjustments which play so large and unrecognized a part in the misery of countless persons in the modern world.

For the nurse whose future work is to be characterized by a peculiar intimacy of human contacts, obviously an initiation into the newer ways of attacking these subtle problems of mental health is indispensable. Such an initiation, as in the case of tuberculosis, can be approached through the medium of lectures, clinics, demonstrations. Opportunities rarely used for teaching the nature and treatment of mental disorders may be found in the medical services of the parent hospital in the care of neurological patients in the ordinary wards or, even in the case of mentally normal patients, in the phenomena of fever or of recovery from anæsthesia. But for the thorough training in this specialty recommended in our subsequently proposed curriculum it is of the first importance that practical training should be given as well.

A study of 5 mental state hospitals conducting training schools for nurses in several states shows how far these institutions have still to go before they will be equipped to offer safe affiliations.[61] At present they fail to measure up to the basic requirements of nursing education. Two of the 5 schools required only completion of the eighth grade for entrance; 2 others but a single year of high school; the remaining school required a full high school course. For a type of nursing needing the highest degree of intelligent co-operation on the part of the nurse, such a low level of general education and background must constitute a peculiarly grave handicap.

A practice in the mental hospitals which inevitably militates against good education for student nurses is the almost universal custom of giving joint training to nurses and attendants without differentiation until the third year. This failure to distinguish between the two groups in training cannot fail to lower educational standards for the student.

The curricula in several of these schools compare not unfavorably with those of general hospitals of good standing. The conditions, on the other hand, of understaffing, of overcrowding, and of totally inadequate supervision put a premium on the subordination of educational standards to the immediate urgencies of the work. The following table speaks for itself:

TABLE 8

Number of:	Hospitals				
	A	B	C	D	E
Supervising Nurses	3	1	0*	3	3
Charge Nurses	2	3	0*	4	0*
Student Nurses	24	16	28	18	14
Attendants	62	54	178	201	36
Patients	1,893	1,056	1,858	2,192	1,055

* Attendants in charge.

According to enlightened standards of psychiatric nursing, the proportion of nurses and attendants to patients should be not less than 1: 7.[62] It ranges in the given hospitals from 1: 9 to 1: 22. The quality of the supervision is indicated by the fact that in certain of these hospitals attendants are in charge of wards by day and by night, and that the total supervisory force of graduate nurses in the 5 hospitals consists of but 19, only a small proportion of whom are registered. At least for the receiving and acute wards, it is imperative to have in charge nurses not only registered but with special psychiatric training.

We have already, in connection with the tuberculosis institutions, pointed out the overweighting of a specialty characteristic of a 3-year course of training in a special hospital, and have suggested that such hospitals can perform a better service by giving special training to affiliates than by attempting to conduct independent training schools. In the 5 hospitals studied there was indeed some provision for affiliations in the basic services, medical, surgical, obstetrical, pediatric; but the time allotted, varying from 6 to 12 months only, was hopelessly inadequate. Naturally, in institutions of such size, wards for bodily illness will provide opportunity for training in bedside care. Thus, for instance in New York state in the year 1921, one adult death in 22 occurred in a state mental hospital. This fact points to the amount of physical illness in these institutions. Four of the hospitals studied stated that instruction in these wards varied from 3 to 8 months, but as there was no definite assignment to specific services, the value of the training cannot be gauged. In some mental hospitals, it should be noted, the provision of tuberculosis wards or pavilions offers excellent opportunity for training in this special service.

[a] Recommendations of the National Committee for Mental Hygiene.

From this brief summary of conditions at typical mental hospitals it is evident that before the rich clinical opportunities offered by many of these special institutions can be made available to affiliates for the required training in psychiatric nursing subsequently recommended, the management and educational standards must be raised to a more modern level. The requirements of the United States Veterans Bureau should be set as a minimum for affiliation.

Psychopathic hospitals and departments of general hospitals, and such great endowed mental institutions as Bloomingdale Hospital, thanks to the smaller proportion of patients to the nursing personnel and the better quality of psychiatric supervision, already offer admirable facilities for gaining insight and experience in this pre-eminently important field of nursing. It should be clearly understood that such experience with the more marked manifestations of mental disorders should not be viewed merely as qualifying a nurse for the special care of mental cases either at home or in institutions. It should equip her also for the detection of incipient symptoms and of those "vexing twists of personality" which need for their control constructive and understanding therapy. In the words of a psychiatric physician familiar with problems of nursing education:

"A systematic psychiatric training for nurses is a necessity, not a luxury, of their professional equipment. If the nurse of tomorrow is to be a co-worker of the well-trained physician of that date, she must have a preparation thorough enough to enable her to take an intelligent part in the constructive program which they have in common." [63]

12. Conditions of Work

HOURS OF DAY DUTY

As we have seen from our preceding discussions, the demand for nursing service is steadily mounting. Notwithstanding the rapidly increasing supply of public health nurses, 40,000 more are needed in the field today. The deplorable conditions of understaffing and overwork in hospital wards have been made clear in the course of this study. With the erection of new hospitals each year and the enlargement of those existing, the

[63] Is Psychiatric Training Essential to the Equipment of a Graduate Nurse? Esther L. Richards, M.D., Associate in Psychiatry, Johns Hopkins University. American Journal of Nursing, May, 1922. Page 632.

demand for additional nurses in institutions is constantly on the increase. Most urgent perhaps is the situation at the top, the formidable deficiency of women of the high qualifications needed for responsible administrative and educational positions in hospital, social, and public health work.

The practical question which faces us is how to stimulate the supply of students? It is therefore important to scrutinize all the deterrents which may operate to lessen the number of candidates.

EXCESSIVE LENGTH OF HOURS

It is generally agreed that among the chief deterrents have been the long and hard hours demanded by the training schools. It is believed that the failure of recruits to keep pace with the rapidly mounting demand is the symptom of a protest, both conscious and unconscious, on the part of the nurse and the public against the long day still in vogue at the overwhelming majority of hospital training schools.

It is not that the youth of today flinches from emergency service. The nurses who worked 18 hours a day in the field hospitals of the Argonne did not complain of long hours, nor did the students who died at their posts during the influenza epidemic. But that the long day, so generally discarded in women's work, obsolete even in industry of decent standing, should be maintained in the hospitals, without excuse of emergency or special need, by tradition, by inertia, and by the acceptance of hospital needs as the criterion of service, the student sees in a very different light. Peace-time duty, year in, year out, deliberately kept at the emergency pitch, does not appeal either to her devotion or to her common sense. Why should she risk youth and health in the service of an antiquated system whose outworn standards are not yet level with the minimum standards even of ordinary industrial life. To win the sympathies of able and intelligent young women and the families from which they come, the first need is to scrap a system in which, as they feel, the student's young energies are more or less frankly exploited as a hospital economy.

Before proceeding to any discussion of the hours of student duty, it may be well to consider the distinctive demands of hospital nursing service and the difficulties of the hospitals in meeting them.

THE NECESSITY FOR 24-HOUR SERVICE

The problem of the hospital in regard to hours is essentially that of the continuous industry. Like any continuous process the hospital service must run 24 hours a day. It can no more shut down at night than can, say, the blast furnace. The primitive way of meeting the demand for 24 hours' unremitting service, in the hospital as in industry, has been the two-shift system, the 12-hour day and night. This is without question the easiest solution from the administrative point of view, and, with whatever abatements of hours off, it is still in vogue at the great majority of schools. Even where the 12-hour day has yielded through provision of relief hours to 10 or 9 hours, the 12-hour night has remained as a matter of course; and where the 8-hour day is actually established a 10-hour night is often still required. The true 8-hour system is in effect in only a fraction of the country's most progressive and modern-minded hospitals; there is, nevertheless, cause for encouragement in its recent growth.

THE NECESSITY FOR 7-DAY SERVICE

Like the blast furnace, again, the hospital nursing service must run 7 days a week. Whatever free time the student is able to obtain must be secured to her not by an expedient so simple as a day of rest on Sunday but by a carefully adjusted system of reliefs.

IRREGULARITY OF THE WORK

A further administrative difficulty arises from the fact that it is impossible to regularize the demands of nursing service from hour to hour. At some hours inevitably the work will press, and at others slacken. A graphic representation would show for every hospital two points of special pressure in the 24 hours, a "peak of the load" morning and evening during the hours of heaviest routine care. This situation is not easily met by the ordinary 3-shift system; it necessitates the service of a larger force of nurses at these special times. The 8-hour day duty must accordingly be so adjusted that the majority of day nurses shall always be on duty at the hours of special pressure.

A GROUP ABOVE THE AVERAGE

In respect to hours of duty, as in other matters already pointed out, the hospitals included in the present study are by no means typical. They not only for the most part represent training schools of advanced educational procedure, but include a number of institutions generally known as pioneers of the 8-hour day for student nurses. One of these hospitals was established on the 8-hour system, and has never varied from it. No school employing the worst practices prevalent in regard to hours is included in the group. Of the hospitals here studied, 9 hours, exclusive of meals, has been found to be the maximum working day for student nurses on general wards. An extremely high proportion, nearly 50 per cent, have adopted the 8-hour day.

How far these figures run above the average is clearly indicated by a study of training schools made by the United States Bureau of Education in 1921.[64] In 1918 only 232 out of 1,612 schools or 14.4 per cent had established the 8-hour day. In 1920 it is highly encouraging to note the remarkable increase of these figures to 539 out of 1,667, or 32.3 per cent. While well below the 50 per cent of 8-hour schools shown by the group in our study, the tendency shown towards the introduction of the 8-hour day throughout the country is very marked. By comparison with these general conditions, however, the criticisms applying to our special group of hospitals must be far more strongly applicable to the rank and file.

A COMMON BASIS OF COMPARISON

Table 9 shows the 23 hospitals of our study grouped according to actual hours worked per day, exclusive of meals and class work. Such a common basis of comparison is made necessary by the variety of hospital practice in reckoning hours of student duty. Thus some schools include class work and meals in time on duty, others include only meals, while the majority consign both class work and meals to the student's free time. In order to compare the actual working day at the various hospitals studied, we have strictly excluded class work and meal times so as to obtain in each case the actual hours of effective service.

[64] U. S. Department of the Interior, Bureau of Education. Bulletin No. 51, 1921. Statistics of Nurse Training Schools, 1919-1920. Page 4. (Advance Sheets from the Biennial Survey of Education in the United States, 1918-1920.)

Compared on this basis, about two-thirds of the hospitals in the group operate on an 8- or an 8½-hour daily schedule.[65] The ten 8-hour hospitals include 2 university training schools but consist for the most part of training schools connected with large private general hospitals with a national reputation for advanced methods. Two large city hospitals manage to maintain a schedule of approximately 8½ hours, as do also 3 small private general hospitals and 1 special hospital of high academic standards. The remaining third, including 2 municipal hospitals and several hospitals under religious auspices, require 9 hours' daily service. The weekly hours should be noted in connection with the daily hours of duty. Thus the 8-hour day may mean at different schools from 51 to 56 hours per week; the 8½-hour day may mean from 54 to 57 hours per week, etc.

TABLE 9

HOURS OF DUTY IN 23 TRAINING SCHOOLS

Daily Hours	Number of Hospitals	Weekly Hours	
		Minimum	Maximum
8	10	51	56
8-8½	6	54	57
9	7	57	60
Median 8-8½		54	

RELATION OF MEALS TO THE DAILY SCHEDULE

Owing to the varying practice of hospitals in reckoning meal times, a "9-hour schedule" and a "10-hour schedule" in hospital parlance commonly amount to the same thing. The so-called 9-hour hospital requires 9 hours' actual service, excluding meal times; the so-called 10-hour hospital follows the older practice of counting time for two meals (one hour) as time on duty. With the adoption of the 8-hour standard, time for meals is uniformly excluded, and the 8-hour schedule means accordingly 8 hours of effective work. One exception is found in the advanced position taken by a university hospital which is attempting to include time for one meal in the 8 hours' duty.

* Throughout this discussion all hours of duty stated will exclude time allowed for meals and class work.

Whether or not time for meals is included in the student's schedule, it must be emphasized that the half-hour allowed for each meal by general hospital practice is too short a period for the health and well-being of the students. Still more inadequate is the 20 minutes allowed for the first meal of a strenuous 9-hour day by one hospital of more than fair reputation. Such meal times, certainly, as fall within hours of duty should not be less than one hour long if they are to afford the relaxation and relief needed after the continuous strain of ward service.[66]

THE RELATION OF CLASS WORK TO THE DAILY SCHEDULE

Class work, at the majority of hospitals studied, is additional to the hours of duty required, except during the preliminary period. During the parts of the year when instruction is given, it ranges in amount from a weekly average of about 2 hours at the schools giving least instruction to about 5 hours at the schools offering most.[67]

As a school reduces its hours of ward duty, it is generally found to increase the time devoted to class work. Most 8-hour schools, in other words, assign more time to instruction than most 9-hour schools.

TIME OF CLASS WORK

These figures show the time devoted to class instruction in the training schools to be certainly meager enough, if any educational program is to be attempted. Slight as it is, it levies, with the preparation it requires, a heavy tax upon the energies of students already impaired by a day's work on the wards. While notable advance has been made in holding classes at more reasonable hours, they are still too often placed in the evening. Professional instruction offered at such a time to tired and sleepy girls is little better than a mockery. A better arrangement places the class work in the afternoon, but even so

[66] On public holidays several hospitals allow a full hour for dinner.
[67] The average has been obtained for each school by dividing the total hours of the curriculum by the possible days of instruction during the entire course of training, and multiplying by 5. Instruction is omitted for 3 or 4 months during the summer and on at least 2 days each week. While these omissions have been reckoned in the case of each average, varying periods when class work is omitted during the last year of training have been necessarily disregarded for lack of definite data, and the figures as given are consequently somewhat lower than would be averages drawn from the number of weeks of actual teaching.

the mental and physical freshness of the students has been spent on the major part of the day's ward service. It is hard at best to combine mental work with physical exertions. But if the training schools were in fact as they are by profession primarily educational institutions, they would see to it that instruction should be offered at such times as to make it an opportunity and not a penance. To insure this, classes should evidently be scheduled as near as may be to the beginning of the day.

The experience of one university school suggests the possibility of concentrating on classroom study in certain periods of the year when students would be entirely free from the fatigue of ward duty, and of concentrating on ward duty at other periods without interruptions for classes. Such alternating work in theory and practice, which has brought the best results in graduate courses in public health nursing, may well prove, with necessary modifications, the best solution for undergraduate training also.

TENDENCY TO INCLUDE CLASS WORK IN HOURS OF DUTY

Signs are not wanting of a tendency, slight indeed as yet but significant, towards including class work in hours of duty. At one hospital, class instruction fell within required hours. Several small private general hospitals with limited curricula, operating on a 9-hour basis, allow time in their scheduled duty for a daily average of about half an hour's class work. A recently established hospital with a fairly complete curriculum and a highly modern equipment shows the tendency towards a reasonable reduction of students' work by its inclusion of any time spent in classes *beyond one hour* in hours of duty.

Fainter indication of the movement may be seen at a large 8-hour hospital in New England which "sometimes," according to its own statement, allows time for class work during the regular hours of student duty. An encouraging instance of change is shown in the action of a distinguished training school which has done effective pioneer service for the 8-hour day. This school had already at the time of our visit reduced all junior ward duty to 7 hours in order to allow more time for class work and study, and was planning in the months immediately following to include all classes of its crowded and thorough curriculum in the 8 hours of student duty. The benefit of such a step to the students' work and its reaction on the educational standards of the schools can scarcely be over-estimated.

"It would be a mistake," says a leading hospital superintendent in a recent article, "to disregard the widespread demand that the 8-hour day be so arranged as to include the time devoted to study and instruction." [68]

TIME OFF DUTY

Failure to Provide One Day's Rest in Seven

As in other continuous industries, it is impossible for all workers in the hospital to have a day of rest on Sunday. Where this is the case in the industrial world the common rule is to give one day of rest in seven. It is probable that such a full day's rest is more urgently needed by the pupil nurse than even by the worker in industry because of the peculiar combination incident to her work of nervous strain with continuous physical exertion, the abnormal atmosphere in which she spends her days, and her inability to escape the atmosphere of her work when the day's task is done.

In spite, however, of its cardinal importance to the student, the difficulty of the hospitals in arranging a full day's rest has led in practice to the compromise of giving two half-days off duty weekly. For the needed repair of the week's fatigue, these two half-holidays are not in any case so valuable as the continuous breathing space and freedom from tension afforded by a whole free day,—a break in all probability of 36 hours. But on closer examination the supposed substitute proves to be by no means an equivalent to a day's relief, even in hours. All hospitals, even those on an 8-hour schedule, require 6 hours' work on these so-called half-holidays. Nothing could mark more strongly the grip of the 12-hour system on the hospital mind than the fact that this system, even when superseded in other respects, dictates the basis for the assignment of half-holidays: the "half-day" off after 6 hours work is half not of the actual working day but of the abandoned 12-hour day.

A few hospitals included in our study fall short even of the low standard set by the two nominal half-holidays. One 8-hour school actually demands a 7-day week of full time service, without allowance of time off duty, a practice scarcely to be matched in America any longer, even in the steel industry. Three others, two 9-hour and one 8-hour school, require 6 days of full time

[*] Publicity and Progress in Nursing Education. S. S. Goldwater, M.D. The Modern Hospital, February, 1921. Page 106.

service and **6** hours on the seventh day.   At the former two, the nominal half-holiday is assigned on a week-day; at the third, on Sunday.   This grudging allowance of 2 hours a week off duty is the more regrettable at the third school because of the enviably high reputation it bears for nursing training.   At one New England hospital it is stated that the allowance of two half-holidays has cost the students the 8-hour day: with their introduction of these half-holidays the authorities felt it necessary to revert to the 9-hour schedule.

Practically all hospitals of our study make an effort to provide a few free hours on public holidays.

NOTIFICATION OF TIME OFF DUTY

If students are to derive such benefit as is possible from their very limited time off duty, it is important that they should receive notification of their half-holidays sufficiently early to be able to plan for them in advance, and to some extent, at least, keep up normal social and recreational contacts with the outside world.   A holiday announced too late for such planning is a holiday robbed in many cases of more than half its value. The student, tired mentally and nervously often more than physically, in need of change and refreshment, is simply left at a loose end, without time to make connections with her friends and plan the amusement that she craves.   Such is the case when, as happens in no less than 5 out of 13 schools reporting on this point, students are notified of their half-holiday on the morning of the day itself.   At 2 of the 5, students are not notified of their afternoon off until 11 o'clock of the same day.   Such lack of common consideration on the part of the training school authorities, such lack of system and forethought, works clearly enough a genuine and needless hardship on the student staff, and often defeats the main purpose of the holiday.

A somewhat better practice is found at 2 other hospitals where students are given notice of their half-holiday "usually the day before."   But the only system really satisfactory is that followed at the 6 remaining hospitals of the 13 affording data where students are notified of their half-holidays at the beginning of each week.   This should be proof, if proof were needed, of the entire feasibility of such careful and considerate planning on the part of the management.   There appears to be no reason, except the habit and temptation of living administratively from hand to mouth, why other schools cannot do likewise.   Several, indeed, state that while they give short notice or none at all for the regular weekly half-holidays, they give notice several days in advance of public holidays.

WEEKLY HOURS OF DUTY

Table 10 shows the total weekly hours of actual duty in the 23 hospitals of our study. These totals represent the sum of the daily hours of service for the regular days of the week plus the hours worked on Sundays or half-holidays. It is clear from the table as from the preceding discussion of time off duty that the 48-hour week does not exist for the student nurse. The 8-hour day in industry implies the 48-hour or even the 44-hour week; it has no such implication in the hospital. The 8-hour day in hospital terminology commonly means a 52-hour week; where but one half-holiday is given, it means a 54-hour week. In but a third of our group of hospitals (8 out of 23) are the required weekly hours less than 54. In only 4 others are they as low as 54. Compared with the 8-hour worker in industrial pursuits, the student nurse on an 8-hour schedule works from 4 to 6 more hours weekly. Compared with the average office or clerical worker, she works from 12 to 15 more hours weekly, and in addition, with a 7-day week and but 2 hours less work on her supposed half-holiday.

TABLE 10

WEEKLY HOURS OF DUTY IN 23 TRAINING SCHOOLS

Weekly Hours	Number of Hospitals
51-53	8
54-56	7
57-59	6
60	2
Median 54	Total 23

In about half (11) of the hospitals included in our study, students are required to work more than 54 hours weekly. In 6 hospitals they work from 57 to 59 hours a week. Two of these are very large municipal hospitals; the rest are medium sized or small private general hospitals. Two schools under religious control require second- and third-year students to work a full 60-hour week.[69] Class work and study added make the total a formidable one.

---

* Juniors in these hospitals work 54 hours a week on the wards.

ADHERENCE TO SCHEDULES OF HOURS: SUPERVISION

The preceding discussion of hours of duty has been based on the statements of the training schools as to their plans for the working day. It is obvious that emergencies must arise, unforeseen and unavoidable stresses, when any hospital with the best will must find it impossible to adhere to these stated programs. Of overtime caused by genuine emergency there can be no reasonable criticism; response to such emergencies is indeed a legitimately important part of the nurse's training. But when the stated schedule of student duty is lightly regarded or even ignored, not for emergency's sake but because of administrative slackness and lack of system, or from understaffing of the wards, overtime must be unqualifiedly condemned.

The vigor of a hospital's policy in the matter of adherence to schedules may be gauged by its system of time-keeping, or the method of supervision by which it seeks to regulate the coming on and going off duty of its students. More than two-thirds of the hospitals included in our special study keep systematic records by a method of time slips or daily written reports by supervisors. In contrast to these systematic and satisfactory methods, four schools, somewhat lax in other details of management as well as this, require only oral reports through supervisors, and three leave the whole matter of time-keeping to the discretion of the student nurse herself.

It will be evident that the last plan penalizes the responsible and conscientious student who will not leave her patients until she is relieved, while it leaves the thoughtless and inconsiderate student free to keep her waiting, without discipline or check, for coming late. Whatever system is adopted, the supervising authorities should have exact information as to whether or not the schedule is maintained, and should be effective enough to enforce its maintenance. They should on the one hand protect the student on duty by enforcing promptness from her successor, and on the other hand they should safeguard professional standards and protect the public by seeing to it that less conscientious students do not stop work at the stroke of the clock.

HOURS OF DUTY IN SPECIAL SERVICES

In certain important respects our picture of hours of duty in student training has been too optimistic even for the picked group of our special study; it has failed to take account of at least two important elements of strain. One of these is the uncertainty of hours and the prevalence of overtime in special services.

In certain special services, notably the operating room and the obstetrical department, hours of student duty tend to be longer and more irregular than on general wards. Even in hospitals where strict observance of schedule is the established rule, these departments are not infrequently treated as exceptions. This is due primarily to the inherent nature of the services, which are often inevitably of the emergency type, and hence make demands at unusual hours upon the staff. Moreover, owing to the irregular and intermittent character of the work, in which high pressure alternates at times with slackness, and the difficulties consequently involved in arranging schedules for these services, hospital authorities have been slower to feel the need of putting them on an 8-hour basis. Again, the necessity of assuring students sufficient practice with the limited clinical material at hand often prevails, in smaller hospitals especially, over the desirability of establishing shorter hours.

Operating Room

Four hospitals of our group state frankly that they do not attempt to maintain the same hours in the operating room that they do on other services. Two 8-hour hospitals of generally high standing and progressive practice nevertheless report respectively an "8- or 9-hour day" and a 9-hour day in the operating room. A third hospital, running on a 9-hour schedule in the general services, states that it requires 12 hours' duty or longer from students in the operating room. An even worse example of excessive hours is furnished by a special hospital, nominally on the 8-hour system, but otherwise of low educational standards, where student service in the operating room reaches the average of 15 or 16 hours daily. "The 8-hour day is secured in the rest of the hospital at the cost of the operating room students," was the comment here of the supervisor in charge of the operating room. The same staff, moreover, is on call at night. As an instance of the criminally dangerous extremes to which such unregulated service may be carried, a case was cited in which under special pressure of work a student remained on duty for 39 hours with only 3 hours free time during the entire period.

Overtime

Unfortunately, moreover, it is not only in the minority of hospitals which admit a difference of schedule for operating room duty that the strain of long hours in this service is necessarily heaviest. Overtime owing to special pressure of work is the besetting difficulty of the operating service. Thus a certain distinguished hospital made recently a special effort to reduce operating room hours, which had run from 7 a. m. to 7 p. m. with 2 hours off duty, to the 8-hour day established in the rest of the hospital services. At the time of our visit, however, it was still found impossible to regulate the work according to schedule, time on duty was still irregular, and long hours on some days alternated with short ones on others. At one operating room visited operations were over for the day, but the work left for the students must have required at least an hour's overtime work. In the main operating room on the previous night, students supposedly free at 6 p. m. were reported on duty until 11 p. m. Total weekly hours had at least been greatly reduced, but these weekly hours according to actual records still ranged as high as 66.

The Solution

In contrast to these instances of overtime and overstrain in operating room duty we may cite the example of certain hospitals in which regular hours are strictly enforced in spite of any emergencies attendant upon the service. These have adopted the only fair solution, namely the system of so staffing the operating room with graduates and paid assistants that students are not alone responsible for the running of the department. Students according to this plan are on duty, as they should be, for their own training, and not to carry the responsibility of the service. They can thus be set free at the end of duty hours, and need not be, except for the benefit of their own experience, on call at night. Especially at two of our best known municipal hospitals the staff is so organized that the students are not essential to efficient service. "At any time," we are told at one of these, "the graduate nurse in charge takes over the work of the student nurse, releasing her for any period necessary for attendance at classes or lectures." At the other, a graduate nurse coming on duty at 8 p. m. relieves any students who may still be in the department.

Obstetrical Department

This plan of organization also offers the only safe basis for student duty in the maternity service. Though but one hospital of the group studied stated that longer service than the 9-hour day of its other departments was required in the obstetrical service, namely from 9 to 12 hours, it is well known that this service also is peculiarly liable to irregular hours and overtime work.

Methods of Insuring Adequate Experience

In both operating room and maternity services, some of the best modern hospitals measure experience not by length of assignment but by requiring the student's presence and assistance at a certain number of operations and deliveries. Others meet the difficulty of insufficient experience during the hours of day duty by calling upon the students at night to supplement it, but allow a corresponding time off duty the following day. Even hospitals which depend on student nurses to staff the operating room and are therefore forced in emergencies to call on them at night, irrespective of their own experience, generally allow an equivalent amount of free time on the next day.

RATIO OF PATIENTS TO STUDENTS

Another source of strain too little considered in estimating the burden of the student's daily schedule is the number of patients assigned to her charge. This must vary to some extent with the type of hospital, since the number of patients a student can properly care for depends upon the nature of their illnesses. Municipal hospitals, for example, with large chronic services can safely assign more patients to the care of one nurse than can hospitals with predominantly acute services. Five patients, however, are generally held to be the maximum number that a student in the great majority of cases can satisfactorily tend.

Of the 16 hospitals reporting on this point, one-half maintain this standard ratio of 5 patients to 1 student nurse; 2 small hospitals of the number were able at the time of our investigation to reduce the number of patients to 4. The other 8 hospitals exceed this ratio: 4 assign on the average 6 to 8 patients to 1 student and the remaining 4, 10 to 11 patients. It will be abundantly evident that an 8-, 9-, or 10-hour day are terms of very different import according to whether the student is in charge of the standard number of patients or of twice that number; whether adequate time is allowed her for her duties, or whether she is driven by the constant pressure of "getting the work done." Unfortunately it is at the great municipal hospitals where long hours are still the rule that conditions of under-staffing and overcrowding especially tend to increase unduly the ratio of patients to students. Such hospitals are 3 of the 4 quoted above as showing the worst ratios.

ANNUAL VACATIONS

Need of Vacation in Training

For a young woman on duty practically every day of the year, working long hours in an abnormal atmosphere, her free time largely given up to class work and study, the question of vacation assumes a critical importance. It is on this that the student must depend to wipe out the cumulative fatigue of the year, to afford much needed recuperation. It is to this that the school must look, if only from the narrowest self-interest, to refresh the student's physical and mental energies, and to help repair the "staleness" and loss of interest already noted as a common symptom of the latter part of the training course. One month would appear to be the minimum time allowed to make such recuperation reasonably possible.

Length of Vacations Allowed

Yet even in the superior group of our study, only one hospital allows as.much as 4 weeks each year for vacation. About half of the schools allow a meager 2 weeks; 10 allow about 3. We must not forget that we are dealing here with more than average standards: among the rank and file of the country's schools the shorter period is undoubtedly allotted by a far larger proportion.

Three others of the schools under immediate consideration vary the vacation from year to year of the course. One of these takes the view that the students need more vacation with each additional year of training, and accordingly allows 2 weeks during the first year, 3 weeks during the second, and 4 weeks during the third. The 2 remaining schools, evidently taking the opposite point of view, give 4 weeks' vacation during each of the first two years and apparently none at all during the third. By a further variation in practice another school connected with a university hospital gives the largest annual allotment of its 7 weeks' total vacation, namely 3 weeks, in the second year. Still another leaves its 7 weeks' total vacation to be divided as need arises among the three years of the course. An allowance for travelling of 1½ days yearly, in addition to its annual vacation of 3 weeks, is made by one school; an allowance for sickness of 1 week for the entire course, in addition to its annual vacation of 2 weeks, is made by another.

Notice of Vacations

In contrast to their frequently late notification of weekly half-holidays, it is gratifying to note the prevailingly considerate practice of the training schools in giving notice of vacations one or two months in advance. Students at some hospitals are encouraged to request the time that they prefer. At one municipal hospital, dates for vacations are selected by the students according to seniority. In contrast to this general attitude of thoughtfulness is the practice of 2 hospitals which give only two days' notice of their annual vacations to students residing in the same city, though they inform students living at a distance "in advance."

RELATION OF HOURS TO HEALTH

The direct relation of working hours to health is significantly indicated by certain figures gathered by the National League of Nursing Education. "From a number of hospitals selected at random," it is stated in Bulletin No. I of their Committee on Education,[70] "it was found that in those with the longer working day, the sickness rate was from 4.8 to 12.8 days per year, while in the 8-hour hospitals none went above 4.8." Facts of common knowledge to the nursing profession, given in the same Bulletin, substantiate from a wide range of experience the testimony of these figures. The lowered vitality due to fatigue, with its sequelæ of disease, is especially emphasized:

"The conditions pupil nurses suffer from are those commonly associated with lowered vitality and resistance. Tonsillitis probably occurs most frequently. Minor infections are also common, but pneumonia, and other serious infections are not at all infrequent. Students suffer a good deal from

[70] National League of Nursing Education, Committee on Education. Bulletin No. I. The Case for Shorter Hours in Hospital Schools of Nursing. Page 11.

heart lesions, nervous and digestive disorders, and a large proportion of them are more or less anæmic. During the last year a great many student nurses have had influenza and many have died of it. Superintendents of nurses have repeatedly noted that when nurses were overworked and tired they were much more likely to take the disease and to have it in a severe form." [71]

Short of actual illness, symptoms of nervous fatigue and overstrain are noted by the Bulletin as common among students:

"Many pupil nurses who never are considered ill enough to be taken off duty show symptoms of overwork and overstrain which are unmistakable to experts. They lose their freshness and buoyancy, they become easily irritated and depressed, they lose their interest in their work and often, especially on night duty, their faces look worn and haggard, showing that their youth and vigor are being prematurely sapped." [71]

RELATION OF HOURS TO WORKING EFFICIENCY

Such fatigue and overstrain must obviously and gravely affect the student nurse's efficiency. Indeed the lowered labor efficiency proved by universal industrial experience to be associated with long hours holds as true in the nursing profession as in industry. The same unfavorable verdict on the work of the long day is heard today from the hospitals as confronts us in the long record of industrial history.

Output

It is a well-known fact that long hours in industry lead to lessened and inferior production. On the other hand the reduction of hours does not reduce proportionally the output of the worker, but leads by the reduction of fatigue to an increased activity generally marked enough to balance or overbalance the curtailment of working time. The well-known relation of working hours and efficiency accepted by enlightened business men throughout the world makes it the stranger that modern institutions like hospitals still countenance schedules of hours long discarded in industry if only on the ground of productivity. The slower pace and greater loss of time of the student nurse working on the 12-hour or even on the 10-hour schedule as compared with the student nurse working on the 8-hour schedule is recog-

[71] Op. cit. Page 11.

nized by a consensus of experienced opinion among hospital authorities. The student suffering from the unavoidable fatigue of the longer day is less swift and deft in her movements, less alert, less energetic in her attack on work than the student working on the shorter schedule. "The statement is often made," says the Bulletin of the National League of Nursing Education already quoted, in speaking of the experience of various hospitals in introducing the 8-hour system, "that the lowering of the sickness rate and the gain in working efficiency almost if not completely makes up for the reduction in working hours." [72] "As a rule it takes only a short time," says the League's Committee on Education in a second Bulletin, "to show improvement in the health and working capacity of the student group." [73]

Quality of Work

But it is not only the amount of work accomplished that suffers by the maintenance of the long working day, or the student's health alone that is endangered. It is a question also of the public safety. The well-known relation of fatigue to accidents and spoiled work in industry has rarely been invoked in respect to nursing service. Yet the analogy is in fact a close one.

Fatigue, according to industrial testimony, may show not only in lessened quantity of work but also in deteriorated quality, that is, in errors, spoiled work, and, especially, in accidents. Even so in nursing, as fatigue sets in not only does the pace of work grow slower and lag behind the schedule, but co-ordination may be impaired, attention and observation dulled, memory unreliable; "serious mistakes occur" to quote once more the League of Nursing Education,[74] "which would not happen if the nurse were not half-dazed with fatigue. The nurse is always held responsible when things go wrong, and often she is made to suffer severely for an oversight or a slip when the conditions she is working under are mainly or entirely responsible." The shorter work-day saves the student from a false and unjust position; it is also an important means of safeguarding the public.

[72] Op. cit. Page 20.
[73] National League of Nursing Education, Committee on Education. Bulletin No. II. Suggestions for Establishing the Eight-Hour Day in Nursing Schools. Page 9.
[74] National League of Nursing Education, Committee on Education. Bulletin No. I. The Case for Shorter Hours in Hospital Schools of Nursing. Page 13.

RELATION OF HOURS TO EDUCATION

It might as well be frankly admitted that, with the longer schedules of hours still generally in vogue, it is impossible for the school to redeem its educational promise; excessive hours of service leave neither time nor energy for sound educational work. We have already pointed out the futility of expecting any adequate class work from students after a full day's ward duty even at hospitals with the most advanced schedules. But of what avail at any time of day are the finest instructors, the most modern equipment, for students in the chronic condition of overfatigue we have described above? "The pupil nurse is always sleepy,"—to quote again the League of Nursing Education's Bulletin: [75]

"She sleeps in her hours off duty, she often sleeps in her lectures and classes, she sleeps in church and even at times in the concert and theatre. When she sits down to study, it is always a struggle to keep awake. Often all the time she should spend in recreation is spent in resting and sleeping."

And further:

"With the present system of long hours good educational work is impossible. Any teacher who is accustomed to working with pupil nurses will testify that in spite of their interest and willingness, they can rarely do justice to their class work. They are simply too tired to concentrate for any length of time, even when the work is presented in the most interesting way. Even young women who are naturally good students find themselves unable to grasp things as readily, to remember as well or to reason as clearly as they did in school or college."

A PRACTICABLE REDUCTION

What are the objectives desirable in the reform of hours of duty? As ultimate aims, surely, nothing less than the 8-hour day with inclusion of all class work in duty hours; the 44-hour week with one full day's rest in seven. But not even the most ardent advocates of reform would press these changes all at once. With the immediate adoption of the 8-hour day, however, the reduction of weekly hours to 44 should be brought about as soon as possible.

[75] Op. cit. Page 12.

A potent obstacle to change is the fear of expense. We have no wish to minimize the financial difficulties of the hospitals. Some additional expense, at least initially, in shifting to the 8-hour system should doubtless be frankly admitted. A somewhat larger nursing staff will need to be secured. What should on the other hand be strongly emphasized is that both the increase and the expense are very much less than commonly supposed. No exact figures of comparative costs are available. Yet it may well be that the ultimate gains of shorter hours will outweigh the losses even financially.

Three elements of economy, too little considered, enter into the savings to the hospital of the 8-hour day: first, the increased efficiency of health and vigor; second, the lowering of the excessive sickness rate generally associated with the long day; and third, the reduction of the present high turnover among probationers. The cost of sickness, and the almost total loss of the hospital's expenditure on students giving up training after the first few months, must certainly go far to offset the cost of a somewhat increased staff.

"As to the percentage of increase," says Bulletin No. II of the National League of Nursing Education,[76] "experiments in several hospitals show that, where no other assistance is brought in, the number of additional nurses may vary from no increase at all to 33 per cent, running as a rule probably about 15 per cent."

EIGHT HOURS BY LAW

"The legislature of California has done for student nurses what the conscience of those who controlled nursing schools would not do, and the student nurses now have a 48-hour week. . . . Nurses in the East do not want the state to compel a 48-hour law for students, but they do earnestly desire compulsion through public opinion."

So spoke a prominent superintendent of nurses at the 1917 Convention of the National League of Nursing Education.[77] The California experiment of shortening student hours by law was undertaken in 1913, it will be remembered, in the face of united opposition from the hospitals. The more valuable should be

[76] National League of Nursing Education, Committee on Education. Bulletin No. II. Suggestions for Establishing the Eight-Hour Day in Nursing Schools. Page 4.
[77] National League of Nursing Education, Proceedings of the 23rd Annual Convention, 1917. Page 58.

their present testimony to its success. According to this evidence, the new system has done all that its advocates could hope. With the "marked improvement" as summed up by the National League of Nursing Education,[78] our discussion of hours of duty may appropriately close:

    (a) The health of the nurses is better; less time is lost through illness and fewer breakdowns occur.
    (b) The nurses feel more fit for their work.
    (c) They have more time for class work and study, and the general grade of their class work is improved.
    (d) They have more time for outdoor exercise and recreation, and they are on the whole happier and more contented.
    (e) The number of applicants has increased and the applicants are on the whole of a better type.
    (f) It has been possible to provide a better course of training in such schools and this helps to attract the better qualified women. The curriculum of study adopted by California schools is well in advance of that in other states, for the sole reason that California has shorter hours of duty and so can give more attention to the educational side of the work.

Night Duty

The distinctive value of night duty is generally recognized to consist in the training in individual responsibility and initiative it affords. Graduate nurses who are asked whether night duty was of value in their past training usually reply without hesitation in the affirmative. Night duty, they feel, gave them the first sense of mastery of their calling. In night duty they escape the excessive deference to the authority and opinions of others. In night duty the young nurse first learns to depend on herself, to feel her own capacity in emergencies. With this sense, a greater interest in training and a quickening of ability naturally follows.

Yet this recognition of the value of night duty cannot obscure its high cost. The nurses who would be most unwilling to have lost the experience are unanimous also in thinking it dearly purchased, at the expense of physical and emotional strain. The

[78] National League of Nursing Education, Committee on Education. Bulletin No. I. The Case for Shorter Hours in Hospital Schools of Nursing.

first night when she was left alone on the ward! The whole first period of night duty! It lives in the nurse's remembrance as a time of fiery trial, when the dawn never seemed to come and time went on leaden feet, when every patient might die, seemed likely to die before morning, when the chance kindness or reassurance of a passing interne or supervisor was greeted with profound gratitude. To the last, even for the older experienced student, night work remains peculiarly taxing.

In any discussion of the rôle of night duty in student training, it must constantly be borne in mind that its real and important benefits are gained at a cost disproportionate to that of day duty in physical and nervous strain. This surtax on energy makes it important that night duty should be safeguarded by careful and deliberate planning; and in especial that its assignment should be guided not by the routine convenience of the hospital but by the educational benefit to the student. To secure the maximum educational return at the minimum expense to the student—this must be the constant objective of a wise training school management. But as organized at present, night duty would seem deliberately aimed to sap the health and spirits of the students. In the interest of health and education, the following precautions are primary.

Since the various hospital services show essential differences in educational value for training, it is evident that for night duty students should be carefully assigned to those offering the most valuable nursing experience. The total time devoted to night duty should not be disproportionately long to the entire course of training; it should be, indeed, no longer than is strictly necessary to assure the special educational values aimed at. The several periods of assignment to night duty, moreover, should be neither too long nor too frequent; and beyond any question the hours of night duty should not exceed the 8 hours now increasingly accepted as the maximum length of day duty. In addition, it seems more rather than less necessary than in day duty that students undergoing the rigors and solitudes of long periods of night duty should be assured of the relief of a weekly holiday. Furthermore, it would appear a mere matter of course that provision should be made for such sleeping quarters as will afford students on night duty both quiet and privacy for sleep in the daytime, and that they should not be awakened to attend classes until after adequate rest. Finally and emphatically, students assigned to night duty must in any reasonable scheme have been in training a reasonable length of time, must be given adequate supervision, and must be placed in charge of a manageable number of patients.

With respect to night duty we shall find the schools of nursing again pursuing various policies, varying from a full recognition of the primary recommendations summarized above to a total disregard of them. With respect to night duty we must reiterate that the inclusion of a large number of superior schools in our study results in a more optimistic picture than the great majority of schools would afford. The abundant evils disclosed in this small group would be far greater in the great majority.

COMPARATIVE EDUCATIONAL VALUE OF SERVICES DURING NIGHT DUTY

The comparative values in training of the various hospital services during day duty tend to be accentuated from the point of view of night duty. Thus the less active services, offering least opportunity for nursing experience during the daytime, are still less active during the night when patients not acutely ill are generally sleeping. Chronic services, of negligible value to students at all times, are especially barren at night; the surgical service is likely to lack the major part of its educational value during the hours of sleep when neither dressings nor treatments are given; of the private service, which is predominantly surgical, the same is true. The medical service, on the other hand, of paramount importance to student training in the daytime by reason of its variety and acuteness, offers an even heightened opportunity in some respects at night. A similarly emphasized value may be seen in the obstetrical service. For it is common knowledge that all vital processes are at their lowest ebb during the night, when crises of all sorts are known to occur. If, then, the special value of night duty in student training lies in the responsibility it entails and the development of independent judgment and action through the necessity of meeting critical situations, the services in which these situations most commonly arise, namely, the medical and obstetrical, should evidently be the special fields of the students' assignment to night duty.

ACTUAL ASSIGNMENTS OF NIGHT DUTY

At all the hospitals studied, however, actual practice shows no trace of these considerations. By policy or need, however unwilling, all wards are staffed at night by student nurses, irrespec-

tive of the value the services offer. In the assignment of undergraduates to night duty as shown in Graph 2, by far the greatest proportion of their time is seen to have been spent in services
other than medical or obstetrical. The average proportion of
time devoted to medical and obstetrical night duty together, at
six representative hospitals amounted to only one-third of total
night service compared with two-thirds consumed by surgical and

GRAPH 2

AVERAGE PERCENTAGE OF NIGHT DUTY ASSIGNMENTS IN MEDICAL AND OBSTET-
RICAL SERVICES COMPARED WITH TIME IN OTHER SERVICES, EXPERIENCED
BY STUDENTS OF 1 CLASS IN EACH OF 6 SCHOOLS OF NURSING

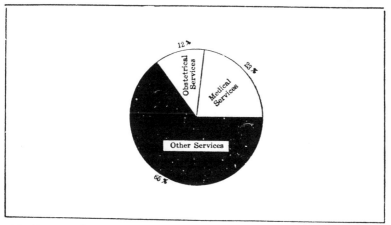

all other services. Individual schools as shown in Table 11 range
from a maximum of only 42.5 per cent for medical and obstetrical
night duty combined to a minimum of 17.5 per cent. Such figures
follow naturally from the fact that the majority of the hospitals maintain predominantly surgical, private, or other special
services.

Further analysis of the results of this predominance of other
services, from a more detailed study of the figures forming the
basis for Graph 2, offers added interest. Hospital 2, a large
municipal hospital, shows a disproportionately large part of
night duty spent in the nervous and mental wards because of
the high ratio of beds here devoted to this service. It is obvious
that night duty in these wards must exact a heavy nervous and
physical toll without affording commensurately valuable training.
Hospital 5 has a large and highly-reputed pediatric service (devoted largely to orthopedic children's cases) and a large private

service, but neither of these can be considered particularly rich in opportunity for student nurses on night duty in proportion to the time they demand. Hospital 21 is a maternity hospital maintaining an almost exclusively private service, and training in obstetrics is given to all students; in common, however, with most special hospitals of this type, the short time allowed for general medical service in an affiliating hospital prevents the possibility of well-rounded training, even during night duty.

This failure to assign students to services promising the best educational return is further illustrated by the records of indi-

TABLE 11

PERCENTAGE OF NIGHT DUTY SPENT IN MEDICAL AND OBSTETRICAL SERVICES COMPARED WITH TIME SPENT IN OTHER SERVICES BY STUDENTS OF 1 CLASS IN EACH OF 6 SCHOOLS OF NURSING

Hospital No.	Medical	Obstetrical	Medical and Obstetrical	Other Services	All Services
1	29.1	10.2	39.3	60.7	100
2	23.6	3.6	27.2	72.8	100
5	11.9	5.6	17.5	82.5	100
6	19.8	22.7 *	42.5	57.5	100
9	20.2	16.4 *	36.6	63.4	100
21	24.4 *	16.7	41.1	58.9	100
Average	23	12	35	65	100

* Affiliated service—proportion of night duty estimated by affiliating school.

vidual students. These show that some nurses actually complete their course without having had any experience whatever of night duty in the services of primary value for training. Thus a municipal school of high standing graduated a fifth of its senior class (14 out of 67) without night duty in medical service. At a training school of the highest reputation, maintained by a privately supported large general hospital, 9 students out of a class of 21 had no medical experience in night duty, 8 had no obsterical experience, and 3 had no experience in either service. In respect to the medical service matters are even worse at a smaller prominent school where half of the graduating class (15 out of 31) were allowed to complete their course without medical night duty.

Bare statement of such facts as these shows the crying need of a readjustment of the assignment of night duty to the ends of student training. But if potential educational benefit to the student is to be made, as it should be, the basis of assignment, it is clearly necessary, to meet the administrative needs of the hospital, that graduate nurses be provided in sufficient numbers for the general staffing of the wards at night in services of no special educational value in training.

TOTAL LENGTH OF NIGHT DUTY TIME PLANNED BY THE SCHOOL

We have seen, then, that the assignments of night duty show no evidence of effort on the part of the training school authorities to make the students' experience fruitful in compensation for its essential physical cost. Night duty seems to be traditionally taken for granted as a matter of routine nursing service without deliberate educational design.

In the matter of length of night duty experience, on the other hand, each school studied presents a definite plan. A study of the figures given by 21 schools (see Table 12) shows the time planned to be, however, largely unstandardized. From minimum to maxi-

TABLE 12

Total Months of Night Duty Planned by 21 Schools of Nursing, Showing the Proportion of Schools in Each Group *

Number of Months Planned during Training	Number of Hospitals	Percentage of All Hospitals
5	6	28.6
6	10	47.5
8	3	14.3
11	2	9.6
Total	21	100.0

* Two hospitals did not report on this point.

mum the allotment of time considered desirable or necessary by the several schools varies from 5 months to more than twice that time. The shortest total period of night duty planned for by any school is 5 months, and only 6 schools planned for this period. The largest group of schools, 10 in number, planned for 6 months, 3 for 8 months, and 2 for 11 months of night duty, during the 3-years' course.

In other words, according to these various plans, students are to spend from about one-seventh to almost one-third of their entire course in night duty, the largest group being destined so to spend one-sixth of their entire course. It is obvious that the extreme variation in planning this service affords no clue to the amount of time actually needed by the student to obtain its essential value for training. The total lack of any consensus of opinion as revealed by these figures suggests indeed unavoidably that each school plans to devote to night duty as much of the student's time as can be spared from the other services rather than as little as need be spent to derive the maximum educational benefit from a type of duty inevitably taxing.

Yet it would seem a matter of elementary human economy that the total duration of this arduous duty should be fixed by some standard plan corresponding to the essential demands and benefits of the service rather than by the varying needs of individual hospitals. If 5 months, as planned by 6 of the schools reporting, is a period adequate for the ends of training, the expenditure of student energy and vitality involved in the plans of the 15 others is excessive by a margin of from 1 to 6 months.

As a matter of fact, the minimum present practice as shown by the 5-months' period is probably far beyond the needed duration of adequate training in night duty. The question of waste in the existing system is illuminated by considering what proportion of night duty is spent in services of real educational use. As shown by Graph 2, the average time spent by the student nurse in services of primary value is but a third (35.0 per cent) of her total night duty. The remaining two-thirds is in effect educational waste. According to Table 12, the average duration of night duty as planned at 21 schools was 6 months. If but one-third of this time was educationally fruitful, we have here, roughly speaking, an average waste of about 4 months. The remaining 2 months or about 9 weeks comprises on the average all services of essential value to the student in the present arrangement of night duty. Two months would indeed seem a sufficient total length of time for night duty experience. With the reorganization of training emphasized throughout this report which would allow time for intelligent study and discussion of cases, the shorter period of night duty would yield a greater educational benefit than the long periods of duty now commonly assigned.

ACTUAL DURATION OF NIGHT DUTY SHOWN BY RECORDS OF STUDENTS IN 6 SCHOOLS

In order to compare the time planned for night duty with actual practice at the training schools, an analysis was made of the records of the students of one graduating class at each of the 6 representative hospitals already listed in Table 11. As shown by these records, the actual experience of students at the several hospitals tends markedly to outrun the time planned for night duty, excessive as we have seen this to be.[79]   But the conspicuous showing of our analysis is not the tendency of student experience to exceed the hospital plan, striking though this is.   However great the variation in plans for night duty might be, however general the tendency to exceed even the time planned, we should assume at least that the assignments of night duty for students of one class would be relatively uniform.   Such uniformity, especially in a peculiarly taxing service, would seem to be a matter of essential fairness.   We have already seen the extreme variation in the assignments of members of one class in the same hospital to the various services.[80]   The outstanding revelation of the night duty records is again the chaotic condition of actual practice, the extreme and bewildering variation in length of service between students actually in the same class.   Graph 3 shows the experience of students in 6 schools which have had the minimum, median, and maximum weeks of night duty in their respective classes.   The extraordinary range of this experience leaps to the eye in the graphic representation, which gives an idea, as typical as it is striking, of the diversity of actual service very generally found among the students of any single class.   In a prominent school (No. 2), maintained by a municipal hospital, for example, experience of night duty ranged in one class from a minimum of 16 to a maximum of 39 weeks; in another school of high reputation (No. 6), from a minimum of 13 to a maximum of 30.   In all 6 schools of our special study the differences between the minimum and maximum student experience range from 16 to 23 weeks.   In practically each school, that is to say, the student having the maximum experience had twice as much night duty as the student having the minimum experience, with the remainder of the class ranging variously between these extremes.

It may indeed be urged that some allowance should be made for a certain variation in individual student experience because of differing needs of individual students for the training in responsibility that night duty offers.   In no educational plan, however, could such excessive variation as we have cited exist— a variation greater than in almost any other hospital service —without making for unequal benefits for some students and undue hardships for others.

[79] For some hospitals a complete record of time spent in excess of time planned is not obtainable.   This is due to the fact that some of these hospitals have work in affiliation for which information was not forthcoming with regard to duration of night duty planned.
[80] See Graph 1, page 198.

GRAPH 3

THE MAXIMUM, MEDIAN, AND MINIMUM WEEKS OF NIGHT DUTY EXPERI-
ENCED BY STUDENTS OF 1 CLASS OR REPRESENTATIVE SECTION OF A
CLASS IN EACH OF 6 SCHOOLS OF NURSING, DURING TRAINING

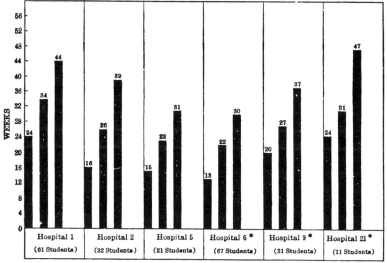

    * The records of time spent in night duty during affiliation were not obtainable; the total for these schools is therefore somewhat higher than stated here.

LENGTH AND FREQUENCY OF THE SEVERAL ASSIGNMENTS OF NIGHT DUTY

The total night duty experience is naturally never given in one continuous period, but is broken into various shorter assignments, interspersed during three years of training. The length and frequency of these several assignments to night duty also present great variations among all the schools studied. As in industrial occupations the question remains open whether short periods of alternating night and day duty are less injurious to the human system and more acceptable to those concerned than longer alternating periods which do not demand as frequent readjustments of habits of living. Two large schools maintained by municipal hospitals have adopted the plan of numerous 2-week periods of night duty; 8 schools of varying types have periods ranging from 4 to 6 weeks; of the total 23 schools, the largest group, 9 in number, have assignments 2 months in length. A university school is trying out the more flexible plan of two 2-week and two 2-month periods, while 2 schools under religious administration have two assignments of the unwarrantable duration of 3 months each. A maximum period might reasonably be set at 1 month.

The length of these assignments is of special significance when it is realized that students are seldom given the regular weekly holiday during night service. Only a negligibly small group of schools allow students a weekly night off, away from the school. A large general private hospital which plans night duty assignments of 2 months each defends this practice of depriving students of their weekly holiday on the rather ironic ground "that the time may not be spent in going home, lest the student become fatigued." It must be said to the credit of this school, that at the end of the assignment of night duty it gives one half day free for each week that the student has been on night duty. Three other schools, 2 maintained by large municipal hospitals, and 1 by a large general hospital, also give a corresponding time off at the termination of the night duty assignment. Ten schools give 1 to 2½ free days at the end of the night duty period, as "change time." But in none of these instances does the time allowed equal the time lost in weekly holidays that have been forfeited during night duty. Two schools with assignments of 2 and 3 months in length respectively allow 2½ and 3 days off at the end of night service, and, in addition, 1 night for each month while on duty. Two schools allow time off neither during nor at the end of night duty, a severe penalty indeed for this difficult service. Only 2 of the schools have a more generous policy of giving 1 night off a week during night duty and 2 days "change time" in which to recuperate from the strain of the work.[81]

LENGTH OF INTERVALS BETWEEN ASSIGNMENTS

The intervals of day duty between the several assignments of night duty should be of such length as to permit the student to make the proper physical adjustment, if she is to derive the maximum educational benefit from both day and night services. The proper intervals between assignments to night duty cannot as yet be dogmatically laid down since no common agreement has been reached except within broad limits, as to the time required for normal adjustment between day and night duty.

[81] The conduct of time off during night duty in schools of nursing is in marked contrast to ordinary industrial practice in which 2 nights off a week are usually given during night work, that is, always Sunday and usually Saturday nights.

An interval of 2 months would seem, in the meantime, a fair estimate of the minimum desirable time.

With a view to determining the prevailing practice in the training schools, a study was made of the intervals between assignments of night duty of 153 students in 6 schools. This examination showed that over a quarter (27.9 per cent) of these intervals were less than 2 months and 11.5 per cent of them less than 1 month. Two schools maintained by large municipal institutions of many wards requiring a numerous night staff, naturally show a high proportion of short intervals between night duty assignments, 43 per cent and 29.5 per cent respectively being less than 2 months. A comparatively small maternity hospital shows the highest proportion of the shortest intervals between assignments, 29.1 per cent being less than one month—a consequence, in this case, more probably of poor planning than of actual necessity. If this cross section may be taken as fairly representative of hospital practice, it is certain that a large percentage of student nurses are subjected in these inadequate intervals to an unwarranted hardship.

HOURS OF NIGHT DUTY

The inclusion of a disproportionately large number of superior training schools in the group visited by us is shown by the high proportion having 8 hours' night duty. The 8-hour night, made possible by using 3 shifts, obviously represents the best practice. It is as yet wholly exceptional. A recent inquiry on hours addressed by the League of Nursing Education to about 1,000 schools of nursing connected with hospitals of more than 50 beds brought out highly damaging facts with regard to the hours of night duty. Of 504 schools reporting (exclusive of California where 8 hours is compulsory by law), only 189 had the 8-hour day. Only about a third of these or 64 schools stated that they had in effect the 8-hour night.[82]

Graph 4 shows the length of night duty in 23 schools visited.[83] Approximately one-fourth of these, that is 6 schools, had adopted the 8-hour night system. Eight hospitals, or 35 per cent, still subjected students to the usual 12-hour night, with relief only

---

[82] National League of Nursing Education, Proceedings of the 26th Annual Convention, 1920. Page 99.

[83] The graph represents the total hours of actual duty per night, including a brief period for the midnight meal allowed by all hospitals. In a few hospitals, where the hours are broken by a period of temporary relief, the total hours of duty are given, excluding the relief period.

for the midnight meal.   In industry similar hours for night work among unskilled men workers recently provoked vigorous protest from an enlightened public opinion.   For women workers in industry the 12-hour night is an anachronism.   What then can be said in defence of the 12-hour night for student nurses, working often under conditions of lonely responsibility and emotional strain, and undergoing this experience for its educational benefit?   The 9 hospitals between these extremes, as shown in

GRAPH 4

COMPARISON OF HOURS OF NIGHT DUTY WITH HOURS OF DAY DUTY IN 22 SCHOOLS, SHOWING PROPORTION OF SCHOOLS IN EACH GROUP.

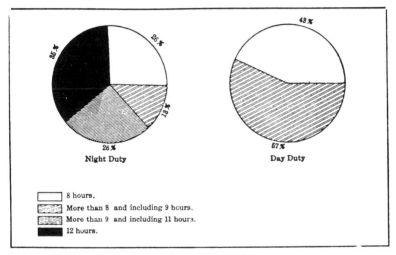

Night Duty   Day Duty

☐ 8 hours.
▨ More than 8 and including 9 hours.
▨ More than 9 and including 11 hours.
■ 12 hours.

Graph 4, apparently represent transitional stages between the 12-hour and the 8-hour schedule.   It cannot be urged too strongly that these advances towards better practice should be carried further until the 8-hour limit for night duty is reached.   Graph 4 shows also the relative duration of hours in day duty and in night duty at the 23 hospitals studied.

According to general hospital practice, the student on night duty is relieved for a brief midnight meal.   All but 4 of the 19 hospitals reporting on arrangements for the night lunch state that a specially prepared hot meal is served to students on night duty.   Often, according to the evidence of students, the quality of the food served is decidedly inferior to that served at regular meals. At three of the other schools the supervisors and students prepare a hot lunch for themselves. The one remaining school, connected with a famous general hospital, provides the student when she goes on duty in the evening with a basket of lunch which she eats at her post during the night.

PROVISION OF SLEEPING QUARTERS FOR STUDENTS ON NIGHT DUTY

The student's ability to meet the physical strain of night duty must depend to a considerable extent on provisions made for undisturbed sleep during the day. Such provisions on the part of the training school authorities would seem a primary safeguard for health and efficiency. Yet in only 6 out of the 20 schools affording data are these elementary precautions effectively taken.

Six schools make no provision at all for insuring quiet or privacy for night nurses during the day. In 5 of these hospitals, moreover, the majority of the students sleep in double rooms occupied jointly by roommates, and in one the majority of students are housed in dormitories. Under such circumstances adequate sleep for student nurses is quite plainly out of the question.

Eight schools post a card on the doors of rooms where night nurses are sleeping. As all of these 8 schools provide for the most part double rooms for students, and as the girls on day duty must come in and out, there is very doubtful assurance of quiet sleep. The posted card, moreover, does not keep out maids coming in to clean the rooms.

Only the 6 training schools already referred to follow the standard plan of providing a separate building or a separate floor in the nurses' home for night nurses. Even this arrangement is open to objection in so far as it involves the necessity of students' repeatedly having to move their effects from room to room. Only 1 of the 6, a university training school, makes definitely the ideal provision that students shall have the privilege of retaining their own rooms while housed in separate quarters during night duty instead of having to remove their entire belongings from one room to another. One school indeed stated that it had abandoned the plan of separate quarters in favor of the practice of posting a card on the door, because the students so much disliked to move. It can be quite readily understood that students having to suffer the inconvenience of frequent moving might prefer

THE HOSPITAL SCHOOL OF NURSING 439

the risk of disturbance in their own rooms. But certainly, unless assurance of uninterrupted sleep is possible under some other plan, separate sleeping quarters should be provided and insisted on, and their importance for health in the long run should be impressed on the students. Unfortunately, under the inelastic system of management too often prevailing in the nurses' home, routine is held more important than quiet rooms for sleep. In several cases known to the writer in schools of high reputation, students on night duty seeking permission to sleep in empty rooms quieter than their own were peremptorily refused by the superintendent of the school.

PROVISION FOR CLASS HOURS FOR STUDENTS ON NIGHT DUTY

But adequate and unbroken sleep is not only of prime impor-. tance to health during the strenuous weeks of night duty; it is important also in the interest of the student's education. Her alertness to the educational opportunities on the wards at night, her mental receptivity and power to profit by class instruction in the daytime, are in large part dependent on her freedom to satisfy the primary need of sleep. The mistaken policy too often followed in the schools of allowing class work to infringe on the 8 hours' rest indispensably required by the student on night duty cannot be too vigorously condemned.

All 23 schools studied provide class work for students on night duty, but much of it is given at hours and under conditions that go far to nullify its potential benefits. Like the class work given to day nurses, it is given in addition to the regular hours of duty. To receive class instruction with any real profit after a fairly continuous day's work is a serious drain on the energies of any student, however ardent; to attempt to receive such instruction after from 10 to 12 hours of night duty is a task so nearly impossible as to rob the instruction of much of its value. Two-thirds of the hospitals studied (15 out of 23) hold classes either in the early morning or in the early afternoon, which means that students must cut short their needed hours of sleep. The contention that class work can thus infringe upon sleep only once or twice a week is rather a reflection on the meager amount of class work offered than an extenuation of so ill-advised a schedule. Seven hospitals give their classes after 4 p.m., thus allowing sufficient time for night nurses to obtain their 8 hours' rest.

Not only do excessively long hours during excessively long periods of time characterize night duty, together with insufficient sleep, but the common understaffing of wards further limits its educational opportunities, and increases the physical burden of the service. It has been estimated that the ratio of patients to students on the general wards at night should not be higher than 10 patients to 1 student. The training schools studied generally exceeded this desirable ratio. Indeed the ratio of 10 to 1 is a rare minimum; the average, as shown by Table 13, is twice as high, and the maximum in 3 out of 16 hospitals reaches as high as from 30 to 40 patients to a single student nurse. As shown in Table 13, one-half of the 16 schools reporting on this

TABLE 13

RATIO OF PATIENTS TO ONE STUDENT NURSE ON MEN'S AND WOMEN'S GENERAL WARDS IN 16 SCHOOLS OF NURSING *

Number of Patients	Number of Hospitals	
	Men's Wards	Women's Wards
8- 9	..	1
10-11	..	..
12-14	3	5
15-19	5	4
20-24	1	1
25-29	4	2
30-34	2	2
35-39	1	1

Median:
Men's Wards   22
Women's Wards   19

* Seven schools did not have records on this point.

point apportion from 12 to 22 patients to 1 student nurse on the men's general wards during night duty. The remaining schools assigning from 22 to 40 patients to 1 nurse (that is, 35 and 40 both in men's and women's wards) are in large municipal hospitals with a great number of chronic wards which obviously need least nursing service at night. In the women's general wards the proportion of patients to nurses ranges somewhat lower than in the men's wards, but still greatly exceeds the standard ratio. One institution reported an assignment of but

8 women patients to the care of 1 student nurse at night, while at the other extreme, a maternity hospital assigned 36 patients to a single student. Nineteen patients to a nurse represents a mid-point between these extremes on women's general wards at night. In schools in which the wards show so deplorable a lack of nurses, it is self-evident that the demands of nursing routine can leave little opportunity for study, and often even insufficient time for the nursing care required.

LENGTH OF TRAINING BEFORE FIRST ASSIGNMENT

The charge of an excessive number of patients during night duty is a special hardship to the student having her first assignment. The unnatural conditions of working at night, the added emotional strain resulting from the conscious responsibility of being alone, with often inadequate supervision, in charge of a large number of patients, renders the practice of assigning students only a few months in training to night duty a needlessly severe ordeal.

Only 4 schools require the students to be in training 9 months before a night duty assignment; 15 schools require 6 months or less of previous training; 6 schools specify only 3 months or less, and 2 of these only 2 months.

Nine months suggests itself as a reasonable minimum length of training before students should undertake the difficult readjustments required in night duty. This period seems none too long for the young student's preliminary initiation into the strange life of the hospital and her mastery of the routine details of day duty.

SUPERVISION DURING THE NIGHT

The lack of adequate supervision is one of the most deplorable features of night duty work. It means not only that the student has no actual instruction during this long period of her training but that she is often charged with responsibility beyond her due. Especially on her first assignment to night duty, when the strain of unwonted responsibility is greatest, adequate supervision is bitterly needed. In many small hospitals students are left totally alone at night in charge of wards with only the superintendent to awaken at need. Of 21 hospitals visited by us and reporting on this point, 12 provide only a single night supervisor to oversee all student nurses. As her supervision duties embrace the entire hospital building, she may easily be out of reach at the very crises when she is most needed, and which students in consequence must face as they best may alone. Six hospitals make somewhat better arrangements by providing one assistant to the general night supervisor. The best system in practice among the hospitals observed, that of assigning a student as junior nurse during her first night assignment, to assist a senior, was found at only 4 hospitals.

In the maternity hospital already cited, students were assigned to night duty in the nursery, until very recently, after being in the hospital only from 2 to 4 weeks. During this assignment they served as assistants to a senior nurse for short shifts during the night. While on this duty they slept on couches in an alcove leading from the nursery, and in the words of the superintendent of nurses the practice was recommended "because it teaches the nurse to waken briskly, and be wide awake instantly when called for duty. It trains her to sleep lightly, as going to sleep expecting a call." Such Spartan practices, of doubtful value in any case, are examples of the unnecessary burdens often laid upon beginners. Surely the essential hardships of night duty can be trusted to offer sufficient "discipline" without adventitious and avoidable trials of the young student's strength and will. It should be the object as it certainly is the interest of the training school authorities to assign night duty to all students but especially to beginners, under such safeguards as shall release its full value for training while reducing to a minimum its standing risk of physical and emotional overstrain.

LIVING CONDITIONS

The primary importance of the living conditions provided for the students in hospital training schools was long unrecognized. It is therefore highly encouraging to note that while many factors remain to be remedied, and while lack of funds still often results in poor if not unmistakably bad physical equipment, there is at least gaining ground a recognition that for the best interests of both students and hospitals, normal living conditions must be provided. Against the old crowded and often insanitary arrangements progressive superintendents of schools have long contended. One such superintendent, known to the writer, on assuming direction of a well-established school with a university connection, labored for over a year before she succeeded in getting sufficient funds to abolish from the nurses' residence the old abomination of the "double-decker" bed for two persons, placed in this instance in rooms which were small for a single bed and one person.

But while, even a few years ago, in plans for new hospitals or additional wings, the nurses' residence was a quite secondary consideration, it is now increasingly seen to be one of the important features of hospital construction, and the provision of better living conditions a legitimate factor in attracting students of good calibre.

"Coming from the care of patients," says, for instance, a recent article in the "Modern Hospital," "the nurse on entering the home should step into a different atmosphere. There should be nothing to remind her of sickness." [84]

It would appear self-evident that the exacting character of the student nurse's work and her long hours of duty make it the more necessary that her hours of rest should be made genuinely restful, that the machinery of her life should, so far as may be, move without friction, and that her limited opportunity for relaxation, recreation, and exercise, should be furthered and not frustrated by her conditions of living. Normal surroundings in her hours off duty should offer her the means of escape and relief from the institutional and professional atmosphere in which she spends the larger part of her waking hours.

Finally, if the traditional hospital system of military or monastic control and routine obedience can be replaced by one of free co-operation in which some individual spontaneity and initiative can flourish, there can be small question of the value of such a more modern policy to the student's development and happiness in her work.

It is indeed too late in the world's history to invoke the monastic and military ideal, and in dealing with the present student body, hospital and school authorities may as well recognize first as last that they are dealing with a group of young women entirely similar to those in any other modern vocational training, with the same mixed motives of ambition, financial need, and devotion to ideals which animate girls and women entering other professions or occupations.

Entering the nurse's training is no longer an entire consecration. That the student body has changed in tone and motive from the earlier pioneers seems not only unquestionable, but

[84] The Nurse's Residence. Edward F. Stevens, Stevens and Lee, Architects. The Modern Hospital, April 1922. Page 322.

reasonable to expect. The students are as a group younger. They share necessarily the questioning spirit of the age. With the swing of the pendulum from the extreme repression, the excessive subordination of the past, they will probably show an extreme reaction towards independence and self-assertion, at least in their time off duty. That they respond less hopefully to progressive ideals or to a progressive educational guidance, there is no ground at all for believing. It is for this reason all the more desirable that unreasonable rigidity, such as still survives from an earlier era in many training school rules and conventions concerning discipline, dress, habits of life, social intercourse, and the like, should yield to a more modern accent in education.

LIVING QUARTERS

Of all the desiderata for normal home life which shall yield the student the maximum amount of recuperation and development, the basic needs have to do with housing conditions. According to general custom among the hospitals studied, living quarters are provided by the training school without expense to the students, whether at the home hospital or during affiliation.

The first essential, unquestionably, is that these living quarters should be detached from the hospital buildings, out of range of hospital sights, sounds, and smells, so that the home life of the students may offer the refreshment of a change of scene as complete as possible from that of the atmosphere of their work. Of 22 hospital schools studied in our special group, this essential of detachment was met in all but 4. Though all had students' living quarters in fairly close proximity to the hospital, in only 2 cases were they under the hospital roof. In these 2 the nurses' home occupies a separate wing but can be entered only through the main hospital building. In 2 other cases a scarcely less bad arrangement makes an actually separate home placed behind the hospital accessible only through the hospital itself.

The remaining 18 schools provide living quarters ranging from admirable up-to-date nurses' homes with all modern conveniences of equipment, and attractive furnishings, to old-fashioned run-down buildings lacking essential comforts, or make-shift student lodgings in made-over private houses or flats. In some cases small family houses or apartments have been used from the beginning in place of any dormitory; in others, family houses have been used as overflows as the school increased beyond the capacities of the original nurses' home. In the latter case, especially, they are too often incompletely converted to their present use, with results of genuine hardship or inconvenience to their inmates; thus, frequent instances were found by our observers where students must pass through other students' rooms to reach bath, toilet, or wardrobe; many of the rooms were ill-lighted and gloomy, and the atmosphere was generally forlorn and unhomelike.

In one training school 5 remodelled cottages added to the original dormitory provide a restful and convenient home life for the students' free hours. These cottages are family houses, refitted and attractively furnished, each one in charge of a matron and cared for by a maid, with sitting room for the use of the students and the entertainment of their friends, and with kitchen and laundry equipment at their convenience. Meals, however, are eaten in the common dining room of the main building.

PRIVACY: THE SINGLE ROOM

Even in the more institutional life of the dormitory, it should be possible to fulfil some minimum conditions of quiet and privacy, at least for sleep. The ideal arrangement is the single room, with its assurance of freedom from talk, noise, and the possible friction of other personalities. To the student in training whose working life is spent among people, needing constant adjustments and contacts, the freedom and relaxation of such privacy is peculiarly valuable.

No training school of the group studied has as yet provided single rooms for all its students. More than half of the schools still have more double rooms than single. The archaic dormitory system still survives in 9 of these schools. Most of the dormitories are furnished with 3 beds, some with 4, 5, or 6, while in 4 dormitories the number actually rises to 10 apiece! On the other hand, a distinct tendency towards the provision of single rooms is discernible in the newer buildings. One large school has built nothing but single rooms in its recently added "New Home;" in one of the great municipal schools eight-ninths of the student rooms are single. In a number of others, double rooms constitute only a small majority. The double bed is fortunately obsolete. In all the schools of our study, double beds were found in but two rooms.

TOILET FACILITIES

It would seem unnecessary to stress the importance of adequate toilet facilities for students whose training should make a scrupulous personal hygiene not only a matter of health and comfort but a point of professional pride. In such a calling as the nurse's the most punctilious personal cleanliness and daintiness should surely be made not only possible but easy and convenient.

In the majority of nurses' quarters provision of toilet facilities is indeed fairly satisfactory, especially in the newer buildings. In these, stationary wash basins are customarily installed in each room. In houses where wash basins are found only in the general toilet rooms the proportion is generally 1 basin to 4 or 5 persons. Among several unpleasant exceptions, one case was found where the toilet provisions for 14 persons consisted of 1 basin and 1 tub. In the matter of bathtubs, the showing is considerably worse. While a number of schools provide a tub to each 4 or 5 persons, and one, even more liberally, 1 tub to 3, there are other instances where 1 tub must serve 8, 10, 14, 16, and even 22! These are not always by any means exceptional cases of makeshift quarters. In one very large school where the entire student body is housed in a single building, there is an average ratio of 10 persons to a tub. At another school the ratio is 14:1 in the main building and 22:1 in the annex. With a group of people living on schedule, whose bathing must be done within short time limits if at all, such a dearth of toilet facilities puts a premium on going unwashed. For girls going on duty at 7 a.m. or to breakfast at 6:30, it means rising perhaps as early as 5 o'clock. How can the student, we may reasonably ask, be expected to take seriously the teaching of personal hygiene and immaculate cleanliness in the hospital, when conditions in the nurses' home deny her the rudimentary decency of a daily bath?

In contrast with these insufficient bathing facilities, provision of toilets in the nurses' quarters is generally adequate. At three schools only were exceptions found: one house had but 1 toilet for 14 or 15 persons; two others have 1 each for the use of 10.

EATING ARRANGEMENTS

In all schools visited the students come together for common meals, even when housed in separate groups. The highly ob-

jectionable practice found in a number of schools of serving the
students' meals in the hospital building is to be condemned
since it robs them of even the slight break and change involved
in quitting the scene of their work for the meal hour. As a
general rule, however, a common dining room is provided in
the nurses' home, or in the main building where there are several
homes. Some of these dining rooms are very attractive; one
notably, though seating 300, is furnished with small round tables
holding from 4 to 6, so that a group sense, at least, of privacy
and quiet is preserved. Almost without exception the food
served at the schools visited was good; in several cases its
quality was emphasized as excellent. Table appointments, also,
such as china, linen, etc., were found to be generally satisfactory.
At but one hospital were they criticised as poor, while at several
they were specially commended.

In the matter of service, conditions are less good. If the
short meal periods are to furnish the students what rest they
may, it is obvious that the food should be promptly and comfortably served without effort on their own part. For this reason
cafeteria service, however good of its kind, is unsatisfactory
because it shifts the burden of waiting, on the students already
taxed with hours of standing and hard work. This cafeteria
plan is in practice at a number of the schools; at others regular
dining room service is quite inadequate, while at two or three
only is thoroughly satisfactory provision made.

HOME LIFE

Beyond the obvious necessities of food, lodging, etc., provisions for the comfort and convenience of the students' home
life vary greatly at different schools. There is fairly general
recognition of the need of girls living away from home for sewing and laundry facilities, as well as for kitchen privileges. Only
5 of the schools studied were without conveniences for sewing.
These are comfortably provided in most cases in a regular sewing room, though in some of the smaller schools more casually by
machines kept in hallways or in a less used classroom. One
training school of conspicuously liberal policy provides a seam-
stress, who, in addition to certain hospital work, is allowed to do
sewing for the students at a nominal charge. Conveniences for
laundrying and pressing are also very generally provided. They
are entirely lacking in only one school, though in two others the
laundry facilities consist only of the stationary wash basins,

and in a fourth the slop hopper in the bathroom is most unsuitably used. In most cases a laundry, often specially equipped, is at the students' disposal.

All but 6 of the nurses' homes visited either provide a kitchenette for the students' use or allow them the privileges of a general kitchen. One large school has a kitchenette on each floor of its principal nurses' home. Such conveniences are a very real addition to the students' comfort, not only for recreational use but in cases of emergency when special extra food or simple remedies are required.

RELAXATION AND STUDY

Less material adjuncts but even more important for satisfying the students' needs outside of the hospital are a recreation room, a liberal and convenient supply of books, and a comfortable and quiet place for study. These requirements are not so adequately met.

At a few of the larger schools special rooms fitted up as libraries are used very properly by the students for the preparation of their work. Two others have special studies. At the rest, such work as the students do is done without the inducements of convenience or comfort. They must study in empty classrooms, often poorly lighted for evening work and without provision of table space, or in their own bedrooms.

Books in varying quantities are found in all the homes, but arrangements for their use seem in most cases little calculated to encourage the love of reading. We have referred in an earlier section (see page 290) to the difficulties besetting the use of reference books. Most training schools cannot provide a librarian, and it is a practice regrettably common to keep professional and general books alike under lock and key. While the key is given on request to take out books, the deterrent of getting it, slight as it is, no doubt suffices to bar most of the casual enjoyment of books as well as much of the more serious reading possible in the very limited leisure of the students' lives. Conditions of chronic overwork in many of the schools leave the students at best but little initiative beyond their routine duties; to many of the girls in training, moreover, the use of books is unaccustomed. In the face of these difficulties, the hope of developing any interest in reading must depend primarily on complete freedom of access to the books together with the encouragement of comfortable surroundings.

At the smaller schools the best conditions for reading are found where the books are on open shelves in the students' sitting rooms and are thus always available.

These students' sitting rooms or recreation rooms are found in the great majority of the schools studied. In 7 out of 23, however, nothing of the kind is provided. In one of these the lack of any reception room as well, practically precludes any social home life for the students. Contrasted with this neglect is the abundant provision at 2 large hospitals of sitting rooms on each floor of the nurses' home, at 2 others of roof gardens, and at still another of a tea-room, in addition to a recreation room.

SOCIAL LIFE AND RECREATION

The limited time and energy left the student for social life and recreation, the practical difficulty, with her rigid schedule of hours, of making social contacts in the outside world, makes it all the more important that opportunity should be offered within the training school for such social life and normal amusement as her work permits.

A prime social necessity from the students' point of view, and from the point of view of any thoughtful management as well, is a place to receive their friends. This need is very generally met by the training schools by the provision of reception rooms. In 4 schools, however, such a room is altogether lacking, and in one of them no arrangement is made to replace it. Here, and at another school, students may meet men friends with whom they are going out in the superintendent's office; they apparently have no place whatever for receiving callers. At a third school they are allowed to receive their friends in the general reception room of the hospital. In a fourth training school without a formal reception room, it is the custom to use in its place the very attractive student recreation room at certain times. On other occasions, students must rely on the general hospital reception room, less objectionable for the purpose here than in most hospitals since reception rooms for the patients' friends on each floor leave the students almost undisputed possession of the main reception room.

In all schools but the 2 wholly without provision for entertaining callers, students are allowed to receive their men friends up to 10 p.m. Small hospitalities are permitted in some of the schools: in one tea is served on Sunday afternoons; in another cocoa with cakes or crackers is served every evening to the nurses and any friends who happen to be calling.

SOCIAL RELATIONS WITH THE MEDICAL STAFF

It is gratifying to see that the traditional social taboo against members of the hospital medical staff has largely given way. In but 2 schools out of 13 giving information in the matter is social intercourse between students and medical staff forbidden. In 2 others internes are invited to occasional dances or other social functions, but no personal social relations are permitted. In all the remaining schools members of the medical staff are received on the same footing as other men. The lowering of the artificial social barriers formerly raised between groups of young people thrown together in their work and likely to have much in common seems a recognition of the good sense and dignity of each group which is not likely to affect adversely the strict professional etiquette of their relations on the wards and in duty hours.

AMUSEMENTS AND EXERCISE

Besides frequent informal dancing among the students themselves to the music of a victrola or piano, formal dances are occasionally arranged at some of the schools. More rarely there are plays or glee club concerts, and two of the schools have their own moving pictures.

For exercise, tennis and croquet are very generally provided for, sometimes on the hospital or training school grounds, sometimes in adjacent city parks. In the case of several schools, a neighboring Young Women's Christian Association supplies opportunity for swimming as well as other indoor recreations. Canoeing and skating, picnics and visits to bathing beaches, are spoken of as amusements enjoyed by other groups of students.

DIRECTED RECREATION

The desirability of actual guidance in recreational activities must depend on the type of student at any given school. At many schools of our study, the student body is largely made up of girls with a background of education and culture, advantages of college or travel, experience such as teaching or other responsible work. In such cases recreational direction is manifestly unneeded. Other groups of students, on the other hand, were, in the main, girls of more limited resources in education and social experience. For these the presence of the "social director," employed at certain training schools, would have definite and appreciable value, and might mean much to the students' development. Aside from any direct guidance, the superintendent of nurses has an opportunity of enormous influence in creating the atmosphere and setting the tone of the nurses' home, in stimulating healthy interests and in making the three years of training a broader education than that of mere technical equipment.

In no case can this influence be more potently or helpfully exerted than in the matter of student government. Whether under self-government or faculty control, the aim of any modern system must be admitted to be free co-operation, not the military discipline and automatic obedience of the old tradition. On the superintendent must depend in the last analysis the responsibility for the sympathetic and friendly atmosphere without which no system of government can be really successful.

Methods of discipline in the home life of the training schools visited vary considerably, but there is a visible tendency towards self-government. The system is already established at 4 of the 15 schools affording data, and in 2 others initial steps have been taken towards organizing it. In several others where faculty control is still maintained, the policy is described as "rational," looking towards student co-operation and the development of individual initiative and responsibility.

In some few schools it was found that the authorities still adhered to the traditional rigid type of control. This involved in certain cases at least a petty military discipline, detailed rules for all occasions, and a general policy discouraging to self-expression or spontaneity. In schools where the old system still obtains, our observers ascribed to it the degeneration of *morale*, the slack and disorganized discipline arising quite naturally from a sense of repression and of natural resentment on the part of the students.

Self-government, however, is regarded by many school authorities with a good deal of critical detachment. Even at the schools where it has been tried, the verdict is not one of unqualified success. The students, no doubt reflecting the attitude of the management, are often themselves uninterested in its introduction. In one case at least, they have definitely gone on record against it. At another school with a notably high grade of students but where the superintendent has for some reason appreciably failed to establish cordial and sympathetic relations with them, one student expressed the opinion that the authorities were not in favor of student government and that under such circumstances it could not succeed.

But the point is hardly sufficiently recognized by training school heads that self-government, like other experiments in democracy, is not an end but a means; that it is primarily for the development of the students, not to get perfect or finished results, and that it may sometimes involve a partial sacrifice of efficiency in the interest of education. From this larger point of view, the criticism of the superintendent who said that the system "took too much time" must seem wholly wide of the mark.

It must of course be distinctly understood that the province of self-government cannot extend beyond the personal and home life of the students. Just as in colleges self-government does not and cannot apply to academic matters, so in training schools the hospital authorities cannot abrogate their responsibilities towards the sick, or delegate to the students such matters as ward assignments and ward management.

It must, moreover, be admitted that self-government in the training schools is on trial under circumstances of unusual difficulty. With the decreasing age requirement for entrance, very young and inexperienced girls in the unaccustomed environment of the hospital are in many cases thrown into conditions of peculiar intimacy with men, whether patients or doctors. The many special problems thus created by the youth of these students make the results of self-government where it has been established seem as encouraging as could be expected. It is noteworthy that in the two large schools where it has been most sympathetically introduced both superintendents and students express themselves distinctly in its favor. The authorities in these cases have wisely led in the creation of the public sentiment which alone can assure the success of the system.

13. Conclusions and Recommendations

In the preceding chapters, in giving our findings of fact, we have in general stated the conclusions indicated by these facts. Without introducing fanciful counsels of perfection, we have under practically every topic balanced examples of bad practice by examples of good practice. Just as in the business world, industries exist side by side, using the same raw materials and labor supply, and supplying the same markets, yet in some cases enabled by good management and good will to provide, with profit, wages and working conditions of a standard alleged to be impossible by less competent competitors, so in the hospital world we see a similar phenomenon. Hospitals of practically similar grade and similar facilities, financial and clinical, exist side by side, the one providing by good management and good will excellent facilities for training student nurses in services which in a comparable hospital are totally disorganized and worthless for training. In urging changes, therefore, the appeal is not to an impossibly ideal condition but to a condition already approximated in some hospitals and accomplished in others.

In the present chapter we attempt to sum up the conclusions indicated in the course of the report, and to outline the curriculum and the type of training which is, in our opinion, not only desirable but attainable.

In formulating these conclusions we have been guided by twofold considerations: not only, that is, by the undeniable necessities of good training, but also by the equally undeniable immediate needs of the hospital. To introduce radical innovations into any established human institution is obviously a slow and delicate task. In their business of nursing the sick, the hospitals cannot at once, or even within a short period of time, be deprived of their present labor supply of students.

Changes must of necessity be gradual, and since the great majority of training schools will continue to keep their close relationship with the hospitals of which they are now parts, it is essential to point out how that relationship may be readjusted to meet at least the minimum claims of education. In our subsequent discussion of endowed schools of nursing we may further outline the training available in an economically independent professional school.

INCREASED COST OF TRAINING

Before proceeding to our suggested curriculum, emphasis must again be laid on the fundamental need of recognizing the school of nursing in the hospital as an educational department which definitely undertakes to give students a training calculated to meet the needs of their future potential patients as well as to care for the immediate patients in the hospital. With this understanding, the need for a rounded training covering all services is clear.

The present custom of using the school of nursing to furnish often the entire nursing personnel will not be superseded until hospital boards and the public are convinced of the unavoidable evils and interferences with training which it entails. We cannot too often reiterate that the crux of the matter is financial. Any changes at all, however small in the beginning, mean an *increase in cost.* But it is an increase of cost which is not new or avoidable; indeed this increase has already begun.

Quite irrespective of the recommendation of this Committee the cost of nursing service in the hospital is bound to grow. It has already grown during the past few years, not alone owing to war conditions, but because the shortage of students has led to the slow but steady increase in paid supplementary services to staff the wards.

Once admitted, this paid staff cannot be dismissed or the need for it forgotten. Once a colored maid has effectually in one hospital replaced students in mending rubber gloves, they will not again be assigned to five or six hours a day of mending gloves in the operating room. Once a graduate nurse has in another hospital been assigned to operations after 8:00 p.m., students will not again be kept hours overtime for emergencies.

We have pointed out that the educational needs of the training school have never been rightly exploited or even given due publicity on which to appeal for needed educational endowments. In order to do this most effectively, it is very desirable that the true costs of the training school be a matter of current record in hospital accounting, and that in calculating costs the income from student services be rightfully balanced against the expenses incurred by the training school.

THE NEED OF A PERMANENT PAID STAFF

For the care of the sick in hospitals in the future undoubtedly permanent services of various grades will have to be provided. Besides the yearly quotas of student nurses, a force, varying according to the size and type of the hospitals, of graduate nurses, attendants, ward helpers, orderlies, and clerical assistants must be, and indeed in many instances is already, recognized as necessary.

With the methods of meeting the financial costs of improved training for nurses, this report obviously cannot cope. These costs of the nursing service are bound up in the whole administration of hospitals and cannot be met alone. Such obvious and urgent reforms in hospital management as, for instance, the reclassification of patients (while totally outside the domain of the training school) would go far to simplify the problem of nursing service. Thus, the segregation of chronic and convalescent cases would make possible a far wider use of the trained attendant than is at present possible, and release student nurses for their proper training in acute wards. Full state support for the indigent cases and the steady increase in paying patients, induced by the high wages of war time, but evidently a more or less permanent phenomenon, are both important elements in the reduction of overhead hospital costs.[85] The joint employment of graduate nurses by private patients not needing full-time nursing care would release the student nurse from the educational waste of private duty without entailing expense to the hospital. Hospital cost accounting itself, as is well known, is urgently in need of reform to clarify the causes of hospital deficits. By economic readjustments of which these are single examples, the training school, like other departments of the hospital, would benefit.

The financial needs of the training schools, as they are at present organized, thus appear to be bound up with the whole organization and financial policies of the hospitals, and cannot be solved alone. The essential point is that the indispensable educational needs of the school of nursing must be brought home as never before to hospital authorities and to the public. If public health is purchasable, part of the cost price, never as yet adequately paid, is the school of nursing. That bill has never even been presented to the public. The present moment may well be auspicious to do so, when as never before the nurse is in demand; when public health has become a new reality, a new object to countless persons, and its field agent, the public health nurse, is a world-wide need.

A Proposed Curriculum

In turning now to outline a desirable training and curriculum, we should make plain that no single norm can be dogmatically

* Cleveland Hospital and Health Survey, Part X. Hospitals and Dispensaries. Michael M. Davis, Jr. 1920. Page 868.

laid down for the great variety of hospitals and nursing schools which exist. The aim of this study has been, and its future usefulness should be, rather to make plain the functions of the future graduates of the training school and thus to clarify principles and policies on which training and curriculum should be based. In the complex problems of training which we have analysed, there can be no surer guide than the future needs to be met by nurses now·students, no more trustworthy determinant than the needs of the community which the school of nursing, in the final analysis, exists to meet.

Without dogmatically laying down a detailed program, we may, however, outline the fundamentals, the minimum requirements as they have emerged from our critical examination of the schools.

In outlining the following curriculum, we have not merely projected a scheme *in vacuo*, but have assured ourselves through conferences with training school instructors and administrators that it is a workable scheme. It should supply the basic training which study of the nurse's functions has shown to be indispensable for all nurses. It should suffice to equip the nurse wishing to devote herself to private bedside duty. It should suffice also to afford a basis for further graduate training in the three nursing specialties: private duty, public health, and administration in hospitals or training schools.

DIFFERENCES BETWEEN SCHOOLS

It goes without saying that any curriculum suggested at this time is of necessity in the nature of a compromise. With the widely varying conditions which exist in hospitals at present, the maximum opportunities and performances of some schools fall far below the minimum of other schools. Yet in the interest of even relative standardization, it may be helpful to outline minimum requirements which shall not, as a whole, compare unfavorably with the best training, on the one hand, now offered, or, on the other, set up standards wholly beyond the reach of smaller schools of lesser facilities, clinical and financial.

The value of attempting to formulate even relative standards has been shown by the excellent influence of the "Standard Curriculum for Schools of Nursing" set forth by the Committee on Education of the National League of Nursing Education, 1914-1918. This curriculum, limited in many ways as it appears today, has indeed set some standards of performance by which schools of nursing have been able to measure their work and to which they have with differing measures of success endeavored to attain.

It must, further, be self-evident, that the schools which have been enabled by good management and good will on the part of the authorities to go beyond the suggested minima, should in no way diminish their efforts to advance their standards and performances. Schools for which the suggested minima are at present unattainable should scrutinize their present course and equipment with a view ultimately to reorganizing them.

AFFILIATIONS FOR SMALL SCHOOLS

Through the joint employment of visiting teachers shared by several smaller hospitals, above all by recourse to neighboring educational institutions—the high school, the vocational school, the junior college, etc.—classroom instruction for student nurses throughout the country could be immeasurably strengthened. Provision of a joint board or committee to plan and supervise such educational experiments would be of inestimable value.

We have already expressed our belief that hospitals which are wholly unable to reach these minima, for lack of facilities under their own roofs or by proper affiliation with other institutions, are not fit places for training nurses and should abandon the attempt. With proper safeguarding of patients by the legal requirement of graduate supervision, such schools may have facilities sufficient for giving the shorter and less advanced course needed for the trained attendant which we discuss in a separate section.

ENTRANCE REQUIREMENTS

EDUCATION

One condition for reducing the present three-years' course should be a higher standard of entrance requirements. In many states the only educational requirement for schools of nursing is completion of one year of high school. This means that the student is too ignorant to grasp the essentials of training. Schooling which has ceased at 14 or 15 years is no preparation for a professional training and, as shown in our studies of nurses in the field, fatally handicaps their future usefulness and success. Completion of four years of high school should be the minimum entrance requirement.

That the schools themselves realize the need of adequate schooling as a basis for the training course, is shown by the fact that in various states in which too low a standard is specified by law (viz. one or two years of high school), this standard is voluntarily exceeded by various schools. Of the 23 schools of our study, only 7 merely met the varying state requirements; 15 exceeded the state requirements by from one year to four years; 11 exceeded by three years the requirement of one year of high school.

AGE AND PERSONAL QUALIFICATIONS

During the seven years between 1911-1918 the age requirement for entrance was lowered two years, that is, from 20 or 21 to 18 or 19. In order to recruit students it is important that, with the completion of high school required for entrance, the age of admission to training should coincide with the age of graduation from high school.

Physical examination of candidates is required in the better schools. It would be highly desirable in the interest of a stable student body to supplement this by some method of determining the grade and type of the intelligence and character of applicants.

Hours of Duty

DAY DUTY

In the threefold interest of health, of efficiency in practical work, and of education and study, it is recommended that hours of duty for student nurses should not exceed 8 in one day or 48, preferably 44, in a week. Class work should be included in duty hours and ultimately study also. Instead of the two afternoons off duty now commonly given after 6 hours of work, there should be one full day's rest in seven. Obviously all these changes cannot be pressed at once. With the immediate adoption of the 8-hour day, the reduction of weekly hours and the establishment of one day's rest in seven should be brought about as soon as possible.

Except in cases of genuine emergency, the schedule of hours planned should be rigorously maintained by an adequate system of supervision. In special services where long and irregular hours are inevitable, the employment of a paid permanent staff, large enough to dispense with student service at the end of duty hours, offers the only effective safeguard against overtime. Nor should it be forgotten that the most reasonable schedule of hours may become exhausting if conditions of understaffing are allowed to throw the responsibility of too high a ratio of patients upon the individual student.

NIGHT DUTY

In view of its admitted drain on energy and health, the total length of night duty in the training course should be as short as is compatible with the maximum educational values to be derived by the students. It should therefore be assigned in services most fitted to develop its characteristic benefits, notably in the medical and obstetrical services. It is believed that these characteristic benefits of night duty can be effectively gained in a period of not more than 2 months, and it is therefore strongly recommended that the total length of the service, now 6 months or more at the majority of the hospitals studied, should be limited to 2 months of the entire training course. Separate assignments may not to advantage exceed 1 month, and time should be allowed students between assignments to make the needed physical compensations for the excess fatigue involved in the service. If 8 hours is deemed advisable as the maximum length of day duty, it is even more important that this limit should not be exceeded at night, nor should students subject to the severer strain of night service be further penalized by the loss of their weekly holiday. In order that the burden and responsibility of night duty should not be prematurely imposed upon young students, it is further recommended that it be assigned only after a fixed minimum length of training, say 9 months. Even more important than in day duty is the assurance of a careful supervision, and the maintenance of the standard ratio of patients to students.

REDUCTION OF THE PRESENT THREE-YEARS' COURSE

In our opinion the reduction of the present three-years' course is of the first importance both in order to aid in meeting the increased demands for nursing service of all kinds in all parts of the country, and to aid in recruiting students who may well hesitate to devote three years to a training to which they may be willing and able to give a shorter period of time. The three-years' course not only should be radically reduced by about one-fourth, but can, in our opinion, be so reduced to the advantage of training.

This reduction can be effected by the following means:

By the elimination of services of least value for student training such as private duty.

By the radical reduction of other services in which students now spend time totally disproportionate to the educational value of the service, such as the surgical wards, the surgical supply room, the diet kitchen.

By the saving of time now educationally barren in the first year for lack of theoretical instruction later given to explain the nursing and treatment of the diseases encountered; and finally

By the saving of training educationally barren in the third year through the monotonous repetition of duties.

Against this reduction of time we must however allow for the various necessary improvements in training already noted.

The amount of time lost throughout the course in many schools in ungraded repetition of duties cannot be stated in figures but amounts to a substantial waste which can, as we have indicated, be eliminated by assigning students to progressively graded experiences.

ENRICHMENT OF THE PRESENT COURSE

By providing manual workers and ward helpers the schools will save student time wasted in non-nursing duties now amounting, by conservative estimates, to an average of from one-fourth to one-fifth of their time in most services.

In our subsequent discussion of the curriculum (see page 470) we show that if the students give to study the average daily time thus wasted in non-nursing duties, this time would be amply sufficient, without any other change in training, for the added hours of instruction which are, in our opinion, indispensable for adequate training.

In the proposed curriculum which follows, an effort has been made briefly to restate the general principles on which training should be based and to give, frankly as a compromise and only as a next step in nursing education, a minimum educational program, with a suggested division of services in the hospital.

In order to avoid, so far as possible, a dogmatic allotment of hours, various subjects which are variously subdivided by different schools, are grouped together, no precise division of time for each subject being attempted.

PROPOSAL FOR THE PRELIMINARY TERM

The first four months of training should be devoted to intensive study, for the most part in classroom and laboratory. There should be no regular ward duty. Students should be taken to the wards for concrete application and illustration of their studies, and to enable them to orient themselves in a new and complex environment.

Thus, for instance, in the teaching of nursing procedures, after sufficient time in the demonstration room students will obviously benefit from seeing demonstrations on the wards and themselves getting practice in such simple procedures as they may fittingly perform under supervision. In dietetics, students need a brief period in the diet kitchen in which to gain practice and deftness in actual cookery.

THE LABORATORY BRANCHES

We have sufficiently argued the case for the basic sciences in the chapter devoted to that subject. Here it suffices to reaffirm our belief that at some future date, all of the elementary chemistry and dietetics needed by the student nurse and increasingly given in high schools and vocational schools throughout the country should be required for entrance; that elementary biology, also increasingly a part of high school instruction, should likewise be a requisite for entrance as a basis for the bacteriology taught in the preliminary term.

When students enter with this modest but invaluable groundwork of elementary science, the training schools will be freed from the necessity of crowding four laboratory courses besides other subjects into a period of four months and in the time released will be able more adequately to develop the class work now crowded into the two subsequent years.

ELEMENTARY NURSING

Hospital housekeeping and bandaging are usually given as separate courses, and are here included with elementary nursing only to show the total allotment of time suggested for these allied topics.

The 90 hours suggested for these subjects in the preliminary term are supplemented by classes and quizzes on nursing procedures held in connection with the later instruction in diseases, and also by similar nursing instruction during the summer terms when fewer formal lectures and clinics are given.

INTRODUCTORY SOCIAL PROBLEMS

An introduction to modern social conditions is of inestimable value in giving to the future nurse the right point of view towards her patients. While the short course proposed can only initiate the student into a profound subject, even though supplemented by 15 additional hours later in the year, it may give her at least an elementary grounding in the social problems which underlie her future work. As a part of the course she should be made acquainted with the social service department of the hospital and its work both on the wards and in the dispensary. She should be taken on some visits of observation to the homes of patients, not herself to do work which she is not fitted to perform, but in order to see and to have interpreted to her the family conditions of hospital patients.

Such a course should teach the prospective nurse from the first something of the cardinal importance of preventive work, something of the social aspects of disease, in emphasizing the social background of the patients and the social problems bound up with their welfare.

SCHEDULE 1

PROPOSAL FOR PRELIMINARY TERMS (15 WEEKS)

Subjects	Total Hours	Hours per Week	
		Lecture	Laboratory
Chemistry	60	2	2
Anatomy and Physiology	90	2	4
Bacteriology	45	1	2
Elementary Nursing (including Bandaging and Hospital Housekeeping) * ...	90	2	4
Personal Hygiene	15	1	..
Dietetics and Cookery	60	2	2
Introduction to Social Aspects of Disease	15	1	..
Drugs and Solutions	15	..	1
	390	11	15

* In addition to instruction in the preliminary term, additional hours in nursing procedures are planned for the summer term.

This proposed curriculum for the preliminary term calls for approximately 37 hours of class work, laboratory and study per week.[86]   About 6 hours per week are thus available for practice on the wards, allowing for Sunday and the Saturday half-holiday.

It is suggested that in order to avoid carrying three laboratory courses at the same time, instruction in chemistry be concentrated during the first two months, and instruction in bacteriology during the last two months of the term.

PROPOSAL FOR PRACTICAL WARD TRAINING

GENERAL PRINCIPLES AND POLICIES

As we have emphasized throughout the course of this report, the ward training which follows the preliminary term should be planned to give a progressively graded and integrated experience. It is desirable that students be given the complete care of patients as soon as this may be safely undertaken. Additional experience in special phases of nursing care, such as temperature-taking, charting, medication, etc., may be given by varying assignments during the day or week.

In order to give the student sufficient experience in the general nursing care which is needed by all patients whatever the disease, and hence is common to all services, it is desirable that immediately after the preliminary term a short period of time such as one month be devoted to intensive training in daily care, on medical, surgical, or pediatric wards, respectively.

With the more rapid acquisition of manual skill and dexterity which such concentration affords, the main emphasis may then be devoted to instruction in nursing and treatment of the different forms of disease, without requiring the long-continued monotonous repetition of services now commonly held necessary merely for practice.

Of this instruction in the nursing and treatment of the different forms of disease, case study, medical and social, should be an integral and highly valued part. Teaching and instruction in case records, and case reports by student nurses should be regularly required in ward training.

	Hours
[86] Lectures	11
Laboratory	15
Study	11
	37

SERVICES COVERED IN THE PROPOSED PROGRAM

The Medical Services

It is proposed that the 6-months' medical service include 3 months in general medical wards, men's and women's, to provide experience in the care of all the commoner medical diseases, the greater proportion of which should be acute; these 3 months to be supplemented by a month in the medical dispensary. In the dispensary as wide an experience as possible is advocated, including especially venereal and skin diseases, and tuberculosis.

The remaining 3 months of the medical services should be allotted to communicable diseases, of which one-third should, if possible, be devoted to tuberculosis. While 2 months is a very short time for training in the other communicable diseases (diphtheria, scarlet fever, meningitis, venereal, etc.) these months are effectively supplemented by the training in communicable diseases obtained in the proposed 3-months' pediatric service.

Training in Tuberculosis

In order to give effective training in the central importance of prevention in tuberculosis and the education of patients in hygienic living this training should be given where possible in special wards or, where this can be arranged, in affiliated tuberculosis sanitaria. While at present such affiliations may be difficult to arrange for, there appear to be no insuperable obstacles to establishing them. Indeed, the assurance of a steady supply of students from affiliated schools, even for short periods of service, would assist in solving the difficulty of the tuberculosis sanitaria in obtaining an adequate supply of students. In the meantime, every school of nursing can at least require a good lecture course, illustrated, so far as possible, by demonstrations and clinics.

The Surgical Services

It is proposed that the 6-months' surgical service should include 4 months in the general surgical, gynecological, and orthopedic wards. The 2 remaining months may be assigned to the operating room, or 1 month each to operating room and accident ward. The surgical service should be supplemented by a month in the surgical dispensary. In the dispensary, effort should be made to give experience in the special diseases: eye, ear, nose, and throat.

Pediatric Service

Pediatric training should be given in special wards or in an affiliated hospital devoted to the care of children. It should include both medical and surgical diseases of childhood. In addition to 2-months' hospital pediatric service, one month should, if possible, be devoted to the children's clinic where experience may be had in the care of fairly normal children. In this connection emphasis should be laid on the feeding of well children. Work in the milk-room in preparation of infants' feedings should be included in this period.

Obstetrical Service

This 3-months' training should be given in special maternity wards or in an affiliated hospital devoted to obstetric work, and should include care of both normal and operative cases. If out-patient service is given, the chief emphasis should be placed on prenatal training for students. The student's presence and assistance at a specific number of deliveries should be required.

Training in Mental and Nervous Diseases

At a time when the mental factor in all disease is receiving constantly increasing recognition and emphasis, the nurse should have a thorough grounding in the prevention and treatment of mental disorders. This experience has in most instances to be secured by affiliation. It is proposed that the suitability of institutions for mental and nervous cases offering opportunity for affiliation should be determined by standards set by some central body, such as the National Committee on Mental Hygiene or the United States Veterans' Bureau.

When affiliations prove impossible to secure, the 2 months allotted to training in mental and nervous diseases should be spent in the medical services, where classes and clinics should be held on the modern nursing and treatment of mental disorders, using for demonstration whatever opportunities the hospital may afford. Such are, for instance, neurological patients in the general wards, as well as the mental phenomena in delirium during fever, recovery from anæsthesia, etc.

Relation of Special Services and General Training

It should be made clear that our proposed reorganization of training and division of services follows the tendency, now generally accepted in other professional training, such as engineering, of strengthening the basic fundamentals and reducing the time devoted to specialties.

In nursing education it is important also to bear in mind that in the specialties which follow the basic medical and surgical months, such as the children's service, communicable, and mental and nervous diseases, opportunity is afforded not only for learning those specialties but for the necessary continued training in nursing procedures and care, whatever the disease in question. In reducing the total course and eliminating repetitions of medical and surgical services, we have counted on the reinforcement of training in general nursing skill and experience during the months of experience in special services.

SCHEDULE 2
PROPOSAL FOR DIVISION OF SERVICES

	Months
Medical, including *	
Medical Wards........ ⎫	
Communicable Diseases. ⎬	6
Diet Kitchen........... ⎭	
Mental and Nervous..	2
Surgical, including *	
Surgical, Gynecological and Orthopedic Wards ⎱	6
Operating Room or Accident Room.......... ⎰	
Obstetrical	3
Pediatric *	2
Dispensary, including	
Medical Clinics.... ⎫	
Surgical Clinics.... ⎬	3
Children's Clinics.. ⎭	
Vacation	2
	24

* In addition see under Dispensary.

Under this course the order of services can be adjusted at need, except that the major part of the medical and surgical services are supposed to precede the special services.

COMPARISON OF PROPOSED DIVISION OF SERVICES WITH ACTUAL EXPERIENCE RECORDS OF STUDENTS

Before proceeding to our proposals for theoretical instruction during ward training, it is highly instructive to compare our proposed division of services with the actual experience of students of one class from each of seven hospitals studied, as shown in Table 14 (page 468).

In order to determine the actual disposition of their time, a special study was made by us of the daily assignments during three years' training of about 250 students in these schools. From this study we have already illustrated (see page 137) the chaotic differences in the assignments of students of the same class, as illustrated by the minimum, median, and maximum number of days spent in each service. We may now compare our proposed division of services with the number of months spent in each service by the median girl who typifies the average experience in each school. In order to reduce the figures to manageable proportions and make possible a fair comparison of our proposed plan and the hospital records, we have summarized the months of practical training under the seven services listed in column one.

It might be supposed that cutting down roughly a third of the time of training would reduce the essential services by one-third. That this is not the case is proved by this comparative study of the proposed division of services and the actual experience of students. From this table it is clear that in the shortened course, the surgical services are radically reduced, and private duty and electives in public health and social service (often offered in the third year) totally eliminated. The pediatrical, obstetrical and dispensary services are markedly strengthened. The proposed mental and nervous service is lacking in 4 of the 7 hospitals and longer in only one municipal hospital where it over-balances the training; the length of the medical services in the shortened course compares favorably with that given by 4 of the schools, and is exceeded only by 2 municipal hospitals in which a large chronic service unduly prolongs the time of training, and by one of the university hospitals. The prolongation of medical and surgical services in private duty is eliminated.

It may be said that the group of 23 hospitals studied is too small to warrant conclusions. For this reason it is the more fortunate that we are able to show in the last column of the table the days spent in the several services by a group of 200 students from approximately 100 schools of nursing. These students, graduated in 1919 and 1920 from Teachers College, had received their hospital training during the ten preceding years. Comparison of the shortened course we propose with this column, representing a "control group" of hospitals many times larger than the group studied, significantly reinforces our picture of nursing education as at present conducted. The characteristics

TABLE 14

COMPARISON OF PROPOSED DIVISION OF SERVICE WITH ACTUAL EXPERIENCE RECORDS OF STUDENTS OF 1 CLASS OR REPRESENTATIVE SECTION OF CLASS IN EACH OF 7 SCHOOLS OF NURSING AND WITH ACTUAL EXPERIENCE RECORDS OF A SPECIAL GROUP OF STUDENTS FROM 100 DIFFERENT SCHOOLS.*

Services	Proposed Plan Months in Each Service	Median Number of Months Spent							
		In Hospital No. 1 by 61 Students	In Hospital No. 2 by 32 Students	In Hospital No. 5 by 21 Students	In Hospital No. 6 by 67 Students	In Hospital No. 9 by 31 Students	In Hospital No. 21 by 11 Students	In Hospital No. 23 by 17 Students	By Special Group from 100 Different Schools
Medical †	6	9	13¾	4¼	6	5½	5½	9¼	6½
Surgical ‡	6	14½	7	10½	12	9½	9½	10½	10½
Pediatric	3 ‖	1½	3	5¼	1¼	3¼	2½	3½	2½
Obstetric	3	3	1	1½	4	3	7	2	2¼
Private §	0	1½	¾	5½	3¼	7¼	6	..	3¾
Nervous and Mental	2	1	6½	2¾	..	..	..	..¶	..
Dispensary	2	1	¾	1½	1¼	1	1	1	¾

* Excluded from this table is all time spent in elective services and services which are available for less than half the students of a class. Time spent in practical work during the preliminary term is included in the designated services.

† Medical service includes all training in general medical, skin and venereal, communicable diseases, tuberculosis, diet kitchen, and the proportion of mixed services stated by the school to be medical.

‡ Surgical service includes all training in general surgical, gynecological, orthopedic, operating room, recovery, urological clinic, eye, ear, nose, and throat, and surgical supplies, and the proportion of mixed service stated by the school to be surgical.

§ Private service includes special and nurse's infirmary service.

‖ For purposes of comparison in this stable, service in the children's clinic is included under Pediatric, not under Dispensary.

¶ Service not given.

variously illustrated in the 7 hospitals specially studied are
reaffirmed in the larger group: the excessive over-emphasis on
surgical training and on private duty, the very scant allowance
of time in the dispensary, the total lack of training in mental
and nervous disease. The medical service is longer than necessary in this group also, since the 6½ months of the median experience include no training in communicable disease.

PROPOSAL FOR THEORETICAL INSTRUCTION DURING WARD
TRAINING

Proposals for theoretical instruction accompanying ward work
follow: In these proposals we do not seek to set a rigid curriculum for all schools. We do suggest the total number of hours

SCHEDULE 3

PROPOSAL FOR THEORETICAL INSTRUCTION

	Hours
Nursing in Medical Diseases	45
Elementary Pathology	15
Materia Medica	30
Diet in Disease	15
Massage	15
Nursing in Surgical Diseases, including Gynecology, Operating Room Technique, Orthopedic Nursing	45
Nursing in Special Diseases Eye, Ear, Nose, and Throat, Skin	15
Obstetrical nursing	30
Nursing in Diseases of Infants and Children	30
Nursing in Communicable Diseases, including Venereal, Tuberculosis	45
Nursing in Mental and Nervous Diseases	45
Applied Medicine and Public Health	30
Elementary Psychology	30
Social Aspects of Disease (supplementing preliminary course)	15
History of Nursing, including Ethics, Professional Problems	45
	450

which it is in our opinion desirable to give during the 2 years
of hospital training following the preliminary 4 months. The
curriculum is based on the assumption that during the first
academic year 10 hours weekly, and during the second academic

year 5 hours weekly, that is, only *an average of 7½ hours weekly,* are devoted to class work. During the two summer terms, it is assumed that instruction will be given chiefly in nursing quizzes, classes, and conferences, and no specific allotment of hours is therefore suggested for 6 months of the 2 years, in order to allow free play for the necessary differences of method and facilities in the various schools. Allowing for 30 weeks of instruction each year, a total of 450 hours may therefore be planned for.

COMPARISON OF PROPOSED COURSE WITH EXISTING CURRICULA

The total number of hours in our proposed curriculum may with advantage be compared with the total curriculum hours in the 23 training schools studied. In the following table the inadequacy of the existing instruction is glaringly apparent. Aside from any considerations of method or personnel in teaching, it is self-evident that with so scant an allowance of time for instruction, the manual side of the nurse's service must be greatly over-emphasized at the expense of her classroom and clinic training in the nursing and treatment of disease. Yet a reduction in the length of the course must to be successful be accompanied by more adequate and intensive instruction.

While our proposed curriculum of 840 hours exceeds all but one of the schools studied, the moderation of our proposal and the present educational deficiencies are shown by the fact that, as previously stated, it is based on the requirement of *only 7½ hours' instruction per week or about 1½ hours per day after the preliminary term on 5 days of the week, and presupposes no hours of formal instruction whatever during the two summer terms.*[87]

As we have shown in the detailed and conservative study of time wasted in non-nursing duties the 1½ hours of an 8-hour day so wasted would, if devoted to instruction, suffice to give the added hours needed for the curriculum. Our study of non-nursing duties is necessarily incomplete and includes only the most obvious causes of wasted time. It should be one of the next objects of inquiry on the part of the administration of hospitals to make more complete and more intensive studies of these sources of waste with the object of further reducing it and

[87] This is based on the group of students entering in the fall, as a norm. Obviously the group entering in January will need a different arrangement of hours.

thus making time in the 8-hour day for study as well as instruction.

Excluding from our preliminary term the 120 hours devoted to subjects other than the basic sciences, we find that our minimum of 270 hours for science teaching exceeds the science allowance of all but 3 schools. Yet besides the 2 university schools and one affiliated with a college which naturally give a fuller theoretical course than most schools, 2 other schools assign more than 200 hours to these subjects, and 7 others give more than 150 hours.

HOURS OF INSTRUCTION IN THE SCIENCES DURING PRELIMINARY TERM IN 22 SCHOOLS

Number of Hours	Number of Schools
50- 99	3
100-149	7
150-199	7
200-249	2
250-299	..
300-349	2
350-399	..
400-449	..
450-499	..
500-549	1

Proposed Plan: 270 Hours

Even in the schools in which the hours of instruction proposed by us for the preliminary term are exceeded or approximated, the hours of instruction during the 2 hospital years so far fall short of the minimum which in our opinion is desirable that only one school exceeds the total of 840 hours which we recommend. Only 8 schools of the 22 have more than 600 hours in their total 3-year course, the average being 578.

TOTAL HOURS OF INSTRUCTION IN 22 SCHOOLS

Number of Hours	Number of Schools
300-399	3
400-499	5
500-599	6
600-699	4
700-799	2
800-899	1
900-999	1

Proposed Plan: 840 Hours

Thus it is apparent that, under our proposed plan, not only is the course shortened by 8 months, but the training proposed is richer than that offered at present, except by a very few hospitals. The higher standards of admission and of teaching should operate, as in all other educational institutions, to increase, not to lessen, the number of applicants. The proposed changes should tend to meet the two insistent demands for more and for better trained nurses. If adopted, the shortened course will, we believe, both aid in stimulating an increase in the number of students and produce a type of nurse better trained for modern needs.

V. TRAINING COURSES FOR THE SUBSIDIARY NURSING GROUP

Following our study of a basic course for nurses we have next to offer suggestions for the training of a subsidiary group for sickroom attendance in minor disabilities or illness, or in convalescent and chronic cases. We have in a previous chapter pointed out that to suggest training for this group is not thereby to create any new type or grade of nurse. The subsidiary worker, known variously as practical or household nurse or attendant is already here, in numbers, according to the census of 1920, about equal to the total number of graduate nurses. Included under these names is a chaos of irresponsible and heterogeneous workers among whom the public has no means of distinguishing the experience or training of any individual. Our aim is to evolve from these chaotic conditions some method of identification and some method of attracting girls and women of more refinement and better address than most of those now available.

Capital Need of Regulation by a Licensing System

We repeat here as forcibly as possible the conviction expressed in our previous chapter that success in the employment of the subsidiary group is strictly conditioned by the enactment of state licensing laws which shall set certain minimum standards for all who nurse the sick for hire, just as similar laws regulate the practice of other professions under given designations, such as the doctor, the dentist, the pharmacist, etc., and thus protect the public by prescribing penalties for fraudulent use of the title.

In our earlier discussions we have also given examples of some short training courses for bedside attendants given by various associations, and have expressed the opinion that such courses, needing special endowment, cannot suffice alone to provide subsidiary workers in really adequate numbers. Where, then, shall additional training be provided?

PLACES FOR TRAINING

Just as the care of the sick in hospitals affords to generations of nurses a training and experience nowhere else to be duplicated, so might training and experience be given a subsidiary group in really adequate numbers in institutions where simple routine nursing duties, suitable to their capacities and future responsibilities, must daily be performed. Whether these shall be institutions for the care of non-acute cases only, or such hospitals or departments of general hospitals as are appropriate for training a subsidiary group, is our first consideration.

It has been suggested that attendants should be trained only in places where there are no acutely sick persons, or where such persons are segregated so that there shall be no opportunity to use the attendants for the care of acute cases. But in view of the large numbers needed, such a restriction would appear impractical. To limit the training of the secondary group to places where there are no acutely sick persons would not result in sufficiently increasing the supply.

There are in the United States approximately 400,000 beds in general hospitals. In special hospitals, the largest number of beds (about 300,000) are in hospitals for nervous and mental cases. Here attendants have long been employed and here it is suggested they should more extensively be trained. But it is doubtful, in view of the special nature of these cases, whether girls and women of the type desired for simple bedside care in the home will be attracted to these institutions for training. Moreover, the need of attendants for nervous and mental cases is itself so overwhelming that increasing inducement will undoubtedly be offered to retain within these institutions so far as possible the attendants trained there. It does not appear probable that the supply of subsidiary workers of desirable standards will be greatly increased from this source.

It has also been suggested that tuberculosis hospitals, in which throughout the country there are approximately 50,000 beds, should be used for training attendants. Undoubtedly desirable training can well be given in connection with these institutions. But as sources of supply for subsidiary nursing service in the home, owing again to the special nature of the disease and the need of the institutions themselves, these hospitals seem to us to offer as little promise as institutions for mental and nervous cases. The material proportion of former patients taken for training further precludes the probability of obtaining from institutions for the tuberculous a large increase of subsidiary workers for household engagement.

There remain, among the special hospitals of the country suitable for training attendants, those for cripples, for convalescents, and for chronics. But all of these together number only about 15,000 beds.

It is true that a large additional number of beds, variously estimated at from 150,000 to 200,000, exists in institutions such as homes for children and the aged, etc. The desirability of training attendants in these institutions alone, owing to the restricted opportunities, is open to serious doubt, though they would be of service for part of the training. According to the rulings of the New York State Department of Education, for instance, training in these institutions alone is not accepted as sufficient to admit candidates to examination for state licensing as "trained attendants."

The question arises whether no other places of training are available. In our study of hospital training schools we have seen that, while many schools connected with small hospitals can supplement their teaching and clinical deficiencies by affiliating with other institutions, and can thus successfully round out their classroom and ward instruction, there undoubtedly remain large numbers of other small schools which are not in a position so to affiliate and whose own facilities are too limited to meet even the minimum requirements for a basic course for nurses. It should be considered whether such small schools may not be developed into appropriate places for training the subsidiary group of workers.

Use of the Small Hospital

At present, schools connected with small hospitals, that is, hospitals of less than 50 beds, make up 40 per cent of the approximately 1,800 training schools of the country. It is often said that schools incapable of conducting a training school for nurses are incapable of conducting any educational undertaking. But is this necessarily true?

Undoubtedly, in training the subsidiary workers, primary emphasis should be laid on the fact that any training is itself an educational undertaking, requiring teaching and supervision. But the subsidiary group, not being destined to have the responsibility of caring for acute disease, needs neither the laboratory sciences nor instruction in the nursing and treatment of disease, on the importance of which in the basic nursing course we have laid emphasis. The teaching and supervision of the subsidiary group is therefore of a much more elementary order than that required for the regular school of nursing.

The fear is sometimes expressed that if the subsidiary workers are trained in schools connected with small hospitals, acutely sick patients in those hospitals will suffer. This is a genuine danger to be guarded against with utmost efforts. Only the provision of an adequate number of graduate nurses can safeguard the care of such acutely sick persons as there may be in the institution. With a state licensing law which places the establishment of all training schools under the appropriate educational authority of the state, the adequate provision of graduate nurses must be a required condition in the establishment of schools for subsidiary workers.

LIMITATIONS IN THE USE OF LARGER HOSPITALS HAVING SCHOOLS OF NURSING

Reservation of certain types of small hospitals for training the subsidiary workers is not incompatible with the use also, for this purpose, of larger institutions maintaining schools of nursing, provided that the education of the two groups of students can be successfully managed. Experience indicates that the training of the two groups when carried on in one institution should be kept separate. There must therefore be assurance that the clinical facilities are sufficient and appropriate for each group. Certainly the training of student nurses and of nursing aides should not be carried on in the same wards. This is because of the twofold danger to student nurses and subsidiary workers alike. The practical difficulties of teaching the two groups on the same wards are obvious on the surface. How shall the work be equitably divided? It would undoubtedly be highly detrimental to the education and development of the young nurse—probationer or in her first year—to be assigned to the same wards with subsidiary workers who might be at a later stage of their training. The equitable division of the work offers almost insuperable difficulties. In our discussion of the permanent employment of subsidiary workers on hospital wards we have already pointed out dangers to be guarded against in their assignments. We have noted the impropriety of employing nursing attendants in nursing procedures which they were not qualified to perform, while on the other hand student nurses were deprived of opportunities for learning the procedures in question. Even were the attendant qualified by practice under supervision to assist in the procedure instanced— a lumbar puncture—the educational loss to the nurse in being deprived of opportunity would have been no less great.

On the side of the nursing aide, training in the same wards with nurse students has proved no less unsuccessful. The temptation is almost irresistible to relegate to the subsidiary worker all the manual and disagreeable household tasks, without any of the simple nursing duties which she can rightfully be taught to perform and which give meaning to her training.

And here we find ourselves invoking, on behalf of the attendant in training, the argument and defense which we have previously sought to invoke on behalf of the probationer and student nurse. No more than they can she be merely exploited in the institutions. True, she, like them, must repeat, until perfect, routine duties and tasks in themselves distasteful, must scrub and scour and dust, clean bedpans and wash soiled linen. True, also, that the subsidiary worker, through her necessary limitations, her short course and differentiated sphere, can never have the supreme experience of the fully trained nurse in sharing issues of life and death, in grasping to any such degree as can the nurse the relation of her work to the nature and treatment of disease. But if this training is to attract girls and women of refinement and good address, rather than mere drudges inappropriate to the sickroom, it must give them scope besides these manual duties to get from such care of patients as they are competent to perform the zest of nursing service however humble, a sense of the worth of their contribution which will tend to vitalize training and to satisfy.

The minimum requirements, therefore, in schools planning to train both groups should be:

Adequate, suitable, and separate clinical facilities for each group.

Provision of a special nurse-instructor and supervisor of the subsidiary group.

A sufficient number of registered nurses to supervise the practical experience of the subsidiary group, so that they may not be under the direction of student nurses, and so that the care of patients may be safeguarded.

In seeking to outline tentative suggestions for a course for the subsidiary group we should stress the fact that, unlike the hospital training of nurses, there is here no body of accumulated experience to draw on for guidance. The comparatively few courses which exist are wholly experimental and in the formative stage. Few standards exist as yet as to the length of the course, subject matter, types of practical experience, or content of class work. The most that can be done is briefly to outline the procedure which best commends itself in the light of such experience as has been obtainable.

We have pointed out that the subsidiary worker, like the graduate nurse, may be employed in any one of the three nursing fields, in private duty, in connection with public health organizations, or in institutions. For the nursing attendant as for the nurse each of these three types of work has somewhat different requirements. In view of the still experimental nature of the subsidiary training, it would appear desirable at this time to plan for the fundamentals of training of which there can be no question. Subsequent differentiations needed, let us say, in the hospital or by public health organizations, may be worked out under supervision of the employing agency.

LENGTH OF THE COURSE

In consonance with the principle which has guided our discussion of the schools of nursing, the length of the course for attendants should be as short as is consistent with a thorough grounding in the fundamentals included. In our opinion these fundamentals can be taught in a period of less than a year, or approximately 8 or 9 months.

ENTRANCE REQUIREMENTS

Educational requirements for this training should be less than for the full nursing course. Completion of grammar school or its equivalent, as required by various state laws, would appear to be sufficient. The subsidiary worker can be taught the simpler nursing procedures, the elements of asepsis, etc., household work and cookery, without the educational preparation indispensable for the fuller professional course.

Age requirements for the subsidiary group should be more flexible than for the basic nursing course. Older women, beyond the age of entering nursing training, should be admitted.

Women whose children are grown often desire to take up simple bedside nursing and are well qualified to do so. The minimum age for entrance should be set at 18 years.

PRACTICAL EXPERIENCE

It is asserted with some justice that one great advantage of courses conducted by associations which send their students to hospitals for part of the training is the supervised experience in home nursing which constitutes the final part of the course. In Boston, for instance, during the final 6 months of the Household Nursing course the attendant in training is sent to selected home cases, under the direction of a visiting graduate nurse supervisor. The supervision in the cases observed by our field agent appeared to be satisfactory, and good relations existed between attendant and supervisor. The attendant thus learns to apply in ordinary home conditions what she has learned in wards or in classroom. Her duties include such care of the household as concerns the welfare of her patient. Sending children off to school and overseeing the household may be as helpful or necessary to the convalescence of the mother as actual nursing care.

Whether the course is maintained by an institution or an independent association, it is desirable that the student's home be used as the practice field for training in household economics and cookery, so as to habituate the nursing aide to home conditions in housekeeping. This training, of at least one month, should preferably be given at the beginning of the course.

WARD TRAINING

Suggestions for the types of cases within the institution in the care of which the subsidiary worker may best receive her training are well enumerated in the tentative rules relating to the licensing of attendants published by the New York State educational authorities: [88]

  Chronic and convalescent medical patients.
  Minor operative and convalescent surgical patients.
  Obstetrical patients, postpartum after third day.
  Normal infants after third day.
  Appropriate tubercular patients.
  Convalescent and well children.

[88] Course of Study and Syllabus for the Guidance of Schools for Trained Attendants. The University of the State of New York, Albany, 1921. Page 13.

CLASS INSTRUCTION

ELEMENTARY NURSING

In the elementary nursing lessons for which 60 hours, or 30 periods of 2 hours each, are recommended in the curriculum given below, the general methods of teaching should approximate those used in teaching student nurses. There should be, that is, demonstration by the teacher, "demonstration back" by the student, opportunity to practise, and finally, application of the instruction on the wards. While the nursing attendant will be taught only the simple procedures needed in non-acute disease, her technique should be carefully supervised, and gentleness and consideration for patients be inculcated.

Among the practical procedures taught, the chief should be:

Beds and bedmaking.

Keeping the patient comfortable in bed, and routine care, such as care of mouth, hair, back, etc.; attending to physical needs.

Baths of all types, in bed and out of bed.

Prevention and treatment of bedsores.

Temperature, pulse, and respiration.

Keeping simple bedside chart.

Administration of common medications.

Local applications for inflammations and congestion.

Irrigations of throat, inhalation.

Care of simple infectious conditions.

Enemas, vaginal douche.

More difficult procedures needing a more careful technique and training in asepsis, such as catheterization, are in some courses taught to the subsidiary group. The wisdom of including these procedures is, however, seriously open to question.

Suggestions for a curriculum follow:

	Hours
Elementary nursing	60
Simple cookery and diet for the sick	40
Hygiene	15
Home economics	10
Care of infants and children	10
After-care of obstetrical cases	5
Care of chronic and convalescent patients	5
Care of the aged	5
Care of tubercular patients	5
	155

This program calls for about 4 hours a week of class instruction and demonstration during the course.

A suggestion which commends itself is that instead of having separate lessons on elementary anatomy and physiology, the nursing attendant should be taught in connection with the appropriate lessons in elementary nursing, personal hygiene, and cookery, the necessary details of anatomy and physiology such as structure and function of the body; organs, bones and their relative positions; general description of digestive apparatus; organs involved in circulation and respiration, etc.

Similarly, a few lessons in bacteriology may fittingly be included in the hygiene lessons, explaining origin and growth of bacteria, and their relation to health and disease; the meaning of antisepsis and asepsis; methods of disinfection for sputum, clothing, and dishes; disinfection, sterilization.

For the lessons on simple cookery and diet for the sick an allotment of time next longest to nursing is recommended: 20 periods of 2 hours each.

Hygiene should include besides the bacteriology and physiology indicated, several periods on personal hygiene, on hygiene of the home and on public sanitation.

In the lessons on infants and children, besides teaching symptoms and care in the common ailments of infancy and childhood, stress should be laid on the physical development of the normal child, modification of milk, care of bottles, nipples, etc.

For a suggestive outline both of procedures to be taught and the content of class work, now in effect, the reader is referred to the tentative rulings of the New York Board of Regents already referred to. Obviously, only through process of experiment can these tentative rules ultimately be judged and either prove their worth or prove the need of modification. New courses are being introduced in St. Louis and Kansas City, Missouri, following the Missouri licensing law, which are not yet as fully worked out as the suggestions for the New York course.

The whole subject needs to have applied to it the best thought and practical experience of leaders in nursing education. If they will apply to the evolution of an adequate training for the subsidiary group the same courage and determination which has won its way in nursing education against the heaviest odds, they will have provided for a no less imperative public service which should rightly be under the direction and support of the nursing profession. The regulation and supervision of courses for nursing aides should be under the same state boards of registration as the hospital schools of nursing and all state nurse practice acts should provide for the licensing of nursing aides or attendants as well as for the licensing of nurses. As indicated in a previous chapter, the provisions of the Missouri act offer the best safeguards and should be followed in all subsequent legislation.

VI. THE UNIVERSITY SCHOOL OF NURSING

Thus far in our discussion of hospital training we have referred at many points to the university schools of nursing, with regard both to teaching in the classroom and practical experience on the wards. We have next to consider the special organization, status and value of the university school which in recent years has become an accepted development of American university education.

The superior educational opportunities afforded by the university or the college as compared with those offered by the ordinary hospital school are abundantly evident. On the side of physical facilities, in the first place, the college and university have as a rule the standard plant and equipment for laboratory work in the sciences which the individual training school finds it so difficult if not impossible to command; supplies and material of all sorts are abundant, liberally provided and easy of access; there are extensive libraries and convenient reading rooms. All these facilities are frequently placed at the nursing school's service; where this is not the case they do perhaps as great a service in setting a standard for the new department. On the side of instruction, the training school, unendowed as it is, can rarely afford the best teaching; the college or university connection guarantees teaching by men and women who are not only specialists in their subjects but trained teachers as well.

Thus the standardizing influence of the university, in replacing as it does the inadequate equipment of the training school and the often unacademic grade of its teaching, can scarcely be overemphasized. Hardly less valuable is the effect of the university atmosphere and surroundings on the student *morale*. Ambition reacts to the atmosphere of intellectual competition; the student nurse is stimulated to do her best and take her place with credit among her fellow students of the various schools. She feels, too, a new sense of dignity and of the importance of her work through her recognition as a member of an educational institution.

But the university with its large endowment and liberal educational standards is important not only for physical facilities, level of instruction, and stimulation of *morale;* it is important for the essential character of the training school itself. As a part of the hospital, without separate endowment of its own, it must inevitably be dominated by and subordinated to hospital needs; it must remain in the last analysis a hospital adjunct, not a disinterested educational enterprise. The long struggle, the devoted labor on the part of nursing instructors to make the student's professional training the first objective of the school is doomed to defeat by a system which depends on the training school for an unpaid nursing staff, and in any conflict between education and practical service must always put education last. In strong contrast is the position of the school of nursing which, as an integral part of a university, exists primarily as an educational undertaking.

It will of course at once be evident that the freedom from financial dependence necessary to the fulfilment of the training school's essential purpose can be achieved in other ways than by a university connection. Various types of organization under some independent body, with separate endowment like that of any other educational institution, would be among the means of better safeguarding the educational standards of the school of nursing. It is far from our purpose to suggest as physically possible or even desirable that the country's 1,800 schools of nursing should all be brought under university auspices. Only a minority will probably ever be incorporated into the university system, though it is to be hoped that the precedent set in Minnesota will be followed, by which the separate schools of three or more hospitals have been amalgamated under the university school of nursing.[89] But that this minority will be of capital importance, regardless of its numerical strength, as experiment stations, as pathfinders of a disinterested professional education for nurses, there can be no question.

We have spoken thus far of the direct advantages to the train-

---

[89] While by this arrangement the separate schools retain their individual identity, their definite acceptance of uniform standards set by the university marks an important step towards a central school.

"A similar plan of centralization," writes a leading professor of nursing education in a recent bulletin of the Bureau of Education, "is being developed in Cleveland under the auspices of Western Reserve University. There are obviously many advantages in such an arrangement, and it is believed that nursing schools, like medical and other professional schools, will more and more tend to consolidate their educational work in a few strong schools rather than in many small or weak ones." (U. S. Bureau of Education, Bulletin No. 20, 1921. Developments in Nursing Education since 1918. Page 14.)

ing school of the university connection. But we must not leave out of account an indirect benefit, perhaps not less important— the tapping of new sources of supply for the schools of nursing, the enlargement of the range of recruits attracted to the nursing profession. Much is said of the need, in the new field of opportunity opening before the nursing profession, of an abler and better endowed class of candidates; much of the demand for leaders, women of education and intelligence, who shall help to solve the intricate and complex problems of nursing in the modern world; but it is too often forgotten that the limited educational opportunity and the narrow character of the technical training at present offered by the majority of training schools must inevitably alienate the very type of women in behalf of whom these appeals are made. The larger educational range, the more advanced professional instruction offered by the university school will, conversely, attract a better prepared and more ambitious grade of student. In view of the fact that these schools must be regarded as a special training field for future public health leaders, administrators, and teachers of the nursing profession, this improvement in calibre is of cardinal importance.

EVOLUTION OF THE UNIVERSITY SCHOOL

While, as we have stated, the undergraduate school of nursing as a professional university school is still in the experimental stage, and still a relatively new venture, its roots go back to an earlier time than might be commonly supposed. The first beginnings of the university connection for the training school may be seen in the establishment of university hospitals for the clinical instruction of medical students. It was impossible that the nursing schools should not reap a certain amount of indirect benefit. In abundant clinical facilities, in teaching by the university medical staff, frequently in opportunities offered by the plant and equipment of the university, and not least in the educational atmosphere gained by the association of medical research and medical instruction, the schools of nursing shared, in the most favorable instances, in the privileges of the medical school.

In a few experiments in central teaching already referred to, arrangements made with a college or university to supply teaching in certain preliminary subjects are of interest, as creating another link between the university and the training school, though the work given is in no sense university work.

The first step towards university recognition of the nurses' training was taken in 1899 when Teachers College admitted properly qualified graduate nurses to the junior class, thus giving approximately two years of college credit to three years of hospital work.

Not until 1910, however, was a school of nursing established as a part of a university system. The University of Minnesota, the pioneer in university education for nurses, admitted students of nursing to this school on the same basis from the first as other college students, and gave its graduates a special professional degree. Other universities in some numbers, including Cincinnati, Colorado,[90] Indiana, Michigan, Missouri, Nebraska, and Northwestern, have followed the lead of Minnesota in giving professional training to students of nursing.

Meanwhile the introduction into colleges and universities of public health nursing courses for graduate nurses or senior students, first undertaken by Teachers College in 1910, was leveling prejudice against the student nurse in the university and establishing her right to a place in academic education.

But the movement toward university education for nurses did not stop here. Its latest development is the combined academic and professional course of five or sometimes four years, leading at once to the college degree and the nursing diploma. Since 1916 no less than 13 universities and 3 colleges have agreed to institute such a course,[91] allowing certain credits towards the B.A. or B.S. degree for the technical training course, and organizing two or three preliminary years of academic work which shall furnish some background of general and liberal education to the professional education to follow. By means of this course the young high school graduate, now often left at a loose end between graduation and the admission age of the training school, may in the interim continue her general education in the broadening and stimulating atmosphere of the university; the young woman hitherto obliged to choose between a college education and nursing training, attracted to the nursing profession but alienated by the narrowness of its technical program, may have two years of academic work including liberal courses before enter-

---

[90] Temporarily suspended pending reorganization.
[91] Cincinnati, Columbia, Leland Stanford, California, Colorado (course temporarily discontinued pending reorganization), Bayler, Iowa, Nebraska, Northwestern, Indiana, Minnesota, Michigan, Ohio, Washington, British Columbia, Simmons, Mills, Milwaukee, Downer.

ing upon her specialized training, and may obtain on her successful completing of the course her college degree as well as her
nursing diploma.

ORGANIZATION OF THE UNIVERSITY TRAINING COURSE

STANDARDS

The university nursing school must under ideal circumstances
be by definition an integral part of the university system. It
must be accepted by the university as co-ordinate with other professional schools, and must on the other hand rigidly conform to
its standards. Either through an independent endowment or
from the university it must have a regular, assured income, large
enough to guarantee its maintenance of university standards of
instruction and management. The members of its teaching staff
must all be members of the university faculty; its students must
qualify for matriculation on the same basis of record, certificate,
or entrance examination as other students. They will pay, too,
the same tuition fees as other students. During their period of
technical training in the hospital their services are commonly
considered fair payment for living expenses. Courses given in the
school of nursing must be as a rule not less than 30 hours in
length if they are to obtain college credit, in order to afford time
for a genuine study and not merely a superficial smattering of
the subject. For each hour, moreover, of lecture or classroom
work an hour to an hour and a half of preparation should be
required and allowed.

A somewhat different procedure is necessarily followed at universities which do not admit women to their undergraduate
schools. At such universities it is proposed to require two years
of academic work in prescribed subjects at a standard college as
prerequisite to two years of nursing training at the university
hospital, followed by a fifth year of postgraduate work.

FIELD FOR TECHNICAL TRAINING

But, however excellent the opportunities offered by any university for the didactic instruction of student nurses in classroom and laboratory, it cannot be considered a suitable field for
the organization of a school or department of nursing unless the
available hospital facilities are also of an appropriate type.
These should include primarily a wide variety of clinical mate-

rial, active services in the fundamental phases of nursing practice: medical, surgical, obstetrical, and pediatric, with facilities available, either in the university hospital or by affiliation, for mental and communicable disease. Large chronic or private services would clearly, on the other hand, disqualify a hospital as a suitable field for the technical training of student nurses.

But while ideally a complete and inclusive practice field may be regarded as a prerequisite for the organization of a university nursing school, an incomplete field need not necessarily be a deterrent, so long as the local geographical facilities hold out the possibility of supplementing and completing it. Thus, at the University of Minnesota the school of nursing was organized when the university hospital offered a limited field for training both in number of beds and range of services; but the clinical opportunities of the Twin Cities offered the promise of indefinite expansion. These initial incomplete facilities have been lately amplified by the affiliation of three local hospitals of high standing which have merged their schools of nursing with the university school, and have placed their wards as laboratories for the training of nurses at the university's service. This has added some 1,150 beds to the bed capacity offered by the original teaching hospital, and has extended the range of experience afforded the students from the basic medical, surgical, and obstetrical services to include pediatric, contagious, and venereal disease training, with accident and emergency cases, dispensary work, and the expected addition in the near future of a psychopathic clinic at the university.[92]

A word must be added about conditions of life and work for students in training at the hospital. If the hospital is to be regarded as a suitable practice field, these conditions must measure up to standards of health and efficiency considered desirable by the university: student nurses should be assured of reasonable hours (not in excess of 48 weekly), and in order that all these hours should be educationally profitable, should be relieved by a permanent staff of non-educational routine work. Living quarters should be comfortable and restful, and provision should be made for normal social life and recreation.

[92] The students' field of technical training thus consists of the university hospital, a free teaching hospital with cases chosen for purposes of study; the Charles T. Miller Hospital of St. Paul, a private hospital; the Minneapolis General, a large municipal hospital; and the Northern Pacific Hospital, a beneficial institution, supported jointly by the railroad and the railroad employees.

ORGANIZATION

Of possible types of organization, that type has certain undoubted advantages under which the hospital is owned by the university. Whether in the training school course leading only to a nursing diploma, or the longer course leading also to a university degree, this type gives the university a better control of hospital standards, and enables it to offer the student of nursing, whether in the shorter or longer course, a unified education from start to finish.

Under a widely different type of organization, the university has no hospital of its own, but provides for the technical training of its students through affiliated hospitals in the same city or state. Under this system, the university does not, of course, conduct the hospital school of nursing; it either accepts and gives credit for a school's existing plan of training, or it arranges with perhaps several schools to give special sections of courses upon outlines and under supervision furnished by the university itself.

It will readily be noted that in this connection the standardizing influence of the university school on the hospital can be powerfully exerted. In the possibility of refusing affiliation to hospitals whose instruction in nursing procedures, either in the classroom or on the wards, is below standard or educationally wasteful, the university school has a strong leverage. It should use its power of approval or disapproval freely for in no other way than by the scrutiny and criticism of the grade of teaching provided by the hospital can the educational side of the technical training be sustained against the exigencies of hospital needs.

In such a centralized system, moreover, there must be due recognition of the necessity for constant adjustments between the various hospitals constituting the group so that they may fit without friction into the joint undertaking.

STATUS IN THE UNIVERSITY

Up to the present time, the department or school of nursing of the university has very naturally been organized under some already existing department. Most commonly it has been made a part of the Medical School; in other cases it has been placed under the School of Science (British Columbia), the School of Liberal Arts (Leland Stanford, California), or the College for

Women (Western Reserve). But such organization can be regarded as temporary and transitional only. With the growing acceptance of university education for nurses, it is essential that the new department be given the dignity and autonomy of an independent status. In no other way can it escape subordination to conflicting claims, and be free to develop its own best possibilities. Especially is this true of its incorporation as a part of the medical unit. Instead of being directly responsible to the board of trustees, the school is placed by this organization under the domination of an intermediary group, and made subject again almost inevitably to the encroachments of the hospital service. The results of this policy under the old system led necessarily, as we have seen, to the formation of the training school committee in order to represent other than purely medical interests in the guidance of the school. To start the new experiment of the university nursing school under the auspices once more of a purely medical group is to perpetuate under a new name a system already found wanting. It goes without saying that during their practical training in the hospital, the student nurses must conform to the hospital régime. Where the university school of nursing has no independent status in the university, the establishment of a special training school committee,—representing the medical and non-medical faculty and the hospital trustees, if there is no university hospital,—is often found as valuable as such a committee has proved to be in the ordinary schools of nursing.

The department of nursing should have its own dean or director, a nurse who should be also a college graduate and who should combine with the highest professional qualifications some experience of college or university teaching. Where a university hospital exists, the director also serves in most instances as superintendent of nurses. This twofold office is open, it must be admitted, to serious criticism, as following a harmful precedent in setting up again the conflict of functions so often emphasized, in re-establishing the struggle between education and service. By a far better arrangement the director would remain the educational head and would have as her associate the superintendent of nurses, who should be an administrative officer simply, responsible to the director, however, for the efficiency of the student's practical training. In her own sphere of directing the nursing service exclusive of students, the superintendent of nurses would naturally be responsible to the superintendent of the hospital.

FINANCIAL BASIS

Though students of the department of nursing would be expected to pay the same fees as students in any other department of the university, it is obvious that such fees could not constitute more than a fraction of the cost of maintenance of the nursing school. Funds for maintenance of the new department would naturally be appropriated by state or city universities which may undertake to organize nursing schools. At other colleges or universities a special endowment fund would doubtless be needed. While it is of the first importance that this fund should be an adequate guarantee of good work and unhampered development, it must be borne in mind that the school of nursing will not need in the nature of things to support financially the whole weight of its teaching. While strictly nursing subjects will always be given by the department itself, as well as certain technical subjects not generally offered in the college curriculum, its theoretical work may largely be drawn from other departments. Whether this work is given without charge to the school of nursing, or paid for at a fixed rate, it will in any case constitute a far lighter financial burden than the maintenance of separate courses. Thus students of nursing may obtain their scientific training where laboratory facilities permit under the regular departments of science, their dietetics from the home economics department, their psychology from the department of education, and their social science from the department of economics and sociology. In addition to these, such liberal subjects as language and history which make up a substantial part of the first two years' instruction will naturally be taken under the appropriate departments, side by side with students working for the degree in arts. Some adaptation of these general academic courses to the special needs of the nursing group is in most cases essential, and may probably be best effected, as will be proposed in some detail in our discussion of training courses for public health nursing, by quizzes under nursing instructors who shall attend the courses and give the general work its special professional direction or by special adaptation of courses by the various departments.

FINANCIAL RELATIONS WITH OTHER DEPARTMENTS

The absence of any fixed financial norm in the maintenance of the school of nursing is noticeable everywhere. Some instances of the varying financial arrangements now in practice may be regarded as tentative and experimental rather than as offering any ultimate solution of the relations between the department of nursing and other departments of the university.

At one university, even courses given expressly for students of nursing are in certain departments considered a part of their legitimate work, and consequently charged to their budgets, not to that of the nursing school.[93] But other courses, such as anatomy and physiology, and English, are paid for at an hourly rate by the department of nursing, and appear on its budget. It is not unusual for laboratories and other facilities of the university plant, either in the medical or other schools, to be placed at the disposal of the nursing students without charge to their department; though in these cases such needed equipment as student microscopes is frequently not included in the offer and must be carried to and from the laboratories by the students themselves.

We may say in general that, so long as the students of the school of nursing are not too numerous to be distributed among the existing academic classes, they may be so entered during their collegiate years at the usual fees but without charge to their own department. According to the estimate of an academic authority, the majority of existing colleges could thus care for from 100 to 150 extra students on the basis of their regular fees.

But at many colleges and universities the limitations of plant and endowment are such that their present registration makes it impossible for other departments with the best will to extend any facilities to a new school, however small its body of students. At these a proposed school of nursing must meet the problem of securing an endowment adequate for the equipment of its own laboratories and the endowment of its own teaching. Rather, indeed, than dependence on the uncertain generosity of other departments, it would seem in any case a wiser plan and a better safeguard of the future interests of the school that some system of proportional costs should eventually be worked out by which the nursing department should bear its due part of the financial burden of the teaching and equipment in which it shares, and thus take its position as an economically independent unit in the university.

FINANCIAL RELATIONS WITH THE HOSPITAL

A somewhat more systematic financial adjustment is already in existence between the university school of nursing and the hospital. The system commonly in use takes cognizance of the

* For example, Junior Dietetics in the Home Economics Department.

fact that the hospital must provide for supervision of the nursing service irrespective of the presence on its wards of student nurses in training. Where students of the nursing school receive the benefit of this supervision, the costs are apportioned between the school and hospital budgets in whatever ratio is considered most just. Thus, by the plan followed at one prominent university school, supervisors' salaries are paid half by the hospital and half by the school. Teaching head nurses are for the most part paid by each in the same proportion. Instructors in the classroom and laboratory are paid wholly by the university, with the exception of the "instructor in science and dietetics" whose entire salary is paid by the hospital, on the ground, apparently, that her services would be needed by the hospital in any case. At another well-known university school, on the other hand, the dietitian's salary is apportioned, two-fifths to the school and three-fifths to the hospital.

THE CURRICULUM

For the combined academic and professional nursing course, the program generally agreed on covers 5 years: 2 to 3 college years, namely, of 8 months, and 2 to 3 hospital years of 11 months. Under varying arrangements, the first 3 years are at some universities devoted to college work, and the last 2 to hospital training. At others the first 2 years are given to college work, the 2 following years to general hospital training, and the fifth to specialization both in college and practical work, either in the hospital or in field training. Where students do not wish to specialize, it should be possible, by a larger proportion of summer work, to obtain the college degree and the nursing diploma in 4 years.

It is evident from the foregoing that no fixed norm has as yet been worked out for the curriculum of the nursing school. Broadly speaking, it may be said, however, that the collegiate part of the course is made up of required academic work, including the preliminary sciences. Some study of the humanities, commonly English, history, and modern languages, some work in economics or sociology, one course at least in psychology, and a good scientific foundation for the later professional training may be considered indispensable. If the course is reduced to four years, certain other subjects, such as dietetics, materia medica, and history of nursing, must be transferred, in the interest of relieving the pressure of the later years, to the earlier part of the course.

In this connection it is of interest to note the distribution of time in the college years as illustrated by typical curricula of several prominent university nursing schools. In the cases of 6 universities or colleges, the weighting of the principal groups of subjects was found to be as follows, as shown by the units or credit points allowed.

TABLE 15

University No.	Percentage of Credits Allowed to Principal Groups of Subjects			Years
	Liberal	Scientific	Nursing	
1	70	30	..	2
2	66–68	32–34	..	3
3	49	37	14	2½
4	39–52	48–61	..	2
5 (College)	37	60	3	2
6	7–49	51–93	..	2

It is on the side of the sciences pre-eminently that the university curricula show the most marked advance over the ordinary school of nursing. Instead of crowding into a brief period of from 3 to 6 months' elementary instruction in the several preliminary sciences, besides usually the intensive teaching of practical nursing and various other subjects, the university school can in its 2 or sometimes 3 college years give the student at least a somewhat more adequate scientific basis for her later practical work. On the side of general education, less progress has been made. Science in general claims from a third to a half of the points required for the academic years of the course, the proportion in one case rising to three-fifths. Liberal studies make up in one notable instance above two-thirds, but in three others from approximately a third to a half. In one university school the required scientific studies make up 51 per cent of the total number of points in the first 2 years of the course, the required liberal studies (90 hours of English) only 7 per cent. Forty-one per cent of the total number of credits is indeed assigned to electives, but while these, if directed altogether to liberal subjects, may raise the weighting of the liberal group to 49 per cent (48.7), there is nothing apparently to prevent their being allocated altogether to science, giving us a weighting of 93 per cent science as against 7 per cent liberal studies.

On the other hand, the 5-year course at another university school emphasizes the collegiate education of the student of nursing by extending it over 3 years and for these years assigns two-thirds of the credits to liberal studies such as English, languages, history, economics, or other courses in the College of Liberal Arts, and one-third to science. The plan followed here, in contrast to that of some of the other university schools, assures the student of a certain equipment of general education as a basis for her specialty. At another school the program proposed for a 5-year course allows 3 years of academic work and assigns between 50 per cent and 60 per cent of credits—the equivalent in credits of more than 3 semesters—to liberal studies. The 40 per cent to 50 per cent remaining is solidly devoted to science, all professional nursing subjects being concentrated together with the technical training at the hospital in the last 2 years of the course.

Hospital Training

During the summer between her first and second collegiate years, it is highly desirable, both as a means of eliminating the unfit from the nursing course and of orienting and fixing the interest of the well-qualified students, that each student should spend a period of perhaps a month in hospital practice.

In the summer after her collegiate term the student will enter the hospital as a nurse in training and will be given her technical experience together with her professional instruction during the next two or three years. Here the accepted standards should not only insure a high level of teaching but do away with the short and superficial courses so frequently tolerated in the present curricula of schools of nursing. Courses of less than 30 hours in the principal subjects should not be admitted for university credit, while short series of lectures on subsidiary topics might well be grouped into a single course of standard length.

In the 5-year nursing course the fifth year is generally devoted to specialization. According to the student's preference, she may take up public health nursing, or supervision in the hospital, or advanced specialties in private duty. In any case she will devote about half the time to theoretical work in the classroom and half to practical work; for public health nursing, in field practice under some nursing agencies; for teaching or supervision, in the hospital, where she may gain experience as assistant with the younger classes, as head nurse, or as a member of the office force.

We do not in this section dwell upon the hospital years of the university school of nursing. The practical experience of the student is sufficiently detailed in the earlier chapters devoted to ward and dispensary training. At its best the university affiliation or control leads to a new progressive accent in the applied teaching on the wards, as well as in classroom instruction. One of its main contributions may be seen in the development of the head nurse as teacher, not only in the practical supervision and instruction on the wards, but in the quiz classes by means of which she gives practical adaptation and concrete application to the science classes of the university, or to the lecture courses of the doctors. On the latter our observer comments at one of the university schools visited:

"The classes, conducted mainly by the head nurses, which accompany the doctors' lectures, are a distinct advance over anything which the investigator has seen elsewhere. There is student participation of a high order of excellence, and utilization of the facilities of the hospital in a way comparable to the uses made of it by the physicians in instructing medical students. It had the atmosphere of professional work, yet at no hospital was there greater consideration for the welfare of the patient."

This enlarged function of the head nurse puts an end to her position, too often accepted in the past, as an overworked executive devoting her scanty spare time to a necessarily perfunctory, unsystematic teaching or supervision of the student nurses on her ward. To qualify as she must under the university school organization as a member of the university teaching staff, she must be a trained teacher as well as a technical expert in nursing. So far from allowing her teaching work to suffer through the pressure of her executive duties, she must be relieved if necessary of administrative work in its interest. Even at other than university schools, interesting experiments in such a division of duties are in progress. Thus a leading municipal hospital is trying the plan of placing as head nurses on several wards highly trained young nurse instructors who shall devote their main energy to teaching while in each case an administrative officer shall take charge of all the routine executive duties of the head nurse's position.

Such educational experiments and many others may well be initiated under the university school and stimulated through its influence in other schools. But when all is said of the standardizing and stimulating value of university auspices, it is well to remember that a university connection or even university control is no guarantee of educational competence in ward teaching, and no safeguard against the evils of understaffing. The university hospital which is understaffed uses its students for hospital service instead of instruction no less consistently than other hospitals.

Even in the university schools, then, educational aims are still only slowly making their way. Cases such as we have quoted show the university school falling well below the mark of the best accepted practice. But in many questions of nursing education there is as yet no "best accepted practice," no consensus of opinion. It is precisely here that the university school can do some of its best service to the nursing profession. In its quality of experiment station it can test by practice the value of mooted educational theories and by the results of its experience influence their adoption or rejection by other schools. One important problem awaiting solution is the best method of relating theoretical instruction and ward training in the nursing course. Shall they be concurrent? The value of the close relation between theory and application thus gained is vitiated in large measure by the physical fatigue of the practical training which limits necessarily the value of study. Shall practical application follow or precede didactic instruction? By varying arrangements to be discussed at some length in connection with public health nursing courses, certain schools give separate theoretical and practical instruction, concentrating the students' time for certain weeks or months in classroom and laboratory, and again for a subsequent period of time in the practice field. At one progressive university school, the so-called "block system" is on trial, by which each of the first two years of the course is divided into three terms, and in each year the spring term is almost wholly given over to theoretical instruction and study. More of such experiments are urgently needed, not only to determine the value of dividing and concentrating theoretical instruction and technical training, but to discover, if the general principle is accepted, the most advantageous length of the respective periods. In such educational experimentation the university school may play one of its most valuable rôles.

CREDIT

Credit is assigned by the university for courses in the school of nursing on the same basis as for other college courses. According to the point system generally in vogue at American colleges, a course of 15 hours of class work for one semester constitutes a point; the average credits for a full year's work are from 30 to 36; and the requirements for the bachelor's degree mount up to about 124 points, or generally speaking, 4 years' work.

The basis of credit for technical work in the hospital is less easy to fix. No more than in the case of any other form of specialized technical training would it be advisable to allow this practical experience, however valuable, to mount up to more than 30 points or about one-quarter of the total credits required for graduation. By a not infrequent practice an allowance of one point for each month of supervised hospital work makes up a total of from 22 to 24 points for the 2 years of ward training. A like basis of credit is allowed for field work under public health nursing agencies.

DEGREES

The degree given to graduates of the school of nursing is at some universities the B.S. now used in many instances for certain branches of applied science as well as for pure science; at others the B.N. or G.N. The usual preference seems to be for the general degree, as indicating some general academic training, together with a special professional diploma, rather than the special degree in nursing with its exclusively technical connotation.

VII. POSTGRADUATE COURSES

1. Courses in Public Health Nursing

The educational implications of our study of public health nursing were summarized in an earlier chapter. Our analysis of the functions of the public health nurse impelled us to the conclusion that for this work a basic nursing course is the first requisite, to be followed by a thorough training in the specialty of public health nursing.

In our study of hospital schools of nursing we have discussed the value of the short courses in public health nursing offered to undergraduate student nurses in their senior year. We reached the conclusion that instead of these short courses, which in the schools of our study were taken by only about a quarter of the total number in the senior classes, sometimes without adequate preparation in the necessary basic hospital services, the principles of preventive medicine, and a minimum of social interpretation should be taught to all students in their regular hospital training, leaving for postgraduate training the special courses in public health nursing.

For the graduate nurse after her hospital experience, the minimum time needed to prepare for public health nursing has been found to be one academic year of 8 to 9 months.

So recent has been the development of all formal instruction for public health work, medical and sanitary as well as nursing, that it is scarcely surprising if much diversity of content and method is found in the postgraduate nursing courses. They have been developed in the main in response to specific needs in special localities. They have grown empirically; their directors using such facilities for practice work and for theoretical instruction as opportunity offered. Hence these courses are for the most part still in an experimental and formative stage, methods and subject matter being tested, rejected, or modified from year to year, while standards of minimum requirements are slowly being developed. In a word, we are confronted here with a new educational problem in professional education. The principles and subject matter appropriate for other vocational and professional education may well offer analogies and suggestive precedents. The actual adaptation to the field of public health nursing of these analogies and precedents is now in process.

From a study of the courses existing we may take stock of the main tendencies in the educational field and of the progress towards standardization. We may point out the most important objectives next to be aimed for.

History and Development of the Courses

Pertinent to the discussion of public health nursing courses is a brief review of their history and development. To gauge correctly their present contribution and the possibilities of the future it is important to realize how they originated and how they stand today.

NUMBER OF EXISTING SCHOOLS OR COURSES

During the year 1919-1920, the year in which these courses were studied, there were in existence in the United States 20 schools or courses in public health nursing.[94]

These schools or courses were the following:

California—University of California, Berkeley, Cal.
† Colorado—University of Colorado and Colorado Fuel & Iron Co., Boulder, Col.
Connecticut—Visiting Nurse Association, New Haven, Conn.
Illinois—Chicago School of Civics and Philanthropy, Chicago, Ill.
Kentucky—University of Louisville and State Board of Health, Lousville, Ky.
Massachusetts—Simmons College and The Instructive District Nursing Association, Boston, Mass.
Michigan—University of Michigan, Ann Arbor, Mich.
Minnesota—University of Minnesota, Minneapolis, Minn.
Missouri—University of Missouri, St. Louis, Mo.
New York—University of Buffalo, Buffalo, N. Y.
New York—Teachers College, New York, N. Y.
Ohio—University of Cincinnati, Cincinnati, Ohio.
Ohio—Western Reserve University, Cleveland, Ohio.
†Ohio—Ohio State University, Columbus, Ohio.
Pennsylvania—Pennsylvania School for Social Service, Philadelphia, Pa.
†Tennessee—George Peabody College for Teachers, Nashville, Tenn.
†Texas—University of Texas, Austin, Texas.
Virginia—School of Social Work and Public Health, Richmond, Va.
Washington—University of Washington, Seattle, Washington.
Wisconsin—Wisconsin Anti-Tuberculosis Association, Milwaukee, Wis.
    †Not included in this study.

[94] Of these 20 schools, 16 gave information for this study, 6 being visited by our field agents, while the remainder co-operated by filling out questionnaires sent them.

Of these 20 schools or courses, 4 (in Colorado, Illinois, Buffalo, N. Y., Columbus, Ohio) owing to special local conditions have been discontinued. On the other hand, since 1920 at least 3 new courses have been organized, in the Universities of Pittsburg, Oregon, and Iowa. The temporary or permanent abandonment of courses in some places and the organization of new ones is significant of the general situation in this field—its experimental nature, the urgent need that calls the courses into being, and the instability of the support which is often accorded them.

COURSES GIVEN PRIOR TO 1917

Although the greater number, at least half, of the public health nursing courses have been organized since 1917, the beginning of formal training in this field dates back to 1906, when the Boston District Nursing Association first offered a course in practical training. Teachers College followed next in 1910. In the next year, 1911, a course was begun in Cleveland under the Visiting Nurse Association; in 1913 one in Philadelphia by the Phipps Institute, and in 1914 a course was established by the New Haven Visiting Nurse Association.

It is significant that with the single exception of Teachers College the courses organized prior to 1917 were started by visiting nurse associations or other public health organizations.

The establishment of these earlier courses was in response to the specific needs of the organizations. As we have seen, the nurse who comes to modern public health work without some understanding of the underlying social and economic causes of disease and disability, without some skill in demonstrating and teaching measures of prevention and cure, cannot, however well-equipped for bedside care, succeed. As the visiting nurse organizations have developed from purely palliative and curative work to placing a greater emphasis on preventive and educational functions, aiming to teach habits of health and hygiene, the necessity of supplementing the hospital training of their personnel naturally developed. Instead of allowing their nurses merely to feel their way towards the newer requirements and learn so far as they were able by experience, special instruction in the principles and practice of public health nursing was seen to be the need of the time. The desirability of organizing such instruction was emphasized by the number of nurses who applied to well-established public health nursing organizations for temporary staff experience to prepare themselves for service elsewhere.

In 1906 the Instructive District Nursing Association of Boston first gave a 4-months' course. It was designed primarily to meet the needs of the staff but other nurses were encouraged to attend as a preparation for other fields. In 1912 affiliation was secured with Simmons College and the Boston School for Social Work and an 8-months' as well as a 4-months' course was offered. In 1916 Simmons College assumed with the District Nursing Association joint direction of the course and established a department, later advanced to a school, of public health nursing.

The course now given by Western Reserve University in Cleveland had a somewhat similar evolution. It was begun in 1911 by the Cleveland Visiting Nurse Association, which secured the active co-operation of the sociology department of Western Reserve University, the Associated Charities, and several specialized public health agencies. Five years later the direction and management of the course was transferred to the School of Applied Social Sciences in the University, though the Visiting Nurse Association retains an active part in the supervision of field work.

In 1910 the first course under university auspices was opened at Teachers College. In the beginning there was no organized field work in connection with these courses, but within a few years it was supplied by affiliation with the Henry Street Settlement. This offered a field service which has steadily broadened according to the varying needs of the students.

In 1913 a course was established by Phipps Institute, Philadelphia, in co-operation with the Visiting Nurse Association, the direction of which was later assumed by the Pennsylvania School for Social Service. In 1922 an affiliation was made with the University of Pennsylvania.

In 1914 a course was established by the Visiting Nurse Association of New Haven which still retains responsibility for it. The association has been fortunate in having enlisted for the instruction, the co-operation of professors from Yale University and in the projected Yale University School of Nursing, the public health course would be a part of the postgraduate nursing training.

In 1915 a course was started in Milwaukee by the Wisconsin Anti-Tuberculosis Association.

COURSES ORGANIZED SINCE 1917

After several years of such experimental courses better organization and instruction was seen to be imperative. Not only was better instruction in theory found essential; but it became evident that the training should be given under auspices better adapted to educational ends than an executive agency. The education of nurses is not the primary function of a nursing organization, any more than it is that of a hospital; and under its auspices there is danger that some of the inherent weaknesses and vices of the relations existing between hospitals and undergraduate training schools may be duplicated in the graduate courses for public health nursing. Primarily there is the danger of conducting such courses as mere apprenticeships instead of in accordance with an ordered educational program. Under an executive agency there tend to be other failings: entrance requirements too low to insure good applicants; no standards in teaching; changes in the personnel of the organization which bring about a lack of stability in the responsible teaching force; lack of libraries and teaching equipment.

On the other hand, educational advantages offered by these active organizations are due to their high standards of practical work, their knowledge of what is needed in the personnel, their enthusiasm for the new approach to old problems of sickness and disability, which is invaluable for stimulating a high degree of interest and participation in the students.

The desideratum, then, evidently is to combine with the opportunities for field work offered by the executive agencies the educational impetus and facilities of institutions capable of giving postgraduate instruction, that is, universities or colleges. It is gratifying to find that of the public health nursing courses started since 1917, practically all have been undertaken by universities or schools of social work, often at the instigation of a public health organization. The development of such courses is interestingly illustrated at a western university.

Through the State Anti-Tuberculosis Association an experienced public health nurse was engaged to give a 12-weeks' summer course at the university in 1918. In the fall she was engaged as a regular member of the university faculty to develop a nursing department, but the influenza epidemic intervened and only a series of lectures on public health nursing, as part of the extension division of the university, was given during 1918-1919, together with some special short courses in some of the hospitals of the city. The following summer the 12-weeks' course was successfully repeated; finally in January, 1920, the first 4-months' course was given, and a 9-months' course was projected thereafter.

AUSPICES AND FINANCIAL ARRANGEMENTS

Regardless of what their origin may have been, 11 of the 16 courses in public health nursing were offered by universities or colleges; 3 by independent schools of social work, and 2 by active public health organizations. While the primary responsibility was thus distributed, the financial backing and supervision of the courses was in many instances variously shared. Of the 11 courses given in universities or colleges, 6 at first sight appeared to be entirely supported by the institution. But even among these, supervision of field work was in 3 instances borne entirely by the public health agencies of the city in which the schools were located, and in the 3 other university courses only the director or one supervisor of field work was paid by the university, the remaining responsibility for supervision being borne by the health agencies. The 5 other university or college courses had a definite co-operative arrangement with the organizations providing practice fields for their students. In some cases, the services of officers of the co-operating agencies were given for instruction in theoretical work, in two cases the teaching district for field work was financed wholly or in part by the affiliated health agency, and in one instance even housing for class work was provided.

In the courses under the auspices of independent schools of social work or of public health agencies, co-operative arrangements of sharing responsibilities for the course were also found. The former called on the active practising agencies to provide field work for their students and in some cases to assist in the theoretical instruction; the latter called on universities and other outside agencies for assistance in the didactic work.

While these courses are thus still in an experimental stage with regard to financial as well as other problems, there is a general tendency for the educational institution to have primary financial responsibility and direction of the course and for the active public health agency to assist by providing the field work and frequently field supervision.

TUITION FEES

In no case were fees from students sufficient to cover expenses. There was no standardization in fees. The charge varied with the policies, type and standing of the educational institutions. For example, one state university charged for a 4-months' course

$27.00 to residents of the state and $39.00 to non-residents. In the Army School of Nursing, students having the 4-months' training in public health nursing were themselves charged no extra fee.[95] Undergraduate student nurses in a university school of nursing in one instance were allowed to take the public health nursing course in the university of which their school was a part free of charge except for fees for laboratory work and diploma, maintenance being provided also as usual in training schools. In a number of schools, student nurses from hospitals in the city were given field work without any fee.

Where fees were charged the maximum fee for a 4-months' course was $45, and the minimum was $10. More than half these shorter courses charged less than $30. For 8- or 9- months' courses the fees ranged from $50 to $166, half being under $100. The fee for the longer 2-year courses was $370.

A number of scholarships were offered in connection with practically all the courses to students who gave evidence of aptitude and adequate preparation for this work. Many of these scholarships were made available through the American Red Cross, and some by other public health agencies. In this way postgraduate training was rendered possible for qualified candidates who would otherwise have been barred by financial difficulties.

FINANCING THE SCHOOLS

The funds needed to supplement tuition fees for these 16 public health nursing schools were raised in a variety of ways, according to the auspices under which they were being administered. Of the universities, 5 state and 1 municipal, 4 received their support through legislative appropriation and taxation. The other 2 government-supported universities joined with the Red Cross or State Public Health Association in raising funds for these courses. In one college, endowment and students' fees covered all expenses. In 4 instances the special advisory or executive committee connected with the public health nursing course was responsible for securing the necessary funds, one committee having a special subcommittee for finances. One school of social work had a finance committee to raise the general budget for the school which naturally included all specialized courses. The 2 public health organizations giving training included the expense of the courses in their general budget. In one instance the funds were raised

---

[95] This was met by a special appropriation.

jointly by the dean of the university and the head of the State Board of Health, the 2 organizations having undertaken joint responsibility for the course. A local chapter of the Red Cross had assumed the task of getting the necessary financial support for still another course given by a university.

ADMINISTRATION

Owing, again, to the experimental nature of these courses, their methods of administration also vary widely. A comparatively small proportion were given in special departments devoted to public health nursing.

Among the university and college courses, 4 were in special schools or departments of public health nursing, 2 were in schools of nursing connected with the university hospital or medical school, 2 were in schools or departments of applied social science, 1 was in the department of arts and sciences, 1 was divided between this department and the medical college, and 1 was entirely in the college of science. The 3 schools of social work maintained separate departments of public health nursing co-ordinate with their other departments, such as those of family welfare, of child welfare, or of community service. The 2 public health agencies had both established special educational departments to conduct these courses with a director in charge responsible to the chief executive of the organization.

ORGANIZATION OF THE COURSE

In considering the proper organization of a public health nursing course we face again the problem of all vocational and professional education; that is, the balance of didactic or classroom and practical training. We have seen in the hospital the over-emphasis on the non-educational repetition of practical work, to the detriment or even the exclusion of class instruction which should illuminate and interpret the students' practical experience. The public health nursing courses, by virtue of their recent organization and the experience which has accrued from the hospital schools of nursing, should be able better to co-ordinate theory and practice and to offer their students an educational program which shall give due weight to the threefold needs of didactic work, practice in the field, and observation in the field of work not actually engaged in.

THE DIRECTOR

Of all the factors necessary to the development of a satisfactory course, one of the most important is a well-qualified director. It is she who plans the curriculum, assigns and maintains general oversight of both field work and class work, co-ordinating the two. The ideal director should have had training and experience both in public health nursing and also in teaching. She should be a college graduate and she should be familiar with the general aims and methods of university education. The demand for such qualified directors is necessarily in excess of the available supply. Moreover, it should be remembered that most of the directors in charge of the present courses have been drawn from among the older public health nurses with the requisite professional experience whose general education was received when college training was less common than it is today. It is, therefore, not surprising that college graduates are exceptional among them. But it is gratifying to note that not only is the number of well-equipped directors increasing each year but that standards for the position of director are steadily improving.

Duties of Director

For the success of a public health nursing course, there must be a full appreciation of its purpose and problems on the part of those who act as instructors both within the university and in the practice field. Because education for public health nursing is still so new a branch, it is of special importance that the two groups of instructors, those in the classroom and those in the field, shall be well co-ordinated and have a sympathetic understanding of the whole plan of education. It has not infrequently occurred that the university staff, in its desire to give a full theoretical course, has over-emphasized the didactic work at the expense of the practical. Occasionally it has been difficult for instructors and even for the director of the course to appreciate fully the equal importance of field work and the necessity of adhering in the field to the same standards as prevail in the university. It is true also that the organizations offering field work have failed at times in a proper understanding of the educational aims of the work.

The director of the course, as the necessary link between the two groups, occupies a highly strategic position. She has not only the opportunity, but it is unquestionably one of her important functions, to interpret to each group the methods, purposes, and needs of the other. Without such impartial interpretation, misunderstandings and improper balance of the course often result. For this reason, and because otherwise she is inevitably handicapped on one side or the other, the director should have had both academic training and practical experience. Without academic background she cannot know whether the classroom work, the choice of topics and their presentation meet the special needs of the nurses; without practical experience she cannot judge the standards and teaching methods of the organization providing field practice. The director, in addition to her own classroom work. needs to keep in close touch with all the didactic instruction. Through discussions and round-tables she has opportunity to judge the calibre of the didactic work, to learn whether it is of genuine practical value to the students, and whether the subjects are presented from the proper approach.

On the other hand, the director should be no less conversant with the details of the field practice. But it is not unusual to find that she has only a general knowledge of the work of the nursing organizations, and that she has failed to obtain a firsthand knowledge of their methods of work, standards, and achievements. The utmost frankness should prevail between the director and the agencies offering field work. Intelligent criticism of the practice work given to students is obviously of constructive value in relation to the work of the staff nurse.

In connection with the desirable qualifications of the ideal director of a public health nursing course and some of the functions falling to her lot which we have enumerated, it is of much interest to learn some of the main facts in the personal histories of the directors of existing courses.

General Education of Directors

As regards the general education of 12 directors reporting, 7 were graduates of a high or secondary school; and of this number, 5 had had college work, including 2 who had B.A. degrees, one from an eastern college of first rank, the other from a small western college, and 2 who had the degree of B.S. Of the remaining 5 directors, 1 had only a grammar school education, 1 had had but one year of high school, 1 two years, and 1 three years of high school, and 1 a combination of two years' high school and one year of normal school. In considering these figures it must, as already suggested, be borne in mind that the directors are mature women, many of whom had their schooling before college or even high school education was general. It is therefore natural that in the past the preliminary educational equipment has been lower than the professional and personal qualifications. With the desire to supplement the deficiencies of their general education, 3 of the 5 directors who had less than the full high school course had taken extension or summer session work in universities.

Professional Training

Of the 12 directors reporting on their professional nursing training, 9 had had a three-years' course, 2 had had shorter courses—two and two and a half years' respectively—and 1 had had a longer one of three and a half years. Only 4 had had all services covered in our questionnaire.[96] But the services missing were those in which facilities for training have been until very recently lacking. Thus 4 had had no training in tuberculosis, 4 no training in venereal disease, 5 no training in communicable diseases, 3 no training in nervous and mental cases, and 1 no training with male cases.

The hospitals in which they had taken their training were all well above the minimum standard set by the National Organization for Public Health Nursing. The smallest had 75 beds and the largest 620. Only 4 of the 12 had had their work in hospitals of less than 100 beds, while 3 had trained in hospitals of 100 to 200 beds, 3 in hospitals of 200 to 300 beds, and 2 in those of 300 or more.

In addition to their general training as nurses, 9 of the 12 directors had taken postgraduate work in public health nursing, ranging in time from 4 months to 2½ years. That 8 of the 9 had taken at least part of this work at Teachers College is a tribute to the contribution which its Department of Nursing and Health is making to the development of the public health field.

The working experience of the directors, between the time of graduation and registration as trained nurses and their engagement as directors, has been various. Only 7 of the 12 giving information had engaged in private nursing practice, and only 5

---

[96] These services were work with men, women, children, infants, medical cases, surgical cases, obstetrical cases, nervous and mental cases, venereal diseases, tuberculosis, other communicable diseases, and dietetics.

had had institutional positions, 4 of these being of an executive character. Eight had had some public health nursing experience aside from courses taken in this field, the length of service ranging from 1 year and 10 months to over 6 years. It is interesting to note that 7 of the 8 who had had public health nursing courses were among the 8 who had had professional experience in this field. Only 2 directors had had neither a course nor practical work in public health nursing before beginning to teach in this field. Six of the 12 directors had done some teaching—5 in general schools, either city or rural, 1 in general nursing, and 4 in public health nursing. One director had done all three types of teaching, and 2 had done both general and public health nursing teaching. The other work in which the directors had been engaged included many activities in public health, publicity, educational and social work.

General Standing

The professional standing of these women is indicated by their membership in the national and state associations of their profession. All were members of from two to six nursing organizations, and all but one were members of either a national or a state public health nursing association. They were women of mature years, their ages ranging from 31 to 45, with the majority under 40 (7 out of 11 reporting). Their length of service as directors of these public health nursing courses varied for the most part according to the age of the course itself; 4 had been directors less than a year, 4 for 1 year and less than 2, while the remaining 7 (of 15 reporting) had held their positions for 2 years or longer, 3 having to their credit a period of 4 years' service, and 1 of nearly 7 years.

Taking the group as a whole, the directors of these courses show a fairly high average of professional training and working experience which should be valuable as preparation for the teaching of public health nursing. Their general education does not reach as high an average.

Salaries of Directors

The salaries of the directors varied greatly, irrespective of length of service, length or type of experience, or of training. The salaries, as far as they were reported, are as follows:

Monthly Salary	Number
Less than $150............	1
$150 and " " 200............	4
200 " " " 250............	4
250 " " " 300............	2
300 or more...................	2
Total	13

Clearly, some of these salaries are not commensurate with the responsibility of the position or the experience, training, and ability required to fill it. It is to be hoped that with the establishment of standards in the training courses themselves will come a raising of the general standard in directors' salaries.

FACULTY

The faculty of these courses is variously composed of nurse instructors, doctors, social workers, with and without special training in health work, public health officials, and university professors of economics and other subjects. As a matter of fact, the excellence of the course does not seem to depend on the relative numerical strength of these different groups. Thus in both a college and a university course of high grade, the nurse-instructors considerably outnumbered all others. In another university school of similarly high standards only 6 out of 16 instructors were nurses, the rest of the faculty consisting of 4 doctors, 4 university professors, and 2 social workers.

Some of the courses depended almost entirely on a small regular staff for instruction; others had in addition a large number of special lecturers who gave one or two lectures as part of a composite course.

ADVISORY COMMITTEES

In the present formative stage of the public health nursing courses, the advisory committee fulfils an important function. If rightly composed so as to include besides representatives of medicine and nursing, representatives of educational interests and also persons experienced in the current problems and needs of the work, it does much to assure a balanced program. Eight of the 16 schools had advisory committees on which public health nursing was usually well represented. Both this and the special executive committee, where this existed, included representatives of visiting nurse associations, public health officials, doctors, professors of medicine, educators, social workers, and active lay members of public health agencies. In one university course, at least, the advisory committee was composed entirely of members of the faculty, almost all medical men, and the absence of outside members more abreast of public health interests to assist in shaping the course was greatly deplored.

Of the 10 schools with executive or advisory committees, 7 included on these committees the director of the course who should obviously always be a member.

ENTRANCE REQUIREMENTS

GENERAL EDUCATION

In our study of hospital training schools we have emphasized the importance of the educational requirements for entrance, and have pointed out that a professional training cannot be successfully based on less than a high school education. The low entrance requirements of the hospital schools of nursing have not only handicapped their own educational programs, but have handicapped also the postgraduate courses following hospital training. With so large a proportion of the hospital schools still accepting for entrance completion of grammar school or a year or two of high school, the postgraduate courses have necessarily been greatly hampered in their effort to require at least the completion of high school or its equivalent. Compromises of all sorts have had to be made and standards relaxed in many individual instances in the interest of accepting as many students as possible to meet the insistent demands for public health nurses.

The postgraduate courses thus labor under the unfair burden of carrying students of unequal educational preparation, and the establishment of proper professional training is endangered or delayed. On the students themselves the reaction of too low standards of admission to undergraduate training is no less disastrous, hampering them in their future careers or even debarring them totally from their chosen fields.

Of our group of 16 schools or courses in public health nursing 11 required high school graduation or its equivalent, with varying degrees of strictness in interpretation. In 2 of the 11 no educational requirement was made for a 4-months' course taken by student nurses from affiliated hospitals, the high school requirement applying only to admission to the longer courses. Some schools by liberal interpretation of the "equivalent" of a high school education admitted students who would otherwise have been disqualified; others made exceptions for those who had had public health nursing or other unusual professional experience; one had certain definite exemptions in favor of foreign students and missionaries. In one instance educational standards were relaxed only for nurses coming from sections of the country where a particular shortage of public health nurses existed. One university accepted in lieu of a complete high school course a general examination.

Of the remaining 5 schools, 2 demanded only 2 years of high school, while 3 had no general educational requirements but accepted the entrance requirement of the candidates' hospital training school.

Relaxing established standards of admission was reluctantly done and coupled with statements from various directors that certificates would not be granted to students who were admitted without meeting the educational requirements. One university which, while requiring an entrance examination, had been admitting students to its public health nursing course on less than high school graduation, found that students with only grammar school education were unable to carry the work satisfactorily. The danger of having the course taken from the school of nursing and made part of the university extension division led to plans for requiring university matriculation for the public health courses in the following year.

PROFESSIONAL EDUCATION

The requirements in professional education were more uniform than for general education. About half the schools admitted only graduate registered nurses. The majority accepted graduation from an accredited training school in good standing and registration in any state.[97]

Where undergraduate student nurses were admitted, which was in nearly half the courses, only seniors were admitted who had finished at least 2 years of training in accredited schools including the essential services. Three of the schools were

[97] Two schools had adopted the National Organization for Public Health Nursing standard for eligibility to membership. One school required registration in the state in which it was located, one in the student's own state. Two schools specified training in a hospital of at least 50 beds, and one in a hospital of 30 beds. Five schools required that certain services must be included while the rest accepted whatever was required in the state of registration.

affiliated with schools of nursing in offering 5-year programs, in which the fifth year was the 8- or 9-months' public health nursing course. In these 5-year programs, 2 years were given to academic college work, 2 years to general nursing training; at the close of the fifth year a bachelor's degree in addition to the nursing diploma, was awarded. Four schools which did not admit student nurses to their full public health nursing courses gave to seniors from local hospitals 2 months of supervised field work, sometimes accompanied by a brief course in the general principles of public health nursing.

PREVIOUS EDUCATION OF STUDENTS IN 16 SCHOOLS

Such being the varying principles of procedure in the different schools, it is of interest to learn the actual facts regarding the students enrolled during the year of our study. Of 1,055 students enrolled in 16 schools, data were secured on the age, schooling and previous public health experience for 813 students in 15 schools.

Of these 813 students, 541 or just two-thirds (66.5 per cent) had a completed high school education or more; 156 (19.2 per cent of the total number) had done some college work; 51 (6.3 per cent) were college graduates. At the other end of the scale 43 students (5.3 per cent) had not gone beyond grammar school; and a third (33.5 per cent) had less than full high school education.

The proportion of students who had less than full high school education varied from less than one-eighth in one college of high standing to nearly seven-eighths in another school which had no definite educational requirement. Thus there is evident the need of adhering more nearly to established standards, as soon as may be.

One hundred and eighty-eight students, or 25 per cent of the total reporting, had had experience in public health nursing before enrolment. Often the experience had been very brief, amounting to only a few months.

For one of the larger schools more detailed data were available on the previous experience of students. Of 120 students, 33 had had previous public health nursing experience, 16 for three years or more, and only 3 for less than a year. Among these students 28 had come direct from army or navy nursing during the war.

The majority of the students were between the ages of 25 and 35, the largest group being in the early thirties. Though there was a considerable group under 25—some 108 out of a total of 839—these were largely senior student nurses who were for the most part taking the shorter courses. The ages ranged from 19 to 52 years, but the median of 32 years shows that the public health nursing field is drawing its recruits for the most part from women of maturity who are still young enough to possess the vigor and enthusiasm which the profession demands.

LENGTH AND NUMBER OF COURSES OFFERED

For the graduate nurse, after her hospital experience, the minimum time needed to prepare for public health nursing has been found to be one academic year. Shorter courses of 4 months have been and are still being offered to meet the unprecedented demand for public health nursing, and the limitations of the present supply. But the short course is recognized to be merely an emergency measure, in no way capable of giving the balanced theoretical and practical program needed for a professional education. In the opinion of leading educators in public health nursing, the 4-months' course should be as soon as possible superseded as a minimum by the recognized 8-months' course.

The 16 schools of our study varied in the number of courses offered, their length, and the number of times they were given during the year. Nine of the schools offered only one course in public health nursing. Three others gave two courses of varying length, while one had three different courses, two had four courses, and one with exceptional facilities for specialization offered eight, counting a 6-weeks' summer course.[98] In this chapter, 28 courses have been considered in the 16 schools. They varied in length as follows:

Length of Course	Number of Courses
4 months	12
6 months	1
8-9 months	12
1 year and 4 months	1
2 years	2
Total	28

[98] In various schools of the group studied summer courses and institutes were held for nurses in the field. Such short courses are obviously of the greatest value for those who are actively engaged in work and wish to enlarge their experience and keep abreast of the best current practice.

The most usual length for these courses was either 4 months or one term, or one academic year which varied in length from 8 to 9 months. Several schools which were giving 8- or 9-months' courses permitted students to enroll for one of the two terms if it was impossible for them to take the full course.

A number of the 4-months' courses were given more than once during the course of a year. Three of them were repeated once during the year, five were given three times, and one, by means of an overlapping of the first and last months of the two successive classes, was offered four times in the course of 13 months. The one 6-months' course was given twice in the year, and in a few of the 8-months' courses, students were permitted to enter in either the first or second term, so that one and one-half classes passed through the school in one academic year. The 2-year courses were offered by one college as majors in a collegiate course of 4 years and were open to graduate nurses only. If the student had not had 8 months of approved field work to her credit before entering, she was required to take it after completing the course, thus making it in some cases 3 academic years in length.

General Plan of the Courses

Relation of Field Work and Class Work

As we have already pointed out, training for public health nursing like all vocational education depends for its success on the proper balance between didactic teaching and the students' practical field work. We have next to consider the apportionment of time between these two sides of the training and the relative merits of different methods of combining them. Four methods of disposing the time have been tried: giving field work and class work concurrently; giving field work first and class work last; vice versa, giving class work first followed by field work; and finally, having a brief introductory period of field work preceding the bulk of the class work, with the remaining field practice at the end of the course. The importance of the subject and the differences of opinion as to the merits of these methods warrant us in discussing them in some detail.

1. GIVING FIELD WORK AND CLASS WORK CONCURRENTLY

Theoretically the method of giving theory and practice concurrently is best, in affording opportunity for close correlation between the classroom and the field. The classroom lessons are given early application and the questions that inevitably arise in the field can be brought back at once to the classroom to be answered. But practically this method has not proved satisfactory in public health nursing courses. For instance, if the mornings are given over to theory and the afternoons to practice work, students having their field experience with a visiting nurse association get none of the most acute cases in the service. It is the custom of all visiting nurse associations to care for their acute cases in the mornings, especially the maternity cases. If students work only in the afternoons it is difficult to arrange an afternoon schedule which does not include too many visits to chronics, the least valuable service from the student's point of view. Moreover, office conferences are most frequently held in the morning or during noon hours. These meetings the student working only in the afternoon would also miss, and it is by attendance at these meetings that she can best get an understanding of the *esprit de. corps*, the nurses' attitude toward their families, their methods of dealing with family and community problems, their close relationship with the supervisor serving as consultant.

When field work is given in the morning and theory in the afternoon the disadvantages to the student are as great. She gets a preponderance of acute cases and little practice with the non-acute. Prenatal cases, nutrition problems, infant welfare—these all-important types indispensable for the student's training—are usually missed in morning practice work. Many important clinics are held in the afternoon, when the doctors are more available after having cared for their own most acute cases and when the mothers of families who are to attend are freer from household duties. Another disadvantage in giving class work in the afternoon is the fact that the student after spending a busy morning in the district is usually too tired in the afternoon to apply herself to study. As a consequence the class work suffers.

In order to offset these disadvantages some directors arrange to have field work and class work on alternating days, thus insuring unbroken days for each. The uninterrupted day is an advantage, but it is offset by the disadvantage of the interrupted week. The student who spends but two or three days of each week in the district cannot carry her families continuously; on the intervening day they must be attended by a staff nurse. The student does not, then, have the advantage of sufficiently definite responsibility, an important factor in her training. The first duty of the visiting nurse association is toward its patients and if the student is unable to carry the entire responsibility of a district, her work must be more or less planned for her by the supervisor. She thus loses the opportunity of planning her own work. On the whole, under the plan of concurrent training the tendency is to over-emphasize theory. Field work is too apt to be looked upon as an interruption to class work, and hence does not call forth the student's entire enthusiasm.

2.   FIELD WORK PRECEDING CLASS WORK

The advantage in having practice work precede the class work is that the student gets more from her instruction in theory. She has been face to face with the problems of the nursing field; she has seen certain methods fail and others succeed. She has worked out certain methods of approach, and is full of questions that can be brought to the classroom. These advantages, however, are gained at a cost to patient and student alike. This arrangement is, again, a reversion to pure apprenticeship or even less well-guided effort. Obviously, there is waste of student time and probable hardship to the patient in learning merely by personal experience.

As we have seen in our study of the field, certain principles and standards of work in public health nursing have been established. It is these which the student is to be taught in her class work. To allow her to spend a first half-year in the field, without any regular instruction in the theoretical basis of the work, is obviously to put a premium upon the acquisition of wrong habits or of bad technique and to throw away the accumulated experience of the profession.

3.   CLASS WORK PRECEDING FIELD WORK

The method of having class work precede field work, while better in theory and practice than having field work first, is nevertheless not satisfactory. There is undoubtedly a serious disadvantage in having the student wait four months before she comes into actual contact with the conditions of which she is being taught. Young students, especially, with no background of experience, fail to get the most out of the theoretical instruction, and have difficulty in applying it in their later services in the field. This disadvantage can to some extent be overcome by frequent conferences with field workers, and regular visits of observation to public health and welfare agencies and institutions.

In view of the practical difficulties of giving class work and field work concurrently, some combination of the two other methods described is thus clearly desirable.

4. A SHORT INTRODUCTORY PERIOD OF FIELD WORK

Instead of giving all class work preceding the field training, the best arrangement would seem to consist in giving a short introductory period of field experience, lasting perhaps one month, to introduce the student to her prospective work. During this period there should be some regular instruction on the principles of the work and regular conferences. It is found possible to put in as much as 4 periods a week without interrupting the actual service in the field.

After this introduction to the field, the bulk of class instruction should be given, followed in turn by the remaining months of practical experience. Most of the observational work, such as visits to institutions, clinics, etc., may best be assigned during the period of class instruction.

APPORTIONMENT OF WORK IN COURSES STUDIED

In the courses studied the disposition of time between field work and class work varied, but in the greater number of courses it was planned to give didactic and field work concurrently. Sometimes the procedure differed in different courses in the same school. For example, in the general 8-months' course of one school, field work could be taken either before or after the theoretical instruction while in a special industrial nursing course in the same school it was required that the field work follow the first term of theoretical work. In the 4-months' course, which consisted largely of field work, concurrent class work was given in the principles of public health nursing.

Of 19 courses 9 gave didactic and field work concurrently; 3 gave them concurrently during part of the time, but also devoted part of the time to field work alone; 4 gave the theory in the first part of the course and the practice in the second part; 3 permitted the field work either to follow or to precede the theoretical work but not to accompany it.

The relative amount of time given to field and theoretical work is difficult to compute, and is also so largely dependent on the length and purpose of the course that in many cases the comparison is without value. The proportion of hours given to each part of the work naturally varied in the different courses offered. It was usual in the shorter courses to give a great preponderance of time to field work, with merely some concurrent instruction in theory. From Table 16 (see page 521) it appears that, taking all 28 courses of different lengths, in the great majority more than half the hours of the courses were given to field work. The median percentage of hours given to class work in courses lasting 8 to 9 months was 38.6, while for field work the median was 61.4. The median percentage of hours given to class work in courses lasting 4 to 6 months was 32.1, while for field work the median was 67.9.

TOTAL NUMBER OF HOURS

In considering the actual number of hours devoted to either branch of the training we must obviously distinguish between the short and long courses. Analysis of these actual hours in the various courses substantiates the showing of Table 16 that more time is devoted to field work than to class work. The actual distribution of hours is as follows:

TABLE 17

	Minimum	Median	Maximum
Field Work Hours			
4-6 months' courses	192	360	656
8-9 months' courses	384	642	872
Class Work Hours			
4-6 months' courses	15	176	372
8-9 months' courses	270	358	640

FIELD WORK

TECHNIQUE OF BEDSIDE CARE IN THE HOME

In field work the student of public health nursing, like any other vocational student, gains her technical skill. Just as in wards of the hospital she is admitted to clinical opportunities

TABLE 16

PROPORTION OF TIME GIVEN TO THEORETICAL AND FIELD WORK IN 28 PUBLIC HEALTH NURSING COURSES BY LENGTH OF COURSE

Proportion of Total Hours in Course	Number of Courses Giving Proportion of Time to					
	Field Work			Theoretical Work		
	In 4-6 Months' Courses	In 8-9 Months' Courses	In More Than 9 Months' Courses	In 4-6 Months' Courses	In 8-9 Months' Courses	In More Than 9 Months' Courses
Less than 10%	..	..	..	2	..	..
10% and 20%	..	..	..	1	..	..
20% " 30%	..	1	..	3	3	..
30% " 40%	2	1	..	3	4	..
40% " 50%	2	3	3	2	3	..
50% " 60%	3	4	..	2	1	3
60% " 70%	3	3	..	..	1	..
70% " 80%	1	..	..	..	..	..
80% " 90%	2	..	..	..	..	..
90% " 100%	..	..	..	..	..	..
Total	13	12	3	13	12	3

nowhere else to be found, so in the field of public health nursing she may learn at first hand to apply her threefold function of caring for the sick, preventing illness, and promoting health.

The question is sometimes raised why a graduate nurse, after three years' training in bedside care of patients, should need any further instruction in caring for the sick.

In reply we may say that in the first place, as we have seen in our study of public health nursing, the bedside care of the visiting nurse calls for a special technique of its own. The visiting nurse who enters a variety of homes in a single day and encounters many different conditions and types of persons and of illness, is called on for resourcefulness and adaptation to varying home conditions unknown in the hospital. In her field work the student must be taught how and what to observe in the home, how to adjust herself to the resources at hand, how to adapt to changed environment the principles learned in her clinical course.

THE FAMILY AS UNIT OF CARE

Moreover, as we have shown, the bedside care of the visiting nurse is no longer looked upon as a purely curative and palliative function, but is to be utilized as an invaluable avenue of approach in teaching habits of health and hygiene to the entire family. In hospital training the whole tendency is to care for the patient as a single isolated individual, unrelated to his home or social conditions. In public health work there is an increasing tendency to recognize the family as the unit of care and to include in the improvement of health a recognition of the part played by the social and economic conditions of the family.

Now just as during an epidemic good hygienic habits can more readily be taught to the community, so they can be taught more readily in a family where sickness exists or has existed. The family, those surrounding the patient, are in the mood for learning how to keep well. They are in the mood also for listening to the nurse who has ministered to their need.

In order to learn how best to adapt her skill in bedside care, how to teach the family to give care between her visits, and how to capitalize her influence in sickness with the family so as to be successful in teaching them habits of health and hygiene, the student should have good training with an organization doing bedside nursing of high standards.

RELATION WITH OTHER SOCIAL AGENCIES

In field work the student should learn, also, how to plan and execute her day's work in the field so as to meet her varied obligations and perform all manner of services. In endeavoring to arrange for the health needs of her families, she will come in contact with other social field agencies and will need to call upon them. She must learn how to utilize these agencies, turning over to them functions of relief, employment, family rehabilitation, etc., which are not properly within her sphere, yet which she must understand, and with which for the best interest of the family she must co-operate fully. Only through actual experience in seeing such constructive programs for family health formulated and carried out can the student appreciate their varied aspects and learn the best methods of treatment. For her grounding in methods of social diagnosis and treatment she should have experience with the local agency dealing with family welfare, such as the Associated Charities or some similar organization. She should have opportunity to observe the office routine, record keeping, and the use of the confidential exchange, for lack of which nurses spend time worse than fruitlessly, in duplicating inquiries and efforts.

APPORTIONMENT OF TIME AND SERVICES TO BE COVERED

We have seen that the tendency in all the courses is to devote more time to field work than to class instruction. Even in the 8- to 9-months' courses the median time spent in the field is well above 50 per cent of the total course. Yet for a well-balanced program, which shall teach the student the principles needed to guide her in the many diverse problems and difficulties which she is bound to encounter, sound classroom instruction, making the freest possible use of case discussion, should make up half of the total course. The time should be divided about equally between field work and work in the classroom. The time to be devoted to field work should thus be approximately 16 weeks. How this time should be divided cannot be too definitely specified. It must depend on the types and relative merits and defects of the local agencies offering field work.

In planning the time to be spent with the various agencies, the director of the course must keep first in mind the objects to be attained. As a foundation, the student should obtain as comprehensive an experience as possible in general family health work. Just as in the hospital school of nursing we deprecate extreme specialization before the student has been taught the fundamentals of training, common to all services, so in the field of public health nursing the specialties should be taught after the first comprehensive foundation has been laid, including bedside care.

At least 8 weeks should be devoted to training with the nursing agency doing the broadest family health work, usually the visiting nurse association. Experience should be given in medical, surgical, maternity, and infectious cases. The Education Committee of the National Organization for Public Health Nursing which has done much as consultant to standardize the existing courses, points out the need during this period of devoting special attention to such matters as use of household utensils, disposal of used dressings, ventilation and care of the room, diet, isolation and quarantine precautions and disinfection, etc.

Four weeks should be devoted to obtaining experience in such special nursing branches as have not been included in the first 8-weeks' work. This should cover training in school, tuberculosis, and infant welfare nursing. If possible, training should be given in mental hygiene and venereal diseases. For those intending to specialize in industrial nursing or hospital social service, special experience along these lines should be offered.

The 4 weeks' training in these various specialties should be chosen with great care. The effort should not be to give experience with as many different agencies as possible, but to give such as will make up a rounded program. No arbitrary time limit can be set for the various specialized services in all cases. It may, however, be generally stated that less than 1 week's experience with any one agency is not desirable; two weeks is a more satisfactory allotment of time. The student should remain with the organization giving field work long enough to gain a working knowledge of its purposes and methods. She should have an opportunity to test her ability in the given specialty. She should remain long enough for the management to have an opportunity to gauge her ability; to detect and make clear to her both her strong and her weak points and to give real instruction in its methods and aims.

Four weeks should be devoted to training with the local agency for family welfare, such as the Associated Charities or kindred organization. It should be clearly kept in mind that this period is not intended to prepare the student herself to undertake family rehabilitation, but primarily to give her an understanding of the approach and technique of the case worker.

For nurses intending to do rural public health nursing, in view of the special problems of country life, four weeks should, if possible, be spent in a rural district where the student may obtain training in the nursing specialties under the conditions which she will presently have to meet.

OBSERVATION IN THE FIELD

Besides actual practice in field work, valuable experience and insight into the various fields of public health and social work may be obtained by well-arranged visits or periods of observation. All the schools of our study gave their students opportunity to observe local health and social service agencies. In some cases this observation was confined to visits to institutions such as tuberculosis sanitaria, hospitals, reformatories, the juvenile court, institutions for the feeble-minded, or the insane, etc. In other courses, regular periods of time were spent in observing the work of health centers, clinics, open-air schools, and similar health work. Obviously, the value of such observation is again, at least in part, dependent on the interpretive guidance given the student.

FIELD WORK IN 16 SCHOOLS

Some field work was required for every course, but five schools made exemptions for nurses with sufficient previous public health nursing experience, allowing them to take only the theoretical work. Most of these schools required that this previous experience must have been comprehensive and carried on under supervision with an accredited organization, and that it must cover the same fields as were included in the field work of the course. Four more schools which did not exempt experienced students allowed them more elasticity in practice work. This privilege was usually granted only to those with from one to two years' experience. One nurse, for instance, who had had two years' tuberculosis work was exempted from further training in this specialized field, and given more time in infant and child welfare work in which her experience was lacking. The rest of the schools, however, did not make exemptions for any students from the required field work.

The schools of our study varied considerably in the scope of their field work and in the amount of time given to the various specialties. All but 2 of the schools required some generalized visiting nursing, while school nursing was required in every one of the schools, and child welfare in all but one. Tuberculosis work and some social case work were also generally required, 12 of the 16 schools making these two subjects obligatory. In the remaining fields of rural nursing, prenatal nursing, hospital social service, industrial nursing, mental hygiene, and venereal work, there was great variation.

In addition to the required program of field work, a number of the schools permitted students to choose among certain other specialized fields according to the student's particular interest or desire. This elective period usually followed the required work. Some of the schools allowed a fairly wide range of choice; others permitted students only to prolong the time spent in any one branch, in some cases conditioning even this on the student's previous experience. Five of the schools required of all students the same program of field work. A few others permitted some leeway to those with considerable public health nursing experience.

Table 18 shows the distribution in the 10 full courses lasting an academic year of the time spent in practice work.

The time assigned to the various types of field work did n vary greatly in the different courses.[99] Yet the amount of tim devoted to experience in school nursing varied from 8 weeks i. a western university course to 1 week in an eastern course given by a visiting nurse association. Field work in social case work varied from 8½ weeks in a southern course to 2 weeks in a midwestern university course. All 10 courses gave training with a visiting nurse association. The variation of time spent with this agency was from 16 to 3 weeks. But this variation is of less account since the time allotted to the visiting nurse association in some instances included experience in nursing specialties. Thus the course giving 16 weeks included work in child welfare, tuberculosis, and prenatal nursing, while in the course giving only 3 weeks to the agency, additional time was allowed for the specialties: 2 weeks for child welfare, 3 for prenatal nursing, and 4 for rural work which obviously may give experience in all the specialties.

The differences in the time apportioned to different services

[99] Where possible the total time devoted to each service is given. Where this was not possible, the total number of weeks of field work has been stated, the various fields included being indicated in the table.

TABLE 18

TOTAL WEEKLY HOURS OF FIELD WORK AND NUMBER OF WEEKS IN EACH TYPE OF FIELD WORK IN 10 SCHOOLS OF COURSES OF PUBLIC HEALTH NURSING

No. of School	Hours per Week	Weeks in Each Type of Field Work									
		General Visiting Nursing	Child Welfare	School Nursing	Tuberculosis Nursing	Prenatal and Maternity Nursing	Rural Nursing	Mental Hygiene	Social Case Work	Other	All Fields
2	44	3	2	2		3	4		2	1	17
3	35–40	9	4			*			4½		17½
5	24	8	8	6			2		6		30
6	24	16	*	8	*	*					24
8	24–33	*	*		*	*			*		17
9	36	4	4	1½	1½	2				6	19
10	40–44	11		3		*					14
13	12–42	5	6		6				4	15	36
14	16–19	8½							8½	17	34
15	37	5	4	1	3			2	2		17
No. of courses having work in each field		10	8	6	5	6	2	1	7	4	10

* Work included in this field; number of weeks not reported.

were due not wholly to the importance assigned to any one special topic but were frequently due to the differences in local opportunities and the quality of the local agencies. The variation in time assigned to school nursing in different courses may indeed be almost wholly ascribed to the unstandardized quality of this special work.

Where there is no teaching district such as is described later in this chapter, the value of the field work to the students must evidently depend in large measure on the development of public health nursing in the community in which the school is located. In at least two cities no general visiting nursing had been developed, hence no facilities for good generalized training were at hand. In one case the need for such practice for the public health nursing course had been a "considerable factor" in the institution of a generalized service by the American Red Cross.

An important branch of public health nursing which was sufficiently developed in only a few cases to afford practice to students was rural nursing. Only 2 of the 10 schools required rural field work. Of the two practice fields one was intensively studied by our field agent and found eminently fitted to give students insight and experience in the special problems and needs of rural work. In view of these special rural conditions, involving often a wholly different understanding and attack, and in view also of the ever-increasing demand for public health nurses in country districts, the lack of opportunity for training constitutes one of the most serious deficiencies in the public health nursing courses.

The failure of three out of ten agencies to give field practice in social case work is to be noted. Without this practical training in making contacts and learning something of the technique and routine of the social agencies, the public health nurse must be seriously hampered if not totally at a loss.

In one school studied the field practice was so diffused as to be of little benefit to the students, and amounted in fact to little more than observation of the work of a large number of clinics, in various dispensaries or health centers. In the month spent with the health department, the field work again was merely observation, wholly unsupervised.

"Several days are spent by students in the department of vital statistics," says our investigator, an experienced public health nurse and teacher, "and a day or so each with every kind of inspector—milk inspector, meat inspector, hospital and day nursery inspector, contagion nurse (giving doorstep instruction)—the student doing no work and consequently having no supervision."

Obviously the need here was to consolidate the field practice and get it under supervision. It was agreed that among other radical changes proposed for the next year, in place of the scattered visiting of different clinics, students should be given one straight month in the tuberculosis clinic with home visiting of patients, and one month in the same way in the baby clinics.

Broadly speaking, the field work of students observed by our investigators varied in merits and defects along the same lines as the work of staff nurses described in an earlier chapter. Where the students did the best work, they either combined curative and preventive nursing successfully or, on the basis of previous good contacts, were successful in getting the individuals or families visited to put into effect necessary hygienic measures. Where the work of students merited criticism it was either because too much emphasis was laid on bedside care alone or the instructive nursing was barren and unintelligible to the person addressed.

SUPERVISION

In our study of public health nursing we have pointed out the determining influence of the type and calibre of supervision in the field. If good supervision is one of the conditions of success in practical work, it is clearly of at least equal importance in training students. Adequate methods of supervising nurses in their field practice must therefore be a prime consideration of a good course.

An interesting development in the control and supervision of student practice has been the organization of the so-called teaching district. Under this plan a certain section of the city or town is set aside as a practice field: the work of the visiting nurse association of the city or even of the board of health is carried in that district, under careful supervision, by student nurses of the public health nursing course. This supervision is sometimes in the hands of the visiting nurse association, but more often the responsibility is vested in the director of the course with a staff of supervisors working under her. Frequently part of the expense of the teaching district is borne by the visiting nurse association, since that organization benefits directly

530 NURSING AND NURSING EDUCATION

from the work of the district. In one instance studied the American Red Cross bore the major part of the expense.

The section selected for a teaching district is usually one of the poorest and most congested parts of the city. For purposes of illustration we may briefly describe the organization and plan of one markedly successful teaching district connected with a university course. This district has a population of from 60,000 to 70,000 persons.

SUPERVISION IN A SUCCESSFUL TEACHING DISTRICT

The work of students in the teaching district is directly supervised by five instructors. These nurses, all of whom are graduates of the course, have been selected for their ability to teach and to supervise. To each instructor is assigned a number of students, including both graduate and pupil nurses. Seven is the maximum number of students assigned to one instructor. Each student is assigned by her instructor to a subdivision of the district, and as her knowledge and skill develop, she is increasingly held responsible for the work in her particular section.

When students begin their field work, they are taken out one at a time (very occasionally two at a time) by the instructor, who gives the instruction in the home and does the work required, while the student observes. A thorough discussion of the visit follows. On a subsequent visit the rôles are reversed, the instructor observing while the student conducts the visit. This procedure is repeated with different types of visits, such as to prenatal cases, communicable disease cases, and so on, until the student has been gradually introduced to the various types of work usually encountered in the district.

Three times daily the students report at the station, to receive assignments, to plan their work, and to carry out the necessary office details. An opportunity is afforded at these times for conference with the instructors. In this way the instructor is enabled to keep constant oversight of the students' work, and the students have an opportunity for immediate consultation and advice upon problems arising in the families they visit.

Every morning a conference is held by the director, which is attended by all the instructors and students. These conferences, in which the students take an active part, constitute an invaluable part of the training. The program may consist of demonstration of nursing technique, instruction in new procedures, consideration of social or other problems in individual families, or discussion of subjects of general professional interest.

Students thus have the benefit of demonstrations given by the instructors in the homes, of direct supervision of their own work in the homes, of individual conferences three times daily with the instructor in the office, and of group discussion in the morning conferences. By this careful teaching they are enabled to derive the full benefit from their experience in field work.

The nursing technique of the students who were observed gave evidence not only of good supervision, but—even more important—it showed that the students had a knowledge of the principles of hygiene and sanitation. Sometimes nursing work is done in which the technique is mechanical, where the nurse observes the details as they were taught her but does not use intelligence in adapting the underlying principles to the special circumstances she encounters. In the teaching district, however, the reverse was found. In their scrupulous attention to detail in the home, in the beautiful care given the patients even in the most difficult surroundings, in their careful disposal of soiled linen and dressings, in their regard for the patients' modesty and comfort, the students in the teaching district showed that their work was not merely a routine, but was based on an application of the underlying principles of public health and of good nursing.

LIMITATIONS OF THE TEACHING DISTRICT

We have described at some length one of the best teaching districts observed because of the excellence of its organization and methods of supervision. Four other schools had teaching districts, differing in various particulars. We must, however, point out some counterbalancing disadvantages in this plan of instruction. However well-adapted for the genuinely educational guidance of students, and practically indispensable as it is in localities having no adequate practice fields, the teaching district loses by being after all an artificial unit. It is not part of an established community agency and it is therefore deprived of the advantages as well as the disadvantages of such a connection. The student works under conditions which are too favorable and will not be reproduced in her subsequent experience. She does not have contact with such problems as enlisting community support which are inevitably part of the work under an established community agency, a wholesome corrective and stimulus to its methods. Nor does she have the benefit of being part of a large and well-established organization, attending its conferences and hearing the experience of the regular staff. Moreover, in any teaching district which is entirely dependent upon a student staff, unless there is a permanent auxiliary force, there is grave danger of exploiting the students and using them on work which is in excess of that needed purely for their education.

Where there is no teaching district, the public health nursing course must obviously take advantage of such organizations as can offer its students field practice.

In our discussion of public health nursing we have shown various methods of supervision which are utilized. In this general direction the students as well as the staff naturally share. Additional supervision and instruction of the student force is obviously needed. In the courses studied, a school either had field supervisors on its staff or left the supervision entirely to the officers and workers of the co-operating public health nursing agencies. Four schools followed the former plan. Two of them had one field supervisor and a director of field work, in addition to the director of the course, while the other two schools had respectively two and three staff supervisors. Where the organization providing the practice field was definitely affiliated with the school or university giving the course, an effective supervision could best be planned. Often, however, the supervisory arrangements were unsatisfactory. With an already overworked staff or one in which no definite teaching responsibility was or could be assumed, the students were without adequate guidance. Sometimes even with a teaching district the number of supervisors was insufficient, and the students realized their lack of adequate advice and oversight.

In the better organized courses weekly conferences were found very helpful in giving insight into everyday problems. Frequent informal individual conferences with students were also of great value. The greatest difficulties in supervision of field work were found in rural nursing because of the small regular staff and the large districts to be covered.

Theoretical Instruction: The Curriculum

As we have shown, the recency and empirical character of instruction in public health nursing has necessitated a variety of methods in teaching and in the content of the curricula. As the earlier experimental courses have been taken over by universities, colleges, and schools of social work, standardizing of the courses is gradually progressing. They still vary, naturally, with the type of institution under the auspices of which they are maintained. Schools of social work, that is, naturally offer a greater variety of courses on social than on scientific or pedagogical subjects. Besides general sociological courses they offer courses on such special topics as housing, immigration, recreation, social legislation, and industrial problems. The public health nursing course offered in a school of social work is almost inevitably, especially in the early years of its existence, weighted more heavily on the social side than might be desirable in making up a new curriculum. Another public health course, offered, let us say, by a college or university which lays special stress on methods of teaching, may over-emphasize pedagogical methods to the detriment of other phases of the training. Or, again, a course offered in connection with public health agencies may give more than due weight to scientific and nursing subjects.

Further variations in the curricula are due to the varying policy of different schools in attempting to make up deficiencies in the hospital training of their students. In some of the curricula, subjects which are proper only to the undergraduate basic course have been deliberately included, on the ground that making up the most salient defects of undergraduate training, such as the lack of the basic sciences, is at present necessary in postgraduate instruction. In other schools this attempt has been considered mistaken, in view of the impossibility of adequately supplementing in one academic year the various and varied gaps in the previous training of the students, while at the same time attempting to give the necessary basic postgraduate subjects.

To a certain extent, it is true, all the schools labor under the disadvantage of having to include in their curricula some topics which should be taught in the basic undergraduate course, after that course in turn has been freed from the burden of teaching the elements properly required, as we have shown in Chapter IV, before admitting any girl to a professional training. In the outline of a curriculum subsequently proposed for the postgraduate course, we assume on the part of the student a previous training more or less approximating that suggested for the basic undergraduate courses, and do not, therefore, include the subjects therein covered.

The subjects contained in the curricula of public health nursing courses may be roughly divided under four general heads or categories: nursing, social, pedagogical, and scientific. All the varied topics taught in the 28 courses, short and long, analysed in this study fall more or less accurately under these four general heads. Only two subjects were found common to all the 28 courses; namely, public health nursing, its principles, its history, or its scope and special fields; and, as it is usually termed in the curricula, "methods of social case work."

It is evident that in the shorter courses no balanced educational program can be offered and that the field work is merely supplemented, as best it may be, by some general concurrent instruction in the principles of public health nursing. For greater accuracy we must distinguish between the curricula offered by the full course of 8 or 9 months and the shorter emergency makeshift courses of 4 months. In further considering the content of the curricula we shall confine ourselves to the full courses lasting an academic year which alone can be held to give opportunity for adequate professional training.

Taking the 10 courses of a full academic year given during the year of our study, and grouping their curricula under the suggested headings, we find them to range in the percentage of hours devoted to each general topic as follows:

TABLE 19

	Minimum	Median	Maximum
Nursing	6.5	20.5	31.25
Social	16.	32.3	67.9
Pedagogical	0.	7.1	25.
Scientific	10.	34.1	60.7

The extreme variation in the existing courses is made clear by these figures. To show the excessive weight given to one or another of the four component elements of the courses, we may show the division of time in four curricula, each one of which gives the maximum amount of time in a different one of the categories.

TABLE 20

Division of Time in 4 Courses.

Subject	Percent of Total Course			
Nursing	31.25	6.5	16.7	14.2
Social	31.25	67.9	33.3	16.2
Pedagogical	6.25	6.	25.	8.9
Scientific	31.25	19.6	25.	60.7
	100.0	100.0	100.0	100.0

CONTENT OF THE COURSES

The content of the curricula whose distribution of hours we have analysed naturally varied greatly in the different courses, even when presented under the same or similar titles.

Under the heading of nursing are included the general courses on public health nursing, and courses on special phases of the work. Courses on the history of nursing, given in a few instances, are likewise included here.

In the social category are included courses which differ as widely as the radical differences in the current teaching of these topics makes inevitable. In some of the courses, an effort is made to give groundwork of economic theory. In others sociology and its applications are chiefly stressed. In still others, government and governmental functions take the first place. Scattered courses on special social topics such as immigration, recreation, housing, etc., are also included in this group.

Under the pedagogical heading are included courses on educational methods, educational psychology, general psychology, the psychology of public health instruction, etc.

Under the heading of scientific courses we include such of the fundamental sciences as are taught in schools which aim to make up deficiencies in the basic undergraduate hospital training of the students, as well as subjects in themselves appropriate to postgraduate work such as more advanced work in hygiene and sanitation, personal and public, preventive medicine, the administration of public health work, etc.

METHODS OF INSTRUCTION

The nurse students in most instances get their instruction in subjects such as psychology, and educational and social topics in the general university courses. The instruction in these courses inevitably shares the merits and defects of the particular university or school in which they are given. Where, for instance, university classes are so large that students have opportunity to recite only a few times each term, the nursing students who are admitted to the class naturally share in this disadvantage. In one instance in a class on public speaking required of students in various departments of the university, nurse students stated that they had opportunity to speak only three times in three months.

The weakness of the theoretical instruction in these courses is its frequent failure to correlate the subject with the special needs of public health nursing and the student's vocational objectives. Thus, in attending a general class in psychology to which public health nurses were admitted in a western university of good standing, our observer comments on the "extraordinarily wasteful procedure" of teaching this subject without any application to the students' special field.

"If the director of the course," writes this investigator, "could attend at least one class each week in each subject and then have one or two hours of quiz and conference in which she related such subjects as psychology and economics to the students' past experience and future problems, the value of the course would be increased 100 per cent."

The psychology course required of nurse students consists of lectures, attended by about 1,000 students from different departments of the university, a weekly quiz conducted by various instructors, and a two-hour weekly laboratory period. Lectures, quiz and laboratory periods were visited by our field agent. The laboratory work consisted of mirror drawings related to the subject of memory. A written paper was required at the end of the period containing tabulations of the time required to make each of the seventeen trials, etc. In neither lecture, quiz, nor laboratory was there any application of the subject matter to the work of the nurse.

"If a nurse instructor," continues our observer, "could call to the attention of the students the applications of such instruction, it would do much towards cementing the course. The student nurse cannot look forward, see her probable experience, and make the application, and the course fails of its greatest usefulness."

On the other hand in another university course, the director or assistant director attended practically every lecture and class in order to keep in close touch with the class work and correlate it with the special interests and needs of the nurse students. Thus in one class period, for instance, following a general lecture in the psychiatric course given by a leading neurologist and alienist, the topic treated was "The Feeble-Minded." Sterilization may legally be practiced in the state in which this university is situated. The class had visited one of the state institutions and had seen several sterilization operations performed on the criminally insane. Our observer gives as the topic for class discussion "What shall we do about the mentally deficient whom we meet in our work?" and continues: "General discussion very varied followed from the class. There was a consensus of opinion that there can be no hard and fast rules but that each case must be decided on its own merits."

Clearly, where special classes are not created for the public health nursing students, special adaptation is needed of many college subjects to meet the special needs of the nursing group. This does not, of course, mean narrow specialization. Another of our observers in attending in another university course a special class on public health administration comments specially on the broad treatment of the topic by a public health physician and teacher of unusual ability:

"Every point that Dr. E. emphasized," she reports, "was of value to the public health nurse, even though he drew very largely from his experience as health commissioner of ——, and many of his hearers will not engage in city work but will be in rural communities. His presentation of the subject was so broad that it could not fail to establish principles for health work in any community. The other lecturers who have been heard up to the present had given the same careful preparation to their subjects, and enumerated their points with unusual clarity. One felt, however, that they presented the theoretical solutions of nursing problems. Frequently lectures are given in nursing courses by very able people who fail because they do not know the needs of the field."

A Suggested Curriculum

Without attempting now to lay down any one norm or dogmatic scheme for a course in public health nursing, we may, in view of these wide discrepancies of content as well as of hours devoted to the component elements of the course, indicate what in our opinion constitutes a well-balanced course and one which will best contribute to the further education of the hospital trained nurse in her career of public health nursing.[100]

In view of the varying nomenclature of courses and the inevitable overlapping of subject matter, we outline under com-

[100] As already indicated, this course is assumed to be a basic graduate course lasting one academic year. On the completion of this general course, there is obviously room and need for further advanced work of two types: one dealing with leadership in public health nursing and further training in the conduct of the work; the other, with the training of teachers for the graduate public health nursing courses.

prehensive titles what is advocated as the general content of the course, attempting to make no specific or hard and fast divisions.

NURSING SUBJECTS

Principles of Public Health Nursing

This course, which under one name or another was given in all the courses studied, is obviously indispensable. While capable of very varied treatment, with varying emphasis on different phases of its history, scope, and technical aspects, the treatment of this topic should give the student a general comprehensive grasp of public health nursing. It should include the treatment of acute and chronic illness, and the teaching of hygiene and preventive methods in the home. The various relations of the visiting nurse to physicians, health authorities, public schools, hospitals, and agencies of welfare, public and private, should be explained. Special fields of nursing should be taken up so far as possible.

SOCIAL SUBJECTS

Social Case Work

Under this title, a course should be given in what has come to be known as social diagnosis and treatment. The essence of social case work is defined as making adjustments between individuals and families on the one hand and their social environment on the other. Obviously, under this broad definition approach to all the typical social maladjustments is included.

Among the technical procedures to be taught are the process of securing and use of the social history, use of social agencies and social resources available for individuals and families, etc.

Social Problems

Under this general title, a course or courses should be given on various problems of modern society, by the case method preferably. Among these topics are the organization of industry and such industrial problems as unemployment, wages and standards of living, industrial hazards; immigration and the problem of the foreign-born; desertion and illegitimacy, etc.

The Underlying Bases of Social Work

A course should be offered dealing with the underlying bases of social work. The aim of the course should be to provide a background of certain fundamental concepts of biology, psychology and economics in relation to the development of society and social institutions.

Applied Psychology

Under this title a course should be given on the practical applications of psychology to mental hygiene, the understanding of abnormal mental conditions seen most frequently, the nature and process of management of the functional nervous diseases (psycho-neuroses), mental deficiency and constitutional psychopathic states. These topics should be presented broadly, so as to emphasize the importance of instinct in life, its modifications to meet the requirements of society, the defects that arise in the process of modification and their psychological explanation. In presenting these topics, the special approach of the public health nurse to her work should be considered, and every effort be made to create in the student the point of view that regards mental diseases, functional nervous diseases, and mental deficiency as imperfect or abnormal adaptations to actual situations in life.

Principles of Teaching

An introduction to modern educational methods and objectives should be given in close conjunction with the course on principles of applied psychology, with special reference to the organization and presentation of material to adult persons.

SCIENTIFIC SUBJECTS

Prevention and Control of Disease

Under this inclusive heading a comprehensive course is advocated on:

Hygiene and sanitation, giving the fundamental principles of sanitary science and their application to urban and rural health problems, such as water and milk supply; disposal of sewage and garbage, etc.

Public health administration, showing the function and methods of health agencies, federal, state, urban, and rural; use of vital statistics as indices of health conditions in connection with nurse's record-keeping; social and health legislation.

The application of preventive medicine in nursing, showing the use in nursing of modern scientific medical methods in prevention of disease.

Family Nutrition

A course should be given on the feeding of families with special reference to nutritive requirements of its various members, the cost of food in relation to the family budget, economical use of food products, etc.

To cover this program in approximately one-half of the 8-months' course, or 16 weeks,[101] the following allotment of hours is suggested:

TABLE 21

Subject	Weekly	Total Hours	Per Cent of Total
Nursing	5	80	25.
Social	5	80	25.
Pedagogical	3	48	12.5
Scientific	7	112	37.5
Total	20	320	100.0

This program assumes a working week of 44 hours, of which approximately 20 are assigned to class work, 20 hours to preparation and reading, and approximately 4 hours to conferences or visits of observation.

2. Courses for Teachers and Administrators in Schools of Nursing

THE TEACHING STAFF

IDEAL REQUIREMENTS

We have discussed at some length the educational standards of the training schools as related to the curriculum together with the content of courses given, hours allowed, and methods used. But neither a wisely balanced curriculum, nor well-planned courses, nor adequate time allotments, nor the best methods can much avail for the students' education without the sole guarantee of their realization—the presence of a well-equipped and experienced teaching staff. Without such a guarantee the wisest educational plans are doomed to be illusory.

[101] Following the practice of most of the courses studied, a term is assumed to consist of 16 weeks.

In the schools of nursing no less than in other educational institutions, it is desirable first of all that the instructors should be qualified in the subjects they undertake to teach, and next that they be professional teachers as well. In addition, it is important for the sake of an adequate professional background and breadth of view, that they have some range of teaching experience outside of their hospital of graduation. For while the value of appointments made from a nursing school's own graduates may readily be seen in the automatic perpetuation of its methods and standards, its traditions and *morale*, the possible disadvantage of such appointments of persons without other experience should be as obvious, in the equal perpetuation of bad with good points and in the danger of inducing complacency and narrowness.

DEVELOPMENT IN RECENT YEARS

Whatever may be said in this section or elsewhere in this report of the inadequacy of the present equipment of teachers and standards of teaching in the nursing schools, the immense educational progress made in this field in recent years cannot well be over-emphasized. Not so long ago all teaching of theory was given by visiting lecturers, without any attempt on the part of the school to supervise or co-ordinate their work, or was allowed to depend on the scanty spare time of women executives already heavily burdened with administrative responsibilities, such as the superintendent or less often her assistants. By the first arrangement the teaching of the students, however good in special subjects, lacked any unified plan; in the second case the claims of education had inevitably to be subordinated to the more immediate urgencies of hospital service.

The appointment of full-time instructors in the more progressive schools has been a revolutionary step in the history of nursing training, and has marked a signal educational advance. Introduced at first as a dubious experiment, the creation of these full-time positions has been quickly justified. In place of the overburdened administrative head we have now, under the present policy in the best schools, the teacher whose primary business it is to teach. In the fields both of practice and theory, the students reap the benefit. In many cases the instructor in theory has virtually and sometimes in name the position of educational director. Under her supervision outside lecturers are brought into the scope of a balanced curriculum and contribute to a unified training.

In the majority of schools indeed the ideal of the separate full-time instructor may be still unrealized. Yet the idea is fading that adequate teaching can be properly done in a busy executive's spare hours. From the better schools an influence is setting towards the rest by which the teaching of preliminary subjects tends gradually to pass into the hands of trained teachers, within or without the hospital.

The best hope for many schools is the central instruction to which, during the preliminary term, students of co-operating hospitals may be sent, as we have described in an earlier chapter (see pages 293 ff.). Such central instruction may be obtained at already established educational institutions, such as the junior college or technical school or by joint instruction provided at a central place of meeting.

Yet the training schools have still a long way to go. The antiquated but still surviving tradition that a teacher must be able to teach practically every subject in the curriculum makes professional preparation impossible. How can a teacher, even with all that college or university study can do for her, be "expert," as any ideal requirements must demand, in the whole list even of preliminary subjects? The first step towards securing expert instruction is for the schools to moderate their demands upon the instructors.

THE SUPERINTENDENT

Though administrative officers are increasingly freed from teaching duties, the traditional position of the superintendent not only as head of the nursing school but as instructor also, and her continuance on the teaching staff at an undoubted majority of the hospitals throughout the country, makes it important to consider her qualifications as instructor and educator. In any case, whether she herself teaches or no, the superintendent must in the last analysis be responsible for the educational tone of the school and its standard of training. In addition to her heavy responsibilities in administering the complicated and difficult nursing service of the hospital, it is she who must define its educational aims, initiate its policies, plan courses and curricula, engage teachers, and supervise their work. Even where, as in certain advanced schools, the instructor in theory has become educational director, leaving the superintendent free for her executive duties, her educational policy will depend for its effectiveness and success on the broad training, the sympathy, and vision of the head of the training school. Without her intelligent support the instructor will be helpless indeed.

QUALIFICATIONS OF THE SUPERINTENDENT

In addition, then, to the administrative training required by the executive duties of her position, the superintendent should have as educator no less than as administrator a sufficient experience of other hospitals than her own to insure her breadth of view and resource in dealing with her special problems. She should have a technical training of wide and inclusive range, covering certainly all important services. She ought no less to have a thorough academic education if she is to supervise and guide effectively the educational policies of the school. For her duties are not only to carry efficiently the exacting routine and meet the daily and hourly crises of supervision and management, but to maintain the educational outlook and vision which shall enable her to keep her school in line with the rapid development and growth of nursing education.

It will not seem surprising if the qualifications of the rank and file of superintendents, as indicated by a study of the preparation and experience of the heads of 18 schools visited, fall short of these ideal requirements. The requirement of experience is perhaps the most generally met. More than half of the 18 (11) were graduates of other hospitals than those of their present office, all but one with further previous experience outside their hospitals of graduation. The remaining 7, who were graduated from the hospitals in which they were serving, had again had an intervening experience of service in other hospitals. Less than half of the 18 (8) had had any special training for their administrative duties.

The technical equipment of these 18 superintendents studied showed indeed marked inequalities, but the omissions were for the most part such services as mental and nervous diseases, venereal diseases, tuberculosis, and communicable diseases which are only now beginning to be available to students of nursing, and which at the time when these women had their training were wholly beyond their reach. More serious occasional omissions were found in infant care (2), in the obstetrical service (2), and in dietetics (3). A wide administrative experience may indeed enable a superintendent to direct such services without personal experience of her own and to obtain the necessary personnel for instruction, provided only her general background and equipment are adequate to the task. It is the varied demands on her judgment in so many and such constantly developing scientific and practical fields that render indispensable a sound basis of general education. It is the lack of this basic education which in many instances gravely handicaps these women, carrying in their dual responsibility towards students and patients a burden scarcely equalled in any other profession.

Academic Education

The academic preparation of the group of superintendents studied shows in even more marked degree the inequalities that we have noted in their technical equipment. Their general education ranged from college graduation to one year of high school. Four were college graduates, and one a graduate of a normal school. With few exceptions they had completed high school, and six had had in addition to their high school course a year or more of college or normal school work. Seven had had no training beyond high school, and several were not high school graduates.

In connection with these inequalities it should be noted that it is by no means only the smaller and poorer schools that show the lack of standardized requirements for their chief position; it is conspicuous precisely in important and influential schools. We must bear in mind, however, that most of the present body of superintendents had their schooling before higher education for women was as common as it is today.

ASSISTANT PRINCIPAL AND SUPERINTENDENT

With few exceptions, the members of the previous group were women of middle age and prolonged experience, most of whom had held their present position for a term of years. Another group, important to consider as members of the training school faculty, not only because they still carry a considerable amount of teaching as well as supervisory work, but because they might naturally be supposed to furnish an obvious field of choice for superintendencies, is that of assistant principals and superintendents. But instead of representing a younger generation, of possibly more thorough education and experience, the 14 assistants from whom data were obtained were scarcely younger than their chiefs (average 37 years as against 42), and their educational limitations were more marked. In point of fact, instead of advancing them to independent positions, the tendency is to keep these assistants as subordinates too long either for their own best interest or that of the school.

INSTRUCTORS

Equipment and Training

But the burden of actual teaching, apart from the professional subjects covered by staff physicians or visiting specialists, is largely in the hands of women instructors resident in the school; they are the keystone of the educational arch. There is commonly a "practical instructor," who teaches, as we have seen in an earlier section (see page 232), nursing procedures, and a "theoretical instructor," who teaches the sciences and other preliminary subjects, and who often acts as assistant instructor in professional subjects as well, conducting the quizzes for lecture courses or clinics of physicians or visiting lecturers. We have already emphasized the great educational advance marked by the appointment of these full-time teachers in the nursing schools. Certain differences of organization and assignment of work exist not unnaturally in different hospitals. In some, as we have seen, the superintendent or assistant superintendent carries some part of the teaching; in others, special subjects such as pediatrics, obstetrics, or contagious diseases may be assigned to ward supervisors or head nurses instead of to the regular instructors.

Whatever the details of organization, these instructors should no doubt ideally be both experts in the subjects taught and trained teachers as well. As much as the theoretical instructor the teacher of nursing practice needs an adequate pedagogical equipment, and, to some extent at least, an intelligent knowledge of the subjects included in a nursing curriculum. Contact with the larger world of nursing education by some teaching experience outside the home schools is also needful, as we have said, for a safeguard against provincialism and a guarantee of some breadth of view in dealing with educational problems.

In point of fact we can scarcely expect such perfection of teaching equipment in the schools of nursing any more than in other vocational fields. It was indeed a notable advance in vocational education when Teachers College first began to give pedagogical training to instructors in schools of nursing. To a discussion of this instruction we devote a subsequent section.

A careful study of the qualifications of 34 instructors in 17 training schools revealed indeed a number of women eminently well-equipped for acceptable and successful service, but a far larger number seriously deficient in training and preparation. In so far as general education went, 4 members of the group were college graduates, and of the rest 12 had had some college or normal training. But more than half of the entire group (18) had nothing beyond a high school education to prepare them for their professional work, 6 lacked a high school diploma, and 2 had had but a single year of high school. Of the whole number only 3 had had a few months of postgraduate nursing training; almost half (15), on the other hand, certainly a high proportion as compared with teachers in other fields, had had some pedagogical preparation for their teaching.

It is of course commonly recognized that experience may well replace or supplement pedagogical training, and a majority of the 34 instructors had had at least some experience in other hospitals than those of their present service. Yet 11 had had no such broadening experience, and of these 8 were also without any special training as teachers. The facts must be faced, in conclusion, that more than half of the 34 instructors studied were handling their work without more expert knowledge of subjects taught than they had received in high school or their own nurse's training or had managed to pick up by private study.

When we come to the groups of supervisors and head nurses, many of whom have a definite teaching schedule, and almost all of whom share the responsibility for the personal supervision and instruction of the student nurses, the teaching qualifications are more limited.

Out of a group of 30 [102] supervisors whose personal histories were studied there was one college graduate, and 8 others who had had some college or normal training. Ten more had high school diplomas, and the remaining 11 had either not completed the high school course or had been educated in private schools. Of 13 night supervisors one had had normal work and one a year of college. Seven others were high school graduates. Only 1 of the day supervisors and 3 of the night supervisors had had any postgraduate professional work.

For 95 [103] head nurses the educational records showed that 4 were college graduates, 8 had had some normal training, and 13

[102] 32 listed; for 2 no data given.
[103] 97 listed; for 2 no data given.

others had had one or more years of college. About half of the whole number (46) were high school graduates, 20 had not finished high school, and 4 had attended private schools. Of the whole group, 4 had taken postgraduate professional courses varying from six weeks to six months.

If we make, then, the very liberal assumption that any normal school or college training constitutes a preparation for teaching, scarcely more than one-fourth of the whole number of supervisors and head nurses considered (34) can be thought to be equipped for the instruction which is one of the most important aspects of their work. It is somewhat reassuring to learn from the data reported that a number of these women,—7 supervisors and 11 head nurses,—had been for a longer or shorter time teachers before taking up nursing training. But as this previous experience coincides in the majority of cases with later normal or college training, it does not appreciably heighten the percentage of the whole group fitted for teaching work.

It is clearly realized that in the preceding discussion, whether of superintendents, instructors, or teaching head nurses, no account has been taken of the personal quality which is after all the prime essential, without which the most thorough equipment is incomplete and avails little. How often gifts of temperament or of character have achieved successes denied to women better prepared but not so happily endowed, we cannot learn from statistics. It is certainly to the resource, the zeal, and the devotion of the group of women discussed that nursing education owes to date its best achievements. All credit should be given them for what they have accomplished against almost overwhelming odds.

CONDITIONS OF WORK

The low educational level of much of the teaching in schools of nursing cannot, in any case, be ascribed wholly or even in chief part to the faulty equipment of some of the teaching staff. Certain conditions in many schools militate so seriously against any high educational standards in teaching that the best efforts of some of the ablest teachers, women of high training and capacity, are discouraged and frustrated. By overlong hours, by excessive number of subjects assigned, and by responsibilities other than teaching laid upon the instructors, many of the schools create handicaps against which a very genius of teaching might strive in vain.

To obtain light on these conditions, the programs and personal histories of the theoretical instructors in 7 prominent training schools were intensively studied.

Length of Yearly and Weekly Programs

In these 7 schools the teaching year varies from 36 to 51 weeks, with a usual length, however, of from 40 to 45 weeks. So narrow a margin for recuperation from the year's fatigues as 7 weeks, to say nothing of the single week allowed in the worst instance, should be balanced, at the very least, by a moderate assignment of hours during the long teaching year. What, in fact, is the case?

The weekly teaching schedules show maxima in the several training schools of from 18 to 38 hours, according to the time of year, and medians of from 12 to 24 hours. At 2 schools with exceptionally heavy programs the median hours are 24 and the maxima respectively 30 and 38. The incompatibility of such schedules with good work is a point which need not be labored. It must not of course be supposed that actual teaching can be expected for such excessive hours. A nu nber of them may be spent in merely formal "chaperoning" of lectures given by visiting instructors. Others again are repetitive work, owing to the sectioning of the larger classes. But even repetitive work, if it is not to be merely mechanical, means, as every teacher knows, the expense of vital force for every hour in the classroom. And neither the offset of chaperonage nor of repetition of work can make these excessive hours in the classroom pedagogically manageable or humanly reasonable. A comparison of such schedules with the 12 or 15 hours' work normally required of instructors in colleges of good standing throws a glaring light on the requirements of the training schools.

Number of Subjects

An apparently reasonable schedule of hours may on the other hand be rendered excessive by the inclusion of an unreasonable variety of subjects. Thus in one school where the maximum of weekly teaching hours is 18, these 18 hours include no less than 10 distinct subjects. Six or 8 separate subjects are by no means unusual in a teaching program. The training school instructor is expected to teach more subjects than the high school teacher in a small city, who seldom carries more than 4 or 5 subjects and often only 1 or 2. In addition to her heavy teaching program, she must moreover often give quizzes on the doctors' lectures in several other fields. At one of the schools studied, a teaching schedule running up to the indefensible weekly maximum of 38 hours covered 7 teaching subjects and 6 or 7 quiz subjects. Here for the courses she "chaperones," the instructor must also conduct quizzes in pathology, surgical and medical diseases, gynecology, special diseases, mental and nervous diseases, and public sanitation! While this is no doubt a somewhat extreme instance, examples of only less excessive demands on the teacher are by no means infrequent.

Outside Duties

But the seriousness of these conditions of overwork is by no means fully stated with the hours of teaching and numbers of subjects taught. A further tax on the teacher's time and strength is levied by a long list of non-teaching duties frequently assigned her. Common among these additional responsibilities are holding office hours and holding interviews, keeping records and making reports, supervising study hours, preparing and posting class schedules and bulletins, giving out reference books, etc. Where, as in several of the hospitals studied, the theoretical instructor virtually carries the responsibility of educational director, these outside duties are still more onerous. They may include, for example, the interviewing and engaging of teachers, the arrangement of class schedules, the planning of courses, the preparation of lecture outlines, the making and giving notice of all changes and readjustments, the compiling of the annual report, and the planning of the budget for the educational department.

In justice to the training school authorities, it should be said that these undue burdens are laid upon the instructors not so much by design as by necessity. The superintendent of a school of any size must obviously be freed from the burden of clerical duties which in smaller schools she commonly carries herself. Clerical assistance is rarely allowed her in any adequate amount, and she is commonly able to secure the appointment of an instructor only on the basis of her assuming responsibility for a large part of the clerical work of the school.

Of good teaching under such handicaps there can be little question. No deliberate design could more certainly lower the level of nursing school instruction. Instructors of supreme capacity and equipment could not in such circumstances perform any but lifeless and routine work.

Salaries

Even in the matter of salaries, the undefined and unstandardized character of these teaching positions is apparent. There is no established scale such as exists to a certain extent at least in other academic work. The salaries, low at best, ranging all the way from $900 to $1,800 with a median of $1,320, are much higher than their face value in that they include residence, board, and laundry. But they seem to bear little relation to the responsibility or importance of positions or the training and experience of teachers. It happens not infrequently that a college graduate with teaching diploma, postgraduate study, and previous experience is found in a lower-salaried position than a teacher with none of these advantages of equipment. The post of instructor is thus without established professional dignity and offers little incentive in the way of rewards or promotion to ambitious students for the special preparation or advanced training which is likely to be so little regarded.

NEED OF STANDARDIZATION

It is evident from what has preceded that the unstandardized character of the teaching positions as well as the unstandardized equipment of the teachers is the cause of much that is unsatisfactory in the present educational status of the schools of nursing. Reforms in both directions are obvious and urgent. On the one hand the high standard of technical equipment now found in a few instructors should be made in time the general requirement. On the other hand the teachers' qualifications should be given a fair chance by a change in the demands on the teaching positions. They should be freed first from the petty routine duties of administration which might be quite as efficiently performed by an ordinary clerical assistant. Next, the teaching schedule should be standardized both as to hours of work and number of subjects taught more nearly in conformity with the demands found reasonable at other educational institutions. Allowance should be made for preparation of work, and a margin of time for the study and thought which alone makes teaching fresh and vital instead of automatic repetition and routine.

Not least in need of standardization is the matter of salaries already spoken of. The scale should be made to bear its due relation to position and preparation, and should be fixed high enough to seem to the student, as it certainly does not now, a fair return on her investment of equipment and effort.

3. Teachers College and Its Influence on Nursing Education

No discussion of the teaching in schools of nursing, however brief, can be complete without some account of the strongest educational stimulus, the most potent standardizing influence ever exerted upon it, namely, that of Teachers College. The position held by Teachers College with respect to the nursing profession is indeed unique; its service has been incalculable. We have included discussion of its courses on public health nursing in an earlier chapter. While it is no longer the only academic institution offering work in teaching and supervision, its courses have by far the greatest variety and prestige. Without its direct stimulus to the instructors, supervisors, and administrators who have studied there, and its enormous effect through them on the standards of teaching in schools of nursing throughout the country, it is safe to say that the development of nursing education would have lagged far behind its present stage in the evolution of a serious professional discipline from the loose standards of apprenticeship.

In the course of our survey, an impressive proportion of the officers and instructors at the better training schools were found to have taken postgraduate work at Teachers College, including superintendents, assistant superintendents, practical as well as theoretical instructors, and head nurses. Since, then, so many executives and instructors, women of position and influence in nursing education, bear to some extent at least the impress of Teachers College, and show the influence of advanced courses in teaching and supervision, it is important to study the work given there in relation to the profession, and to examine the group of nurses there assembled as illustrative of the coming leaders in the nursing world.

History of the Department

The Department of Nursing and Health at Teachers College was founded some 20 years ago in response to an insistent appeal from certain leading members of the nursing profession, as a direct attempt to meet the need of the schools of nursing for trained teachers and supervisors.

The new department at Teachers College was to furnish both subject matter and technique of teaching. It was also to teach administration, and by doing so put a new emphasis on executive efficiency. No such courses had ever before been offered. Here was a virgin field, a wholly new technique to be developed, with students at that time for the most part unprepared for any academic work. With a view to securing the best material, the course was first opened to a few candidates who were to be not only graduate nurses but women of experience either as training school superintendents or as head nurses in large and important wards. Applicants were required from the first to present evidence of good preliminary education, though nursing students were not required to meet the full matriculation requirements of the college unless they wished to qualify for the B.S. degree. The educational requirements have steadily risen until now the department admits regular students only on the same conditions as other college students; if, namely, they present full entrance qualifications (15 high school units), or are prepared to make up a small high school deficiency after admission. The present professional requirement, no longer including administrative experience, except for courses in administration, is that the student be a graduate of a training school which commands a varied clinical service of at least 50 patients daily and offers satisfactory training in medical, surgical, pediatric, and obstetric services, and that she be a registered nurse.

Every year many students applying for admission are rejected because of deficiences in their educational or professional preparation. Exceptions are sometimes made in the case of women who have shown marked ability in the professional field or of foreign students who come with good credentials. Such women may be occasionally entered as non-matriculated students, but the irregular group they compose is never larger than about 2 per cent of the whole student body.

Student nurses in public health work who come to the college for a few hours a week are non-matriculated students as a rule but are required to have the equivalent of high school education. This is the only group accepted during the regular college year for less than a full year of work. It is interesting to note that while the requirements are held up more and more rigidly each year, the numbers entering the department have steadily increased.

The certificate was at first given for a year's work. The public health group is the only one now in which a certificate can be obtained in one year, the other branches requiring approximately two years after matriculating and in addition to professional training.

At first most of the students entered for a year of work, and
only a few qualified for the bachelor's or the master's degree.
Now almost half of the regular student body in the department
is registered for one or the other of these degrees and this may
involve from one to three and sometimes four years of college
work. A student with a high school diploma coming from a first
class professional school will probably receive the bachelor's
degree in approximately two and one-half years. A student with
a weak professional training, on the other hand, receives less
credit for it and takes longer to obtain the degree. The majority
of those who are able to afford only one year of work to begin
with, plan to return in a year or two to complete the requirements
for the degree. Each year, moreover, sees a larger group making
genuine sacrifices to stay on longer than a single year.

It will be seen that the general effect of the requirements set
up by Teachers College is to put a premium both on sound preliminary education and on sound professional training.

FACILITIES

From the first the department has had but a comparatively
small subsidy. That it has any endowment is due to the generosity of a donor who has the distinction of being the first person
who has ever endowed higher nursing education in the United
States, Mrs. Helen Hartley Jenkins of New York. It has been
built up in the face of lack of funds, imperfect equipment, inadequate facilities of all sorts. Office work is rendered difficult by
lack of space; classrooms and laboratories, whether the department's own or those shared by its students with other departments, are congested and often not well equipped. Yet the work
has gone forward steadily through the indefatigable service of
the entire department staff.

ORGANIZATION

CLASSIFICATION OF STUDENTS

The student body in the Department of Nursing and Health
consisted in the year of our study (1920-1921) of 305 nurses, of
whom 100 were students in training taking a short 4-months'
course. Of the graduate nurses 75 were in the teaching or administrative groups; 90 were entered for the public health nursing courses. The distribution was approximately:

In administration 25
In teaching 50
In public health 90

In addition to these, there were several small groups, such as students taking the combined course with the Presbyterian and St. Luke's Hospitals, students in occupational therapy, and students taking special subjects, altogether about 30 to 35. Almost all of these students were high school graduates, and several had had one or two years of normal school or college work or had even taken a degree. Approximately 85 were registered for degrees at Teachers College.

CURRICULUM

REQUIRED COURSES

For the degree and a diploma in teaching in schools of nursing, the student must satisfactorily complete two years' work, with required courses amounting to 40 points out of a possible 60 or 72.[104] These required courses with their weighting by points are given below:

			Points
Education	6 courses {	4 General 2 Applied to Nursing Schools }	18
Subject-Matter of Teaching	5 courses {	Chemistry (Elementary) Biology (Physiology) Micro-Biology, including Bacteriology } Hygiene (Sanitary Science) History of Nursing	16
General	{ 1 course 2 courses	Supervision in Hospitals and Training Schools .... Social Science	2 4
		Total	40

Two things are striking in this list of required courses: first, the relatively large amount of time given to pedagogy; and, second, the small amount of time given to preparation for the teaching of individual subjects. Both points, indeed, are readily explained. The pedagogical emphasis is a part of the general stress on educational theory at Teachers College, considered by the authorities essential for the diploma in teaching. The lack of thorough preparation in the subject matter of teaching is a nat-

[104] The major in administration in schools of nursing is planned along similar lines, but without required work in science and with a larger amount of time allowed for free electives. Required courses amount to 32 points only.

ural and practically a forced compliance with the conditions of teaching in the training schools.

We have spoken already of the unreasonable number of subjects assigned to the individual instructor. With a teaching program of even five or six subjects, to take a very moderate instance, how can the would-be teacher hope to obtain, or any college or university plan to give, any adequate grounding in so wide a field? The student is driven to seek a general acquaintance with the whole list; on the college, on the other hand, the pressure is imperative to aid her necessity, and meet the existing situation by offering the short courses in many branches, which are in such striking contrast to the intensive professional preparation customary in other lines of work, or to the equipment of the college student for the teaching of two or three subjects, but which are at present indispensable.

For obviously the college cannot far outstrip the conditions of teaching in the schools of nursing, or prepare its students for a demand which does not exist. Few schools can at present afford more than one general instructor. The larger schools employ as we have seen only two, the teacher of practical nursing and the teacher of "theory" or, chiefly, the basic sciences. The teaching division in the Department of Nursing and Health consists therefore of three groups, those who are fitting themselves as:

(1) General all-round instructors in the smaller schools.
(2) Instructors of practical nursing in the larger schools.
(3) Instructors in "theory" or basic sciences in the larger schools.

Courses required for the teaching major are limited to those believed to furnish the indispensable basis for all three groups.

It may of course be said that the work at Teachers College in scientific or nursing subjects is superimposed upon a body of knowledge acquired in the three years of training. But our examination of training school teaching has shown all too clearly the thoroughly inadequate character of much of the instruction offered. The fact must be faced that for the majority of students at Teachers College the college courses are all that can be relied on as a standardized basis for future teaching work.

Even after her postgraduate course, then, what has the future teacher of science to work with? In chemistry, for example, she will have, according to the list of required subjects, but one half-year of elementary chemistry to supplement her own earlier and often meager training school course. The college, in view of the varied subjects in which she must secure some preparation at least, cannot insist upon the two-years' course which is unquestionably a minimum for teaching. The same limitations necessarily control the required courses both in bacteriology and in anatomy and physiology.

ELECTIVES

Elective subjects are added by advice of the department according to the special kind of work which the student expects to take up. A study of various programs of students in both teaching and administration showed that the electives did not in general shift the emphasis of the required subjects, but preserved about the same relative proportion of technique and content of teaching. The elective hours went in large part to cultural subjects, such as English, history, French, Spanish, fine arts, etc. Other subjects taken by these students were of professional value although they will not be taught. Among these were physics elected by 3 of the 6 students in question; nutrition and household administration, in each of which one student elected a course, and speaking, elected by 2 students.

The programs, to sum them up, show a large amount of work in education, both required and elective; a much smaller proportion of courses in subjects likely to be taught, either scientific or nursing; a few border-line subjects, and a wide variation from the intensive work of the professional school in the amount of time spent in fields of culture versus professional value.

The reasons for the pedagogical emphasis and for the cultural studies are persuasive and weighty enough, related as they obviously are to professional need on the one hand and on the other to the personal intellectual hunger of students without earlier cultural opportunities. Yet the most impressive feature of these schedules is their common reflection of the existing dilemma of all nursing education: the necessity, namely, of giving preparation to students along so many lines.

FUTURE POSSIBILITIES

The Department of Nursing and Health at Teachers College has in a short space of years performed an irreplaceable service to the training schools of the country through the better equipment and the invaluable stimulus given to successive classes of nursing instructors. The further development of its courses waits necessarily upon the further progress of the training schools. It may, however, be queried whether, with the growth of teaching standards in the training schools and the changing of the pedagogical situation through the agency precisely of such work as that of Teachers College, it may not be possible to limit somewhat further the requirements in education, and transfer some of the time now spent on technique to the subject matter of teaching. How far indeed is it of value for the nurse instructor to proceed along the same path with prospective teachers in other fields? Comments of students interviewed in our study showed not infrequently a feeling that the time spent in these general educational courses is not all well spent, as the instructors do not seem sufficiently familiar with the special problems of the nursing schools. With the time at the student's disposal so strictly limited, may it not be wise to lay more relative stress on these special problems and especially the problems of adult education?

The existing difficulty, as we have already indicated, is bound up with the whole problem of nursing education. With the raising of standards both of admission and of teaching in the training school, the quality and amount of work in the various college courses can be further advanced. As the schools are able to afford a larger teaching staff, the student of teaching may look forward to greater specialization, and Teachers College to giving her the intensive work appropriate to a standard professional training, now rendered impracticable by the exigencies of the situation.

INCLUSION OF PUBLIC HEALTH NURSING

One important aspect of training teachers and administrators for schools of nursing, which is necessarily a new issue, is their more adequate initiation into the new medical and nursing field of prevention of illness and health instruction. These teachers and administrators are to be the leaders and guides of new generations of nurses. How is it possible for them, it may be asked, to stress the new prevention, the teaching of health and hygiene, if they are not themselves fortified in the principles and practice of instructive, preventive nursing? How shall they teach the minimum of social interpretation of cases, give the medico-social background underlying most physical disability and sickness, and needed for proper training in all phases of nursing?

To make any additions to the already over-crowded programs of postgraduate students is a practical impossibility. We should argue in the direction of reducing rather than of increasing the programs of the group studied at Teachers College, for instance. Yet to give the grounding in principles of prevention and public health nursing which all student nurses should have, some adequate preparation is needed for the future instructors and teachers themselves. The only practicable method which suggests itself is the addition of a four-months' course, combining class work and field work in public health nursing, for all this group.

That such a suggestion would be favored by many who are fitting themselves for administration and teaching was shown by the opinions expressed in interviews with these students.

TYPE OF STUDENTS

The fact should be borne in mind that the nurses entering Teachers College are not as a group in the position of students entering other professional schools. They constitute a peculiar group, with high qualifications of experience and intelligence, but with educational handicaps.

According to the general testimony, the nursing group as a whole is of "average ability," "holds its own with other groups," while the best members of it, by force of their experience and maturity "will outrank almost any group."

The characteristics of the nursing students at Teachers College were marked, according to our observer, herself a college teacher of high standing, with surprising clearness. Most striking was the mental homogeneity of the group, the general uniformity of type. Conscientious, hard-working, ambitious, responsible, these adjectives recurred again and again in the comments of instructors. Intellectually hungry as these students are, almost painfully conscious of their short-comings, their eagerness takes the form of heavy programs (often including as many as eight courses), and of an overwork which sometimes defeats its own ends. The financial sacrifices they make for the work at Teachers College, their ambition and zeal for knowledge command a respect so deep as to rebuke any criticism of their electives, say, in French and fine arts. This eagerness of spirit naturally makes them appreciative and stimulating students, "a joy to teach," as one of their instructors put it. Their fine professional spirit and loyalty, their scientific habit of mind, is everywhere recognized.

But with all their eagerness and devotion, they are constantly handicapped by their limited preparation and their lack of background. Their defective training shows in their weakness in dealing with and organizing material, their generally noted lack of the power to synthesize. The conditions of their training, especially in the old type of training school with its excessive discipline and rigidity, are perhaps in some measure reflected in a certain lack of initiative and originality. As the old ideal of military discipline in the training schools passes and is replaced by a freer spirit of co-operation among the students, as moreover the larger number of college women among the teachers and administrators brings a more original spirit into the schools, the coming generations of nurses may in turn show a larger initiative and freer development. The defects and qualities of the group as a whole are well summed up in the following comment by one of their most observing instructors:

"The qualities of marked leadership, initiative, originality, the vivid personality, the critical mind, the investigating type of mind, creative ability, these are not common among the nurses at Teachers College, but probably not any more common among other groups of students. It is probably because we need these qualities so much in nursing that we are disappointed when we do not find more people with them. On the other hand, because of their really vital interest in their work, many women of average ability are able to make a much bigger contribution to nursing progress than their previous training and qualifications might seem to promise."

THE LARGER AIM OF POSTGRADUATE INSTRUCTION

Postgraduate courses in teaching and administration modelled on those at Teachers College are being organized in other universities. In such courses a larger aim should be, as it has been at the pioneer college, to set standards for the future leaders of the profession. The student should learn not only teaching methods and material, not only the principles of administration, but the breadth of vision which shall envisage the nurse's training and its problems as a whole, and govern its new adjustments and expansions. From this standpoint, the prime service of such college courses is perhaps the student's emancipation. They rescue her from the isolation and parochialism of her nursing school, and make her realize herself and her training as a part of the educational system of the country.

It is this feeling of enlargement and participation in wide aims, the "chance at enlarged vision," the new "stimulus and outlook in all directions," which is perhaps most often spoken of by students of Teachers College in expressing their sense of the value of their college experience.

Finally, Teachers College has played a valuable part also in stimulating among its nurse graduates regular meetings for discussion and conference on educational problems—a movement which is growing among other teaching groups and which holds, in the opportunity it offers for democratic and purposeful inquiry and exchange of experience, one of the most hopeful promises of educational advance.

APPENDIX

COPIES OF SCHEDULES USED IN THE SURVEY *

1. TRAINING SCHOOL SERIES

Schedule I

ORGANIZATION OF TRAINING SCHOOL

A.   I. Legal name of school...
   II. Address: City...................State ....
  III. Is the school incorporated?.................Date ....
  IV. Legal name of hospital...
    V. Is the school a department of the hospital?.....................
  VI. " " " " " " a university?.........Of a medical
       school? ....

B. Governing Board or Training School Committee (give exact title)....
   I. ....
  II. What are its functions?.......................................
 III. How many times did it meet during past year?................
     Date of meetings...
  IV. How many members?............V. Give names of members and
    indicate their relation to hospital and position in community.

VI. Name other boards having administrative or advisory powers.

C. Finances for fiscal year ending ....
   I. Is the school endowed?.......Amount of endowment...........
  II. What is the value of the school property?.....................
 III. How is the property maintained?.............................
 IV. What is the charge for tuition?.............................
   V. What was the total amount received for special nursing of private
    patients by students?.......................................
  VI. Is a money allowance made to students?......................
    Give amount 1st year........2nd year........3rd year..........
 VII. What other allowances are made?............................
 VIII. Give itemized statement of receipts and expenditures last year:

* Schedules for Industrial Nursing and Postgraduate Courses not reproduced here.

561

1. RECEIPTS		2. EXPENDITURES	
Sources	Amount	Items	Amount

D. Clinical Facilities:
  I. Type of hospital...
  II. No. of beds...........III. Daily average of patients............
  IV. Daily average of admissions..................................
  V. Average number of days in hospital per patient...............
  VI. NUMBER OF BEDS IN SERVICES UTILIZED FOR TRAINING

Medical Wards		Surgical Wards		Children's Wards	Obstetrical Wards	Communicable Disease Wards	Nervous and Mental Wards	Private Rooms
Men	Women	Men	Women					

  VII. Operating room: daily average operations......................
  VIII. Obstetrical wards: daily average deliveries.....................
  IX. Out-patient department:
      1. Daily average attendance................................
      2. Services ....
  X. TRAINING IN AFFILIATED INSTITUTIONS OR ASSOCIATIONS

Name of Affiliating Institution or Association	Address	Type of Experience	Length of Service	Required or Elective
1.				
2.				
3.				

  XI. If the affiliations are elective, for how many students is each
      available? ....

E. Faculty
  I. Head of school.............................
      1. Title ....
      2. Salary ....
      3. Date of appointment....................

APPENDIX 563

4. Graduate of.............................School for Nurses
5. Year of graduation......................
6. State and year in which registered.......
7. How is the head of the school appointed? ....
8. For what term?...........................
9. How is she removed?....................

II. Staff of school:

GRADUATE NURSES

Name and Degree	Position	Annual Salary	Duties Other Than Teaching	Subjects Taught Classroom Wards	No. Hours per Week

III. INSTRUCTORS AND LECTURERS OTHER THAN NURSES

Name and Degree	Position in Relation to Hospital	Subjects Taught	No. of Hours per Week	Occupation Other Than Teaching in Training School	Annual Salary from Training School

F. I. Are conferences held of entire teaching
staff? ....How often?...........
II. Are conferences held of part of the teaching staff? ....How often?...........

G. I. Obtain two copies latest annual report of hospital.
II. "   "   " last annual budget.
III. " weekly teaching schedule for each member of the teaching staff (Schedule III A).

Schedule II

ADMINISTRATION

A. I. Number of students:

Preliminary Course	1st Year	2nd Year	8rd Year	Total

II. Ratio of students to patients:

	GENERAL WARDS		PRIVATE WARDS		PRIVATE PATIENTS	CHILDREN
	Male	Female	Male	Female		
Day.......						
Night						

III. 1. Total number of graduate nurses employed..................
    2. Ratio of students to graduates...............................

B. Requirements for admission:

    I.

	MINIMUM AGE	MINIMUM EDUCATION
School Requirement...		
State Requirement....		

II. What educational credentials are required?.....................
....

III. Who evaluates the educational credentials?.....................

IV. Who makes the final decision in regard to the eligibility of applicants? ....
....

V. Is student required to sign contract with school?...............
How binding is it regarded?...................................

VI. Are students from other accredited schools given credit in time?..
....

VII. 1. Is a physical examination made before ending of preliminary
       course? ....
    2. Who makes the examination? ....

C. I. Date of beginning of school year.....................
II. Length of course............years.............months.........

	PRELIMINARY	1ST YEAR	2ND YEAR	8RD YEAR	TOTAL
Division of Course (Give No. of Months)...					
Vacation (Give No. of Weeks)....					

564

III. What is the length of the probation period?....................

IV. Dates for admission of classes...........................:....

V. Number in each group admitted during 1918 and exact dates of admission:
....
....

VI. How much time, if any, is spent by each section at end of course without class instruction?...................................

D. Hours of duty:

I. 1. Is the 8-hour system in force?..............................

2. Schedule other than 8-hour system:

	GENERAL WARD	OPERATING ROOM	DIET KITCHEN	OBSTETRIC DEPARTMENT	SPECIAL CASES	PRIVATE PATIENTS
Day Duty Week Days						
Day Duty Sundays						

II. What additional free time is given during week?................

III. How is the time students are off duty checked?.................
....

IV. Are class hours included in duty time?.........................

V. How much time is allowed for:
Breakfast..........Dinner..........Supper..........

VI. Are operating room students on call at night?..................

VII. Are maternity "   "   "   "   "   "   ....

VIII. What is the number of hours on night duty?....................

IX. "   "   " length of term of night duty?.....................

X. "   "   " number of periods of night duty for each student?...

XI. What time off is given during night duty?.....................

XII. "   "   "   "   " at termination of night duty?.........

XIII. When are classes held for students on night duty?..............

XIV. How many months must a student have been in the school before assignment to night duty?.....................................

XV. Who supervises students during the first period of night duty?....
....

E. I. Obtain following information from inspection of records:
Inspection of student's credentials. Make list showing education, age of admission, and previous occupation.

II. Record of hours of duty for one week for one student from each class.

III. Obtain record of night operation for past month, and amount of time thus spent by students who are on day duty.

IV. Obtain same record for maternity cases.

V. Obtain record of time planned for students in different departments.

VI. Make copies of practical experience of each member of present senior class, include illness and vacation; i.e., copy monthly record card or sheet.

VII. How many terms of service are planned for a student in one department?

VIII. What is the relation in time of theory to practice?

F. Obtain two copies of each of the following:

I. School announcement.

II. Any other descriptive material for distribution.

III. Application blanks.

IV. Schedule of 8-hour system.

V. Any other form used for obtaining information re applicant.

VI. Daily time book (specimen pages).

VII. Records of theoretical work.

VIII.   "   " practical   "

IX. Case record.

X. Record of practical procedure.

XI. Efficiency record.

XII. Students' contract with school.

TEACHING PROGRAM OF INSTRUCTORS

[Calendar was enclosed for checking]

SCHEDULE III B

PERSONAL HISTORY OF MEMBERS OF FACULTY

A. 1. Name and address of school where now employed.................
....
2. Name of nurse ....3. Age ....4. M. S. W. ......
5. Are you registered? ....6. If so, give state and year..........
7. Name of present position (specify instructor, supervisor, head nurse, assistant, etc.) ....
8. Length of service in present position ....years..........months
9. Name duties of present position ....

B. I. Did you hold a paid position *before beginning nurses' training?*.....
(Describe last two positions only)

NATURE OF WORK *	LENGTH OF SERVICE	
	Years	Months

* Specify exact position held, e.g., teaching; clerical work; employment in store or factory other than clerical; personal service, such as caring for children; social work; etc.

II. Paid positions held *after completing nurses' training:*
1. Have you done private nursing? ....If so, for how long? ....years
....months
2. Positions other than private nursing:

	NAME OF EMPLOYER	PLACE	NATURE OF WORK *	LENGTH OF SERVICE	
	Institution, Organization, or Individual	City or Town and State		Years	Months
a					
b					

* Give name of position and kind of work; e.g., head nurse, operating room; supervisor, private wards, etc.

C. I. General Education:

	NAME	CITY OR TOWN AND STATE	YEAR OF GRADUATION	IF NOT GRADUATE, NO. OF YEARS ATTENDED
Grammar or Parochial School				
High School				
College				
Other Schools not Nurses' Training Schools				

II. Hospital Training (undergraduate):
  1. Name and address of nurses' training school ....
  ....
  2. Year of graduation ....3. Length of course.............
  4. No. of hospital beds at time you graduated ....
  5. Were pupils sent out of hospital to do private nursing? ....
  6. If so, how long were you thus employed? ....
  7. How long did you spend on special duty with patients to whom
     a charge was made for special nursing?......................
  8. Did your training include work with the following:
     a. Men...........b. Women.............c. Children............
     d. Sick infants under 2 years..........e. Medical cases.........
     f. Surgical cases..............g. Obstetrical cases..............
     h. Nervous and mental cases........i. Venereal diseases........
     j. Tuberculosis.........k. Other communicable diseases (specify
        which) ....
     ....
     l. Dietetic department...................m. Other departments
        (specify) ....

III. Post-Graduate Courses:

SCHOOL OR COLLEGE	CITY AND STATE	LENGTH OF TIME ATTENDED	YEAR	SUBJECTS STUDIED	DEGREE OR DIPLOMA

Nurses' organizations of which you are a member.......................
....
                              Date............................

Schedule IV A

CURRICULUM, SECTION 1

SUBJECTS	Prelim.	NUMBER OF PERIODS				METHODS			TIME OF SESSION		
		1st Year	2nd Year	3rd Year	Total	Lect.	Recit.	Lab.	a. m.	p. m.	After 6 P. M.
Anatomy and Physiology											
Bacteriology											
Chemistry											
Hygiene (Personal)											
Dietetics and Cookery ..											
Bandaging											
Massage											
Sanitation											
Materia Medica											
Clinical Diagnosis											
Medical Diseases											
Surgical Diseases											
Operating Room Technique											
Gynecology											
Obstetrics											
Pediatrics											
Orthopedics											
Communicable Diseases											
Nervous and Mental											
Eye, Ear, Nose, Throat .											
Theory and Practice of Nursing											
Occupational Diseases ..											
Occupation Therapy											
Venereal and Skin											
Hospital Housekeeping .											
Public Health Nursing .											
Psychology											
Ethics											
Professional Problems ..											
Social Service											
Other Subjects											

What is the length of the lecture period?......................Recitation
period?.....................Laboratory period?.....................
Demonstration period?...

Recent changes:

SCHEDULE IV A (Cont.)

CURRICULUM, SECTION 2

To be filled out in conference with instructors.
I. Methods, equipment, and facilities for work in introductory sciences.
  1. Anatomy and Physiology.
    a. Methods of teaching:
      (1) Are formal lectures the rule?.............................
      (2) In how far is subject developed by question and discussion rather than by lectures?.................................
      (3) Do students take notes?......Are these inspected?..........
      (4) Is a textbook used?...........What?.....................
      (5) Are there frequent quizzes?...............................
      (6) Are special reports or papers by students called for?........
      (7) How are directions for laboratory work given?..............
      (8) What records are kept of laboratory work and demonstrations? ....
      (9) Are these corrected?......................................
      (10) Are conferences held with students? ....
      (11) Final examinations: When held?...........................
          How important?...
      (12) What factors determine the student's grade in the course? ...
      (13) Remarks:

    b. Equipment:
      (1) Demonstration material. Note items present, with number where possible:
        Skeleton ....Other bones ......Models ....
        Charts ....Lantern ....Reflectoscope ....
        Lantern slides.........Preserved specimens..........
        Microscopes (number and kind).....................
        Microscopic slides.........Physiological apparatus....
        Dissecting instruments.....Glassware ....
        Chemicals, etc., for chemical side of physiology........
        Are demonstrations of fresh material made?..........
        Do students go to autopsies?.......................
        Is there use of medical or other museums?............
      (2) What equipment is there for laboratory work done by the student?

(3) What financial provision is made for new equipment and up-keep? ....Annual appropriation? ....
Special requisition? ....Is it easy to get what is needed? ....

(4) Library: Books for this department:
  (a) Number (approximate) ....
  (b) General character..
  (c) Used by instructor, much or little....................
  (d) Used by student, much or little......................
  (e) How are books procured?.............................
  (f) Remarks:

(5) Assistance in laboratory:
  (a) What assistance is there in the preparation of laboratory for work of students or in the preparation of demonstrations? ....
  ....
  (b) Is the room free so that preparation may be made for laboratory or demonstration? ....
  (c) What assistance is there in clearing away after laboratory or demonstration? ....
  ....

(6) Room used for laboratory and demonstration:
  (a) Is space adequate for number of students?.............
    Number in working section?........................
  (b) Is lighting sufficient? ....
    Daylight? .... Artificial light? ....
  (c) Is storage sufficient for equipment and supplies?........
  (d) Is equipment well kept?....................
  (e) Water .... Gas ....Sinks ....

2. Chemistry. Is chemistry required for entrance? ....
  a. Methods of teaching:
  Note points in which this differs from method in anatomy and physiology.

  b. Equipment:
  (1) Is this planned for demonstration by the instructor, or for work in the laboratory by the individual student?........
  ....
  (2) Of what does this consist? Note approximate quantity:
    General apparatus such as burners, stands, test-tubes, racks, etc. ....
    ....
    ....
    Glassware..
    Chemicals..
  (3) How are supplies and new equipment procured?............
  ....
  (4) Library, for this department.
  Note same points as for Anatomy and Physiology.
(See I. 1. b. (4).)

(5) Assistance. Note same points as for Anatomy and Physiology.

(See I. 1. b. (5).)

(6) Room used as laboratory:
    (a) Is space adequate for number of students?............
        Number in working section?......................
    (b) Is lighting sufficient?...................................
        Daylight? ....Artificial light?.............
    (c) Is storage sufficient for equipment and supplies?.......
    (d) Is equipment well kept?.............
    (e) Water ....Gas ....Sinks ....
3. Bacteriology.
  a. Methods of teaching:
  Note points in which these differ from those of Anatomy and Physiology.

  b. Equipment:
    (1) Is this planned for demonstration by the instructor or for work by the individual student?........................
    ....
    (2) Of what does the equipment consist:
    Microscopes: Number.............Kind.................
               Immersion lenses.........................
    Demonstration microscopic preparations....................
    Sterilizer.................Incubator......................
    Autoclave...........Glassware......General apparatus....
    (3) How are supplies and new equipment procured?............
    ....
    (4) Library, for this department:
    Note same points as for Anatomy and Physiology.

(See I. 1. b. (4).)

(5) Assistance. Note same points as for Anatomy and Physiology.

(See I. 1. b. (5).)

(6) Room used as laboratory:
    (a) Is space adequate for number of students?.............
        Number in working section?........................
    (b) Is lighting sufficient?...................................
        Daylight? ....Artificial light?.............
    (c) Is storage sufficient for equipment and supplies?.......
    (d) Is equipment well kept? ....
    (e) Water ....Gas ....Sinks ....

4. Nutrition and Cookery.
    a. Methods of teaching:
       Note points in which these differ from those of Anatomy and
       Physiology.

    b. Equipment:
       (1) Is equipment of dietetic laboratory of modern type, with a
           set of appliances for each student or two students?........
           ....
       (2) General description of equipment:
           ....
           ....
           Charts: Are sample cuts of meat and similar illustrative
           material used? ....
       (3) How is new equipment procured?............................
           ....
       (4) Library, for this department:
           Note same points as for Anatomy and Physiology.
                                                    (See I. 1. b. (4).)

       (5) Assistance. Note same points as for Anatomy and Phys-
           iology.
                                                    (See I. 1. b. (5).)

       (6) Room used as laboratory:
           (a) Is space adequate for number of students?.............
               Number in working section?..........................
           (b) Is lighting sufficient?................................
               Daylight? ....Artificial light?.............
           (c) Is storage sufficient for apparatus and supplies?........
           (d) Is equipment well kept?..............
           (e) Water ....Gas ....Sinks ....

II. Methods of teaching the theory and practice of nursing.
    1. Demonstration Room:
       a. Size..... b. Lighting..... c. Maximum number in section......
    2. Equipment:
       a. Is there running water?...... b. Gas stoves?.................
       c. Electric stoves?...
       d. How many desks?............ e. Blackboards? ....
       f. "   " beds? .... g. Cribs? ....
       h. "   " dolls? .... i. Give type of doll.............
    3. Is the supply of the following adequate:
       a. Linen..........b. Rubber goods..........c. Glassware..........
       d. Drugs..........
    4. Is there material sufficient for practice by individual student?......
    5. "   " demonstration by the teacher?.......................
    6. "   "   "   "   " students?..........................

7. Are the students used as subjects for demonstration?..............
   To what extent?..
8. Are the patients used as subjects for demonstration?............
   To what extent?..
9. How much time is allowed each student for practice in the demonstration room?..
10. Is this practice supervised?..................................
11. Who prepares material for class?...............................
12. Who puts away material after class?...........................
13. What textbook is used?...
14. What provision is made for carrying out classroom practice on wards?...
   ....

III. Methods of teaching subject in courses not involving laboratory work or ward practice.
   1. Subject ....
      a. Are formal lectures the rule?..................
         Do students take notes?.......................
         Are these inspected?..................
         Are quizzes based on these notes?.............
      b. In how far is this subject developed in class hours by questions and discussions rather than by lecture method?.............
         ....
      c. Is a textbook used?........What?..........................
      d. Library references given?........
         Use of library: Necessary........Advised......Little........
      e. Are there frequent quizzes?......Weekly......Bi-weekly......
      f. Are special reports or papers by students called for?...........
      g. Final examinations: When held?...........................
         How important?.............................
      h. What factors determine the student's grade in the course?....
         ....

IV. In conference with instructor.
   Note in what respects instructors would change their own courses were it possible.

What is the opinion of instructors regarding the best general program of teaching?

SCHEDULE IV A (Cont.)

CURRICULUM, SECTION 3

Data to be secured from superintendent or head instructor.
I. Records and grading of students:
   1. What records of student's work are kept in office?.................
      ....
      Secure individual's card if available.

2. Note in each case relative importance of practical and theoretical work. ....

....

3. What factors are included in estimating the work of the individual?
 a. For continuance after preliminary period?....................

....
 b. For continuance after probationary period?....................

....
 c. For recommendation after completion of course?...............

....
4. What reasons are stated as adequate for exclusion after preliminary or probationary periods?......................................

....

....
5. If a student fails in certain courses of the preliminary or later work, what is done about making up those failures?.................

....

....
 a. If examination is failed when ward work is satisfactory?.........

....

....
 b. Does such failure delay her date of graduation?...............;

....

....
II. Does announcement of school contain reliable descriptions of work covered in different courses? (If not, secure data if possible.)

III. Are physicians' lectures given with regularity, or are they often deferred? ....

....
IV. How is work lost by illness made up?.................................

....

....
V. If work is lost by emergency calls, is this made up?..................
 How? ....

....
VI. Is any arrangement made, either by allowing credit or adjusting work, for previous work of students, e.g., college courses?...............

....

Schedule IV B
OBSERVATION OF CLASS TEACHING

Training school ....
Subject of course...
Subject of day's lesson................. ,....................................

Class ....
Method ....
Presentation:
....
Students' participation:
....
Interest:
....
Correlation with other subjects or with practical work:
....
Comment:

SCHEDULE IV C

WARD EQUIPMENT

A. I. Service Rooms:
  1. Bathroom: a. Is it clean?...... b. Adequate facilities?..........
  2. Utility room: Are the following present and adequate?
      [List of equipment not reproduced here]
  3. Portable Equipment—Is it adequate?
      [List of articles not reproduced here]
  4. Diet Kitchen:
      [List of equipment not reproduced here]
  5. Linen Closet:
      Supply of linen........Arrangement........Cleanliness........

SCHEDULE IV D

OBSERVATION ON WARDS, SECTION 1

A. Assignment of Staff on Wards.
  Give assignments in detail, listing staff by rank and stating length of
  time in school by years and months. For each member of the staff
  described:
  1. Note especially assignment of following ward duties, i.e., medicines,
      dressings, diets, care of patients, treatments, housekeeping, and
      rounds.
  2. Give diagnosis of each patient cared for in sample wards, stating
      stage of disease by days.
  3. Divide assignments into:
      a. Housekeeping duties.
      b. Nursing duties.
      c. Degree of responsibility incurred.

B. Assignment of each probationer on ward:
1. Housekeeping duties.
2. Nursing duties.

C. Number of assistants other than nurses on these wards:
Day: Orderlies.... Attendants.... Maids.... Cleaners.... Porters....
Night: " .... " .... " .... " .... " ....

D. Supervision:
a. By whom given?..
b. For what apparent purpose?......................................

E. Amount of bedside instruction:
a. Who gives it in nursing care of patients?..........................
b. " " " " study of cases and diseases?.....................

F. What provision is made for carrying out class instruction on the wards?
....

G. Do classroom methods obtain uniformly over hospital?..............
a. If not, give reason...
b. If so, how is this insured?.......................................

H. Charting and record keeping by students. (Obtain by investigation.)
a. Does each student keep record?............
b. How is record kept at night?..............

I. Method of receiving physicians' orders:
a. On charts...............................
b. On order book..........................
c. By verbal order.........................
d. Or both verbal and written..............
    (1) If written, who writes it?.............
    (2) Who signs it?.......................
e. Written reports by students..............

J. Service being given by students which might equally well be done by paid workers (maid or other person), allowing for legitimate experience for student. (Obtain by inquiry and observation.)

List service	Estimate per day
a. Dusting	....
b. Cleaning wards and service rooms.............	....
c. Sweeping	....
d. Disinfection of beds..........................	....
e. Folding and putting away linen...............	....
f. Carrying trays................................	....
g. Setting trays.................................	....
h. Washing dishes...............................	....
i. Making of supplies and dressings.............	....
j. Cleaning of large number of instruments......	....
k. Washing and mending rubber gloves..........	....
l. Constant running of sterilizer.................	....
m. Washing stained linen........................	....
n. Washing gauze	....
o. Pulling washed gauze.........................	....
p. Errands about hospital........................	....
q. Accompanying patient to x-ray room, etc.....	....
r. Answering door bell...........................	....
s. Switch-board operator day or night...........	....
t. Routine work in diet kitchen—beyond needed..	....
u. Experience such as cleaning vegetables........	....
v. Cooking in large amounts for private patients.	....
w. Setting trays.................................	....

OBSERVATION ON WARDS, SECTION 2

A. Study of technique, individual student:
    I. Name of student................................
   II. Length of time in school...........Years...........Months.......
 III. a. Patient: Man....................Woman.........Child.........
      b. Is the patient acutely ill?........................
      c. " " " convalescent?......................
      d. " " " chronic?...........................
      e. Diagnosis ....
      f. Type of treatment given.....................................
      g. List of all articles used:

   IV. Were all articles at hand on beginning treatment, or did student leave
       patient to get them?..
    V. How long did it take to complete treatment?....................
   VI. Did the student work neatly, intelligently, skilfully, and with con-
       sideration for patient?..
  VII. Specify and illustrate..

Schedule V A

EQUIPMENT AND BUILDINGS

A. Nurses' Home:
  I. Is the home separate from the hospital?..
  II. Bedrooms:
    a. Total number for graduates..........
    b. "   "   " students............
    c. Number of single rooms for students..
        "   " double "   "   " ..
        "   " dormitories "   " ..How many beds in each?..
    d. Has each student a bed to herself?....   ....
    e. What arrangements are made to ensure quiet for night nurses?....
    ....
  III. Number of persons to tub....Shower....Wash basins....Toilet....
  IV. Dining Room:
    a. Is the food excellent....Good....Fair....Poor....Sufficient.....
    b. Is the service excellent... "   .... "   .... "   .... "   ....
    c. Are the appointments excellent..Good..Fair..Poor...Sufficient...
    d. What arrangements are made for night nurses' luncheons?......
    ....
  V. Library:

	REFERENCE	PROFESSIONAL	GENERAL	TOTAL
a. No. of books				

    b. No. of magazines: Professional............Popular............
    c. No. of newspapers....d. Is the library used much or little?......
    e. Are the books always accessible to students?...................
    If not, at what times are they accessible?......................
  VI. Are the following rooms provided for the use of students:
    a. Reception room.....b. Recreation room......c. Study room......
    d. Sewing room........e. Kitchenette ....f. Laundry ....

B. Type of student: Characterize the impression made as
  Excellent.......... Good..........:. Fair.......... Poor..........

Schedule V B

GENERAL CHARACTER OF SCHOOL LIFE

A. Type of Student:
  I. Education and general intelligence............................
  II. Age ....
  III. Health and general appearance................................
  ....

IV. Personal qualities and characteristics...........................
....

B. I. Type of discipline and control: Is it rigid and military; rational
and co-operative, directed toward developing student's powers of
self-discipline and recognition of responsibility to others; or
slack, disorganized, and ineffective?

II. Is there a student government association?......................
a. What are its scope and powers?...............................
....
b. What are the rules relating to visitors?........................
....
c. What are the rules relating to the medical staff?..............
....

C. Recreation:
I. How long in advance do students know the dates of vacations?....
........Of half-holidays?............Of hours off duty?........
II. What types of indoor recreation are available?...................
....
Are they used much or little?...............................
III. What types of outdoor recreation are available?................
Are they used much or little?...............................
IV. Clubs and other student's organizations. Describe...............
....
....

D. I. General attitude of students: Is there evidence of harmonious
atmosphere, with confidence between students and teachers, or
evidence of repression and friction?

II. What evidence is there of attempts to develop initiative and independent thinking?
....
....
III. Are there evidences of good school spirit?......................

II. PUBLIC HEALTH SERIES

Schedule 1

PERSONAL HISTORY NURSE

[Same as Training School Series. Page 561]

Schedule II A

OFFICE REPORT: PRIVATE AGENCIES

A. I. Name of Association...
    Address................................Year founded..........
B. Organization:
    I. Types of work.
       1. General visiting nursing:
          a. Specify what kinds of work are included....................
          ....
          ....
          b. What types of sickness are refused or referred to another
             organization for nursing care?...........................
       2. Specialized services:
          a. Infant or child welfare; up to what age?..................
             Specify what kinds of work are included..................
             ....
          b. Antituberculosis work.......Placement......Bedside care...
             Supervision ....Instruction ....
          c. Industrial nursing ....
    II. 1. Total number of visits made during last fiscal year..............
        2. Total number of cases............................
        3. Cost of a visit...
        4. Average number of visits per day per nurse....................
        5. Number of patients paying:
           a. Full cost ....
           b. Part cost ....
           c. Nothing ....
    III. Personnel:
         1. Board of managers: Title....................................
            a. How many are men?...........................
            b. "   "   " women?.......................
            c. How often does the board meet?....................
            d. Does the nurse superintendent meet with the board?........
         2. Nursing committee:
            a. How many members?........................
            b. How often does it meet?......................
         3. What committee determines policies?...........................
         4. What committee controls the budget?........................
         5. Staff:
            a. Superintendent: Name and title...............
            b. Assistant superintendents, how many?..........
            c. Supervisors,   "   "   ....
            d. Staff nurses,   "   "   ....

e. Student nurses (graduate) how many?..........
f.   "   " (undergraduate) "   " ....
g. Attendants or practical
   nurses   "   " ....
h. Nurses employed in clerical
   work (full time)   "   " ....
i. Dietitians   "   " ....
6. By whom are the following engaged and dismissed:
  a. Supervisors ....
  b. Staff nurses.....................................
  c. Clerical workers................................
7. What are the minimum professional and educational requirements for a staff position?...............................
8. Are staff nurses assigned to special services? Describe..........

C. Administration.
  I. Supervision:
    1. Number of staff nurses to a field supervisor:
                      Minimum....Maximum....
    2. How often do staff nurses report to the supervisor in the main or branch office or station?.....................................
    3. Does the supervisor visit in homes, a. With the staff nurse?.....
                      b. Without the staff nurse?..
    4. Are printed or written standard practice instructions used?.....
  II. Conferences:
    1. Are meetings of entire staff held regularly?...a. How often?....
      b. Who calls the meeting?.................c. Who presides?..
      d. Who attends?...
    2. Are case conferences held regularly?.........a. How often?....
      b. Who presides?...................c. Who attends?........
    3. What conferences of other organizations are regularly attended by members of the staff?...............................

  III. Efficiency:
    1. What methods are used to judge efficiency of nurses?...........
    2. a. Are efficiency records kept?..........b. Has the nurse access to her record?...
      c. If not, how is the nurse informed of her standing?...........
  IV. Salaries:
    1. Staff nurses: Minimum....Maximum....Rate of increase.......
    2. Supervisors: " .... " .... " " " ....
    3. What is the length of vacation on salary?....................
    4. Are the following furnished in addition to salary:
      Uniforms.....Board......Lodging......Other allowance......
  V. Hours of work:
    1. What are the hours of work daily?........Sunday?........
    2. Is time spent in record keeping included in working day?...
    3. Is there one complete day of rest in seven?............
    4. Is there a weekly half-holiday in addition?...........
    5. Overtime work: average per week per individual during last month ....
    6. Is night work expected?..........For what cases?............
    ....Is time off allowed for night work?...........
  VI. Recording
    1. How many hours weekly are spent in recording by supervisor?
    ....By staff nurse?.........................
    2. How many clerical workers (not nurses) are employed?.........

APPENDIX

D. What is the superintendent's conception of the function of the Association in regard to the education of:
    a. Patients and families.....................................
    b. Nurses ....
E. Comment by superintendent on education, training, and personality of staff nurses ....
....
....
F. Obtain two copies of the following:
    1. All record forms.
    2. Practice instructions.
    3. Efficiency record.
    4. Annual report for last *two* years.
    5. Publicity material published within the last year.
G. Remarks:

Schedule II B

OFFICE REPORT: PUBLIC AGENCIES

[Same as Schedule II A, with necessary differentiation for public agencies]

Schedule III

I. Account of day's work—This account should include:
   1. General information: Type of community (urban, suburban, rural); industries; housing; etc.

II. Description of activities of the nurse other than home visiting (milk station, dispensary, schools, work with groups, etc.).

III. 1. Method of transportation used by nurse.
    2. Visits:
       a. Summary of day's work (classify and give nature of visits).
       b. Significant visits:
          (1) Purpose: Instruction, nursing care, friendly call, etc.; number of previous visits; diagnosis, if there is sickness; description of actual service rendered.
          (2) Teaching: What was the nurse trying to teach? Methods. Evidence of success or failure. Evidence of previous teaching.
          (3) Social co-operation: Did nurse recognize social problems? Was she interested in them? Evidence of co-operation with other agencies. Evidence of effort to determine effectiveness of agencies. Methods of dealing with relief cases, especially emergency relief.

IV. Description of technical nursing: Summarized from all visits. General appearance of work: thorough, inadequate; careful, careless; tidy, untidy; finished, hurried; etc. If standard instructions are used, did the nurse appear to conform to them?

V. Describe personality of nurse: Note breeding; intelligence; initiative; interest in preventive work; interest in social problems; skill in getting information; approach to families. Relations with families: businesslike, mechanical, brusque, friendly, considerate, sympathetic, sentimental, etc. Her attitude toward her work; loyalty to organization.

584

VI. **Recording:** Comment on character of records and methods of recording. Give approximate time spent.

VII. **Relations** of nurse to physicians and other workers.

VIII. **Remarks:**

Titles in This Series

1 Charlotte Aikens, editor. *Hospital Management*. Philadelphia, 1911.

2 American Society of Superintendents of Training Schools for Nurses. *Annual Conventions*, 1893–1919.

3 John Shaw Billings and Henry M. Hurd, editors. *Hospitals, Dispensaries and Nursing: Papers and Discussion in the International Congress of Charities, Correction and Philanthropy*. Baltimore, 1894.

4 Annie M. Brainard. *The Evolution of Public Health Nursing*. Philadelphia, 1922.

5 Marie Campbell. *Folks Do Get Born*. New York, 1946.

6 *Civil War Nursing:* Louisa May Alcott. *Hospital Sketches*. Boston, 1863. BOUND WITH *Memoir of Emily Elizabeth Parsons*. Boston, 1880.

7 Committee for the Study of Nursing Education. *Nursing and Nursing Education in the United States*. New York, 1923.

8 Committee on the Grading of Nursing Schools. *Nurses, Patients and Pocketbooks*. New York, 1928.

9 Mrs. Darce Craven. *A Guide to District Nurses*. London, 1889.

10 Dorothy Deming. *The Practical Nurse*. New York, 1947.

11 Katharine J. Densford & Millard S. Everett. *Ethics for Modern Nurses*. Philadelphia, 1946.

12 Katharine D. DeWitt. *Private Duty Nursing*. Philadelphia, 1917.

13 Janet James, editor. *A Lavinia Dock Reader*.

14   Annette Fiske. *First Fifty Years of the Waltham Training School for Nurses.* New York, 1984. BOUND WITH Alfred Worcester. "The Shortage of Nurses—Reminiscences of Alfred Worcester '83." *Harvard Medical Alumni Bulletin 23*, 1949.

15   Virginia Henderson et al. *Nursing Studies Index, 1900–1959.* Philadelphia, 1963, 1966, 1970, 1972.

16   Darlene Clark Hine, editor. *Black Women in Nursing: An Anthology of Historical Sources.*

17   Ellen N. LaMotte. *The Tuberculosis Nurse.* New York, 1915.

18   Barbara Melosh, editor. *American Nurses in Fiction: An Anthology of Short Stories.*

19   Mary Adelaide Nutting. *A Sound Economic Basis for Schools of Nursing.* New York, 1926.

20   Sara E. Parsons. *Nursing Problems and Obligations.* Boston, 1916.

21   Juanita Redmond. *I Served on Bataan.* Philadelphia, 1943.

22   Susan Reverby, editor. *The East Harlem Health Center Demonstration: An Anthology of Pamphlets.*

23   Isabel Hampton Robb. *Educational Standards for Nurses.* Cleveland, 1907.

24   Sister M. Theophane Shoemaker. *History of Nurse-Midwifery in the United States.* Washington, D.C., 1947.

25   Isabel M. Stewart. *Education of Nurses.* New York, 1943.

26   Virginia S. Thatcher. *History of Anesthesia with Emphasis on the Nurse Specialist.* Philadelphia, 1953.

27   Adah H. Thoms. *Pathfinders—A History of the Progress of Colored Graduate Nurses.* New York, 1929.

28   Clara S. Weeks-Shaw. *A Text-Book of Nursing for the Use of Training Schools, Families, and Private Students.* New York, 1885.

29   Writers Program of the WPA in Kansas, compilers. *Lamps on the Prairie: A History of Nursing in Kansas.* Topeka, 1942.